Student Guide to

PRIMARY CARE

Making the Most of Your Early Clinical Experience

Student Guide to

PRIMARY CARE

Making the Most of Your Early Clinical Experience

Edited by

David J. Steele, PhD
Professor and Assistant Dean for Curriculum and Evaluation
Department of Family Medicine and Rural Health
Florida State University College of Medicine
Tallahassee, Florida

Jeffrey L. Susman, MD
Professor and Chair
Department of Family Medicine
University of Cincinnati College of Medicine
University Hospital
Mercy Franciscan Hospital–Mt. Airy
Cincinnati, Ohio

Fredrick A. McCurdy, MD, PhD, MBA
Professor, Department of Pediatrics
University of Nebraska Medical Center
Nebraska Health System
Children's Memorial Hospital
St. Joseph's Hospital
Omaha, Nebraska

HANLEY & BELFUS, INC. / Philadelphia

Publisher: HANLEY & BELFUS, INC.
              Medical Publishers
              210 S. 13th Street
              Philadelphia, PA 19107
              (215) 546-7293; 800-962-1892
              FAX (215) 790-9330
              Website: http://www.hanleyandbelfus.com

Note to the reader: Although the information in this book has been carefully reviewed for correctness of dosage and indications, neither the authors nor the editors nor the publisher can accept any legal responsibility for any errors or omissions that may be made. Neither the publisher nor the editors make any warranty, expressed or implied, with respect to the material contained herein. Before prescribing any drug, the reader must review the manufacturer's current product information (package inserts) for accepted indications, absolute dosage recommendations, and other information pertinent to the safe and effective use of the product described.

Library of Congress Cataloging-in-Publication Data

Student guide to primary care: making the most of your early clinical experience /
[edited by] David J. Steele, Jeffrey Susman, Fredrick A. McCurdy.
      p. cm.
    Includes bibliographical references and index.
    ISBN 1-56053-545-8 (alk. paper)
     1. Primary care (Medicine)—Handbooks, manuals, etc. I. Steele, David J. (David Jay),
    1948– II. Susman, Jeffrey. III. McCurdy, Fredrick A., 1944–

    RC55 .S784 2002
    616—dc21

                                                            2002068783

STUDENT GUIDE TO PRIMARY CARE:
MAKING THE MOST OF YOUR EARLY CLINICAL EXPERIENCE   ISBN 1-56053-545-8

Last digit is the print number: 9 8 7 6 5 4 3 2 1

Printed in Canada

Contents

Contributors

Wendy L. Adams, MD, MPH
Assistant Professor, Department of Family Medicine,
University of Nebraska Medical Center, Omaha, Nebraska

Dale R. Agner, MD
Chief of Medical Staff, Fifth Medical Group, United States Air
Force Regional Hospital, Minot Air Force Base, North Dakota

Saira Mir Asadullah, MD
Clinical Assistant Professor, Department of Internal Medicine,
University of Illinois College of Medicine, Peoria, Illinois; Mason
District Hospital, Havana Medical Associates, Havana, Illinois

Suzanne J.G. Cornwall, MD
Assistant Professor, Department of Family Medicine, University of
Nebraska Medical Center, Omaha, Nebraska; University Medical
Associates–Summit Plaza, Bellevue, Nebraska

Mark H. Ebell, MD, MS
Associate Professor, Department of Family Practice, Michigan
State University College of Medicine, East Lansing, Michigan

Cynthia R. Ellis, MD
Associate Professor of Pediatrics and Psychiatry, Munroe-Meyer
Institute for Genetics and Rehabilitation, University of Nebraska
Medical Center, Omaha, Nebraska

Paul W. Esposito, MD
Associate Professor, Department of Orthopaedic Surgery,
University of Nebraska Medical Center; Children's Hospital,
Omaha, Nebraska

Andrew Faraci, MD
Department of Internal Medicine, University of Nebraska Medical
Center; Omaha Veterans Administration Medical Center, Omaha,
Nebraska

Brian J. Finley, MD
Associate Professor, Department of Family Medicine, University of
Nebraska Medical Center; Nebraska Health System; Erhling
Bergquist Hospital, Omaha, Nebraska

Bruce C. Gebhardt, MD
Associate Professor, Department of Family Medicine,
University of Cincinnati College of Medicine, Cincinnati, Ohio

Dennis P. Goeschel, MD
Department of Family Medicine, University of Nebraska Medical
Center; Nebraska Health System, Omaha, Nebraska

Jeffrey D. Harrison, MD
Associate Professor, Department of Family Medicine, University of
Nebraska Medical Center; Nebraska Health System, Omaha,
Nebraska

William Henry Hay, MD
Clinical Assistant Professor, Department of Family Medicine,
University of Nebraska Medical Center, Omaha, Nebraska

Virginia M. Helget, RN, MSN, CIC
Infection Control Specialist, Department of Health Care
Epidemiology, Nebraska Health System,
Omaha, Nebraska

Julie A. Hobart, MD
Assistant Professor of Clinical Family Medicine,
Department of Family Medicine, University of Cincinnati
College of Medicine, Cincinnati, Ohio

Keith B. Holten, MD
Associate Professor, Department of Family Medicine,
University of Cincinnati College of Medicine, Cincinnati, Ohio

Russell J. Hopp, DO
Professor of Pediatrics and Medicine, Department of Pediatrics,
Creighton University School of Medicine, Omaha, Nebraska

C. Gerald Judy, MD
Assistant Professor of Pediatrics, Section of Pulmonology and
Cystic Fibrosis, Department of Pediatrics, University of Nebraska
Medical Center; Nebraska Health System; Children's Hospital,
Omaha, Nebraska

Joseph Kiesler, MD
Assistant Professor, Department of Family Medicine,
University of Cincinnati College of Medicine, Cincinnati, Ohio

Amy E. Lacroix, MD
Assistant Professor and Director of Adolescent Medicine,
Department of Pediatrics, University of Nebraska Medical Center,
Omaha, Nebraska

Carol A. LaCroix, MD
Assistant Professor, Department of Family Medicine, University of
Nebraska Medical Center; Nebraska Health System; University
Medical Associates, Omaha, Nebraska

Louise M. LaFramboise, PhD, RN
Assistant Professor, College of Nursing, University of Nebraska
Medical Center, Omaha, Nebraska

David R. Mack, MD
Professor, Department of Pediatrics, University of Ottawa Faculty
of Medicine; Children's Hospital of Eastern Ontario, Ottawa,
Ontario, Canada

Christopher C. Madden, MD
Sports and Family Medicine, Longs Peak Family Practice,
Longmont, Colorado; Team Physician, Niwot High School, Niwot,
Colorado

Fredrick A. McCurdy, MD, PhD, MBA
Professor, Department of Pediatrics, University of Nebraska
Medical Center; Nebraska Health System; Children's Hospital; St.
Joseph's Hospital, Omaha, Nebraska

Kristine L.S.P. McVea, MD, MPH
Associate Professor, Department of Family Medicine,
University of Nebraska Medical Center, Omaha, Nebraska

Jim D. Medder, MD, MPH
Associate Professor, Department of Family Medicine, University of
Nebraska Medical Center, Omaha, Nebraska

William C. Minier, MD
Assistant Professor, Department of Family Medicine, University of
Nebraska Medical Center; Nebraska Health System, Omaha,
Nebraska

Arvind Modawal, MD, MPH, MRCGP, DTMH
Assistant Professor, Department of Family Medicine, University of Cincinnati College of Medicine; Consultant Geriatrician, University Hospital Geriatric Evaluation Center, Cincinnati, Ohio

Gerald F. Moore, MD
Professor, Section of Rheumatology, Department of Internal Medicine, University of Nebraska Medical Center, Omaha, Nebraska

Michael J. Moran, MD
Associate Clinical Professor, Department of Pediatrics, University of Nebraska Medical Center; Medical Director, Children's Advocacy Team, Children's Hospital, Omaha, Nebraska

Patrick Morgan, BS, BA
University of Minnesota, Minneapolis, Minnesota

Debra E. Mostek, MD
Assistant Professor, Section of Geriatrics and Gerontology, Department of Internal Medicine, University of Nebraska Medical Center; Active Academic Medical Staff, Nebraska Health System, Omaha, Nebraska

Arwa Nasir, MBBS, MSc (Peds)
Clinical Assistant Professor, Department of Family Medicine, University of Nebraska Medical Center; Nebraska Health System; Clarkson Family Medicine, Omaha, Nebraska

Laeth Nasir, MBBS
Associate Professor, Department of Family Medicine, University of Nebraska Medical Center; Nebraska Health System, Omaha, Nebraska

J. Scott Neumeister, MD
Assistant Professor, Department of Internal Medicine, University of Nebraska Medical Center; Nebraska Health System, Omaha, Nebraska

David V. O'Dell, MD
Associate Professor, Department of Internal Medicine, University of Nebraska Medical Center; Nebraska Health System; Omaha Veterans Administration Medical Center, Omaha, Nebraska

Audrey Paulman, MD, MMM
Clinical Assistant Professor, Department of Family Medicine, University of Nebraska Medical Center; Nebraska Health System, Omaha, Nebraska

Paul M. Paulman, MD
Professor and Predoctoral Director, Department of Family Medicine, University of Nebraska Medical Center; Nebraska Health System; Nebraska Methodist Hospital, Omaha, Nebraska

Sheryl Pitner, MD, MPH
Assistant Professor, Department of Pediatrics, University of Nebraska Medical Center; Nebraska Health System; Clarkson Family Medicine; St. Joseph's Hospital, Children's Hospital, Omaha, Nebraska

Jane F. Potter, MD
Harris Professor of Geriatric Medicine; Chief, Section of Geriatrics and Gerontology, Department of Internal Medicine, University of Nebraska Medical Center, Omaha, Nebraska

Layne A. Prest, PhD, LMFT
Associate Professor and Director of Behavioral Medicine, Department of Family Medicine, University of Nebraska Medical Center; Nebraska Health System; University Medical Associates, Omaha, Nebraska

W. David Robinson, PhD, LMFT
Assistant Professor and Associate Director of Behavioral Medicine, Department of Family Medicine, University of Nebraska Medical Center; Nebraska Health System; University Medical Associates, Omaha, Nebraska

Debra J. Romberger, MD
Associate Professor, Section of Pulmonary and Critical Care Medicine, Department of Internal Medicine, University of Nebraska Medical Center; Nebraska Health System; Omaha Veterans Administration Medical Center, Omaha, Nebraska

Jose R. Romero, MD
Associate Professor, Section of Pediatric Infectious Diseases, Department of Pediatrics, University of Nebraska Medical Center; Associate Professor, Departments of Pediatrics and Medical Microbiology and Immunology, Creighton University School of Medicine, Omaha, Nebraska

Amy L. Ruane, EdS
School Psychologist, Coeur d'Alene School District, Coeur d'Alene, Idaho

Mark E. Rupp, MD
Associate Professor, Section of Infectious Diseases, Department of Internal Medicine, University of Nebraska Medical Center; Medical Director, Department of Health Care Epidemiology, Nebraska Health System, Omaha, Nebraska

Maria M. Sandvig, MD
Volunteer Associate Professor, Department of Family Medicine, University of Cincinnati College of Medicine, Cincinnati, Ohio

Connie J. Schnoes, MA
Munroe-Meyer Institute for Genetics and Rehabilitation, University of Nebraska Medical Center; Nebraska Health System, Omaha, Nebraska

John L. Smith, MD
Assistant Professor, Department of Family Medicine, University of Nebraska Medical Center, Omaha, Nebraska

James H. Stageman, MD
Associate Professor, Department of Family Medicine; Program Director, Residency Training, University of Nebraska Medical Center, Omaha, Nebraska

David J. Steele, PhD
Professor and Assistant Dean for Curriculum and Evaluation, Department of Family Medicine and Rural Health, Florida State University College of Medicine, Tallahassee, Florida

Andrea F. Suslow, MD
Instructor, Section of Geriatrics and Gerontology, Department of Internal Medicine, University of Nebraska Medical Center; Nebraska Health System; Thomas Fitzgerald Veterans Home, Omaha, Nebraska

Jeffrey L. Susman, MD
Professor and Chair, Department of Family Medicine, University of Cincinnati College of Medicine; University Hospital; Mercy Franciscan Hospital–Mt. Airy, Cincinnati, Ohio

Thomas G. Tape, MD
Associate Professor, Department of Internal Medicine, University of Nebraska Medical Center; Nebraska Health System; Omaha Veterans Administration Medical Center, Omaha, Nebraska

Richard P. Usatine, MD
Associate Clinical Professor, Department of Family Medicine; Assistant Dean of Student Affairs, University of California, Los Angeles, UCLA School of Medicine, Los Angeles, California

Ed Vandenberg, MD, CMD
Assistant Professor, Section of Geriatrics and Gerontology, Department of Internal Medicine, University of Nebraska Medical Center; Nebraska Health System; Acting Chief of Geriatrics, Omaha Veterans Administration Medical Center, Omaha, Nebraska

John J. Vann, MD
Omaha Children's Clinic, Omaha, Nebraska

Cynthia L. Van Riper, MS, RD, CDE
Discipline Director for Nutrition, Munroe-Meyer Institute for Genetics and Rehabilitation, University of Nebraska Medical Center, Omaha, Nebraska

Mary A. Wampler, MD, MPH
Medical Director, Occupational Medicine Clinic, Methodist Health Systems, Omaha, Nebraska

Douglas H. Wheatley, MD
Associate Professor, Department of Family Medicine, University of Nebraska Medical Center, Omaha, Nebraska

Preface

Picture the following scene: You are a first- or second-year medical student. Like many medical schools, yours has modified its curriculum to provide students early opportunities to get into the real world to see patients. In addition to your course work in anatomy, biochemistry, and pathophysiology, you find yourself spending an afternoon every few weeks in the busy practice of a community-based preceptor. You still feel a bit self-conscious when you put on your short, white jacket and drape the stethoscope around your neck. Every time you take a patient's blood pressure, you get tangled up in tubing. Beyond the most general of questions, you don't know what to ask a patient about her concerns, let alone have answers for questions she may ask you. You feel like a fraud. It's only a matter of time before everyone figures out what you already know—you know nothing! Back at the medical center, you've had lectures, demonstrations, and small group sessions on basic interviewing and the physical exam. You have interviewed and examined simulated patients. But that's the classroom—that's dealing with fake patients. This is the real world—these are real patients.

Sound familiar? If your answer is yes, then this book is for you! It is intended to be a just-in-time resource for medical students, physician assistant students, and nurse practitioner students who are in the early stages of their clinical training and just beginning to see patients in the ambulatory setting. This book is a survival guide of sorts that should be helpful to you when you find yourself asking questions that begin with phrases such as "How do I...?" or "What do I ask about when...?" or "What should I be on the lookout for when a patient presents with...?" This book has been designed to accompany you to the clinic and serve as a ready resource to help you plan your visits with patients or seek answers to questions that arise in the course of your clinic encounters.

Let's say your preceptor is a pediatrician and one day says to you: "Mrs. Smith brought her 3-month-old daughter, Emily, in today for a well-baby visit. Why don't you go in and get started on the exam? I'll be in in about 15 minutes to see how things are going." Now what do you do? You've seen well-baby exams but you've never done one. This situation is where this book can come in handy. You can take a few minutes reviewing the section on the pediatric encounter dealing with well-child examinations and get an idea about what to cover. Consider another example: Your preceptor is an internist and tells you to do a "quick" history and physical on a patient who is being treated for hypertension. A review of the chapter on hypertension gives you a good handle on what might be included in a targeted history and physical. Here's one final example of how this book might be helpful to you in the clinic: You have just completed a history and physical exam on a patient who is concerned about lower back pain. You feel good about the encounter and the exam, but you want to be sure you didn't miss anything significant before presenting your findings to your preceptor. So, you excuse yourself, go to the conference room in the clinic and quickly scan the chapter on back pain, looking at the "red flags." This review confirms that you have indeed done a thorough and appropriate evaluation of the patient's symptoms.

As you scan the table of contents, you will note that this book is organized into four major sections: Orientation to the Office; Getting Started in Ambulatory Patient Care; Common Signs, Symptoms, and Illnesses; and Common Procedures in Primary Care. Our emphasis throughout is on the common problems, procedures, and activities of everyday medicine, whether that practice is family medicine, general internal medicine, or general pediatrics. You should also be aware that this book is not intended to be a substitute for the more detailed treatments found in the standard textbooks of medicine. We urge you to think of this book as a bridge between the patient sitting in front of you in the office and the wealth of information that is available to you in standard sources. We trust you will find this book helpful as you visit with your patients and gain the knowledge and skills that will enable you to be the kind of physician you've always wanted to be.

David J. Steele, PhD
Jeffrey L. Susman, MD
Fredrick A. McCurdy, MD, PhD, MBA

Acknowledgments

We have accumulated many debts in developing this book. First, we must acknowledge and thank the authors, an impressive group of clinicians and educators. As a group, they bore our nagging, begging, and cajoling about deadlines, format, and length with patience and good humor. We are glad that we can still count many of them as friends!

We also owe a special debt to Matthew Harris for suggesting this project to us and for encouraging us to contact Linda Belfus about publishing this work. Linda has been enthusiastic about this project, and we appreciate the "we can do this" attitude that helped us clear some of the inevitable hurdles that go with publishing any book. Our production editor, Cecelia Bayruns, is a model of professionalism and efficiency, and we wish to thank her for her commitment to this project.

Anne Toews, of the University of Nebraska Medical Center, Department of Family Medicine, served admirably as our editorial assistant. She did everything from stuffing envelopes, to tracking down references, to reformatting chapters, to correcting creative spelling. Thanks from all of us, Annie!

We also want to say a special "thank you" to Ilene Steele. At a point in time when her editor-husband was drowning in a sea of manuscripts, chapter proposals, and correspondence, Ilene stepped forward and volunteered her own considerable organizational skills to getting the project firmly on track.

Jeff Susman acknowledges Sarah May for all her support and also Katie, Dan, and Ben, the joys of his life. Fred McCurdy thanks his wife, Diane, for encouraging him when it would have been easier to quit and go on to something less complex! Finally, Dave Steele offers his personal thank you to "the lovely Mrs. Steele" for her constant support, love, and friendship. What a find you are, Ilene!

Icons Used in This Book

Throughout the book, information has been supplied in side bars to help clarify key points in the body of the text and to serve as easily accessed aids to understanding. These elements are called out in the text and correspond to information in the side bar that is marked with one of the following icons.

 This indicates a brief **Definition** of a technical term or brief description of a physical examination maneuver.

 Red Flags are descriptions, explanations, or warnings about potentially serious conditions that may be suggested by the history or physical examination findings.

 The **Brain** icon denotes hints, reminders, and correlations.

 The **Treatment** icon presents succinct information about treatment options and considerations.

 The **Consultation and Referral** icon is used to provide succinct information about when to refer and the most appropriate referral sources.

1. Survival Skills for Your First Day in the Office

Paul M. Paulman, MD • Andrew Faraci, MD

Synopsis

The information in this chapter will help you adapt during your first visits with your clinical instructor. Early clinical experiences are valuable because they:
- Allow you an opportunity to integrate and practice skills learned in the classroom
- Help you see and understand the application of basic science knowledge to patient care
- Give you an opportunity to develop a one-to-one teaching, learning, and mentoring relationship with a practicing physician
- Offer you the first "real world" medical experience

Getting the Most from Your Clinical Experience

Your Preceptor

Your preceptor has had years of training: college, medical school, and residency. Although this training has provided your preceptor with the knowledge, skills, and experience needed to offer competent medical care, very few physician preceptors have had formal training in educational methodology. Most preceptors learn to teach by experience. Regardless of your preceptor's experience level as a teacher, however, you can do several things to enhance your learning in the clinic. To begin with, negotiate a "learning contract" with your preceptor that covers areas such as:

- Your knowledge and previous experience
- Your preceptor's comfort level with medical student–patient interaction in his or her clinic. (For example, are students allowed to interview patients on their own, perform physical exams, and participate in the care of patients?)
- Your preceptor's expectations of you
- Content areas (what should be learned in the clinic or office)
- Your learning style
- Your expectations
- Your college's expectations
- Logistics (e.g., office hours, dress code, types of patients)
- How you will be evaluated and graded

Learning contracts can be explicit or implicit, but they work best when both parties explicitly discuss these issues. Learning contracts need not be written, but the elements should be understood by and agreeable to both parties. Most learning contracts can be discussed and finalized in one or two 15–30-minute sessions. Negotiating a learning contract before or on your first clinic day is an excellent way to start your clinical experience.

Look for opportunities to meet your learning goals. Formulating a learning contract requires that you think about and set some learning goals for your clinical experience. Tailor your goals to match the learning environment. Your preceptor's office is not the best place to learn about Krebs cycle or histology of the gastrointestinal tract, but it presents excellent opportunities to interview patients, practice physical examination skills, and view the effects of disease processes.

Examine your learning goals as well as those of your school and your preceptor. Be assertive *(Red Flag 1)*. This is the time when all those countless hours of studying pay off. Show them what you know. Expressing interest will open doors to further opportunities; don't stand there and expect lectures from your preceptor. Be available and enthusiastic; you may find unexpected learning opportunities. The patient with the "dull" and mundane presenting complaint may have other conditions or history which are fascinating.

Ask for feedback. Prompt your preceptor to critique your performance and suggest ways to improve. Questions such as, "Dr. Jones, what else should I include in this note?" or "Dr. Smith, how could I perform my abdominal exam more efficiently?" may elicit sound, practical clinical advice from your preceptor.

Observe your preceptor's practice style and adapt to it. Each physician has his or her own manner of dealing with patients and staff. If you learn to adapt your style to match or parallel your preceptor's style, you will likely increase your learning opportunities. However, be aware that there are productive and destructive interaction styles. As you observe and adapt to your preceptor's style, analyze the negative aspects and avoid them.

 1 - Although being assertive is important, you must recognize your limitations and lack of training. Admit your mistakes. It is okay not to know how to ask the right questions or perform the right exam. Preceptors respect your honesty, and it helps them assess the areas in which you may need further assistance.

Adapting to the Clinic

Most medical care in the United States is provided in ambulatory clinics (physicians' offices). These clinics are usually efficient, with well-established routines. These clinics also must generate money to pay for operating costs and salaries. Just as adapting to your preceptor's style enhances your learning opportunities, adapting to the pace and routine of your preceptor's clinic will increase your chances to learn and participate in the care of the clinic's patients. For example, you will work in practices with many patients and in practices with a lower volume of patients. Take advantage of both types by learning efficiency in high-volume settings and fine tuning skills in low-volume practices. In either situation, bring your books and study materials—if your preceptor is tied up with an examination or procedure, you can use that time to review lecture notes or readings.

People in the Clinic

- **Patients.** The most important people in the clinic are the patients. Ask your preceptor about her practice profile and the characteristics of her patient population.
- **Front office staff.** The front office staff greets patients, answers phone calls, schedules appointments, gets charts for the physician, and often handles business, accounting, billing, and insurance issues for the clinic. The clinic's office manager often is included with the front office staff. The manager is in charge of day to day clinic operations. No clinic survives without a well functioning front office. The front office staff can teach you about the business aspects of practice, and they may suggest patients with specific conditions and histories for you to interview and examine.
- **Back office staff.** After patients have been scheduled and greeted by the front office staff, the patient and the patient's chart will be handed over to the back office staff. People in the back office may include nurses (RNs or LPNs), nursing assistants, and technicians who perform x-ray or laboratory procedures. The back office staff

can teach you technical skills, including vital signs, laboratory, and x-ray techniques. The back office staff often knows which patients you should interview to enhance your education. Knowing and working with these staff people is often critical to your success or failure in the clinics. Treat staff as equals, and ask them lots of questions. They often can show you the unspoken, "quick-and-dirty" way to interpret a test, and they can be helpful in orienting you to the behind-the-scenes taboos and unspoken rules of a successful working practice.

In the office, you may meet other physicians and providers, including physician assistants, nurse practitioners, nurse midwives, therapists, or social workers. These providers see patients in association with or under the supervision of physicians. These individuals often will allow you to interview and examine their patients. Take advantage of the learning opportunities they provide.

Adapting to the Patients

Remember that a preceptor depends on his patients for his livelihood, and he may have long, ongoing relationships with his patients. Here are some "Rules of Engagement" to ensure good interactions (and learning opportunities) *(Red Flag 2).*

 2 - All of your clinical activities must be supervised by your preceptor. As a student, you are not licensed to practice medicine. Do nothing to or for your preceptor's patients unless your preceptor is on site. The only exception to this rule is a life-threatening emergency, during which you would render rescue assistance and first aid to the limit of your knowledge and ability.

- Be yourself! Be sincere and, most of all, know that it is okay to be nervous. In fact, it is even okay to admit to the patient that you're uncomfortable. This simple admission can help put you both at ease. It allows the patient to see you with your guard somewhat down and opens the door for the patient to be more open and at ease in return.
- Look professional. Patients respond positively to students who are well groomed.
- Be interested and enthusiastic.
- Identify yourself as a medical student. Use whatever terms (e.g., *student, student doctor*) your preceptor prefers. Being honest with patients is the first step in developing a trusting therapeutic relationship. Some students feel that they are wasting patients' time when they interview them. This view is not shared by the majority of patients. Patients often appreciate the attention students give them. Many patients are rather proud of their role as "instructor" for "their" medical students and the part they play in medical education by working with students. Because medical students bring a fresh perspective to the relationship, students often discover important aspects of the patient's history and examination that were not noted by the patient's physician.
- If you don't know something, say so. As a student, you are not expected to have the same depth of knowledge as your preceptor. Do not try to impress patients by making something up in an encounter. Most patients can tell when you are faking.
- Respect the preferences of the patient. If the patient does not want to talk to you, go on to the next patient. Chances are that encounter would not be fruitful. Most often, the front office or back office staff will have prescreened the patients who do not want to interact with students. Remember, the better the staff knows you and how enthusiastic you are, the easier it will be for them to present you honestly and enthusiastically to patients.
- Maintain confidentiality. You may discuss patient information with other medical personnel only. Otherwise, what you see in the clinic, stays in the clinic. As a health care provider, you must *never* use any information about your preceptor's patients for *any* reason other than

to provide medical care for your preceptor's patients.

- Be aware that patients will tell your preceptor things they won't tell you; this is because most patients have a long-term relationship with their physician. Conversely, patients may tell you things they would not (or have forgotten to) tell their physician.
- Be aware of your limitations and your strengths. You should actively participate in the care of your preceptor's patients (as your preceptor permits) to the limit of your knowledge, skills, and experience. Being overly aggressive or timid in the office can have negative learning consequences for you. When in doubt, ask your preceptor if she feels you should be doing more or holding back in your patient interaction. Your patients have the right to know that you are inexperienced prior to performing procedures on them. Patients have a right to refuse to allow you to treat them.
- Maintain respectful relationships with patients and staff. *All* patients and *all* staff can add to your education. Showing respect, listening, and paying attention to people will improve your learning opportunities.
- Ask questions. Your preceptor may assume you understand more than you do. If you don't understand something, ask questions. If you are uncomfortable with an assigned task, let your preceptor know about your discomfort.
- Ask to be observed. Your preceptor can give you valuable feedback about your performance if he observes you. Ask your preceptor to observe segments of your interview and examinations. Remember, time is money, so it is unlikely that she can spend a large block of time to observe a complete history and physical exam. Nonetheless, let her know you would appreciate being observed even for brief periods.
- Practice your skills. Expertise comes with practice. The more exams, histories, and procedures (such as vital signs) you do, the more proficient you become.

Adapting to the Process of Care

Most patients seen in the clinic will progress through a series of steps in obtaining care. Although you will be involved only in some of these steps, knowledge of all the steps will improve your learning in the clinic. These steps include the following:

- Appointments. Most appointments are arranged at the time of a previous visit or via the telephone, so you will not be involved much in this step.
- Front office check-in. The front office staff greets the patient, readies the clinic chart or file, and updates financial (insurance) and demographic information. You probably will not be involved in this step.
- Back office check-in. The patient is called, vital signs obtained, and chief complaint elicited. The patient is then placed in a room and prepared for the examination. This is an excellent point at which to interact with the patient. You have an opportunity to review the chart, gather background information, perform vital signs, and interview and examine the patient.
- Physician (provider)-patient encounter. You should be involved in this step. Your preceptor may have you present your history and exam findings to him and may observe or demonstrate interviews and examinations.
- Laboratory tests or x-rays (if needed). Your patient may have lab or x-ray examinations. Participate in these examinations. Clinic lab and x-ray procedures offer an excellent opportunity for you to learn basic lab tests and blood drawing. The technical staff in your preceptor's office is usually enthusiastic about teaching you these procedures.
- Back office checkout. Your preceptor will dismiss your patient, write prescriptions, and arrange for a follow-up visit if necessary. You should participate actively in this process.
- Front office checkout. Your patient will return to the front office to have outside lab, x-ray, or consultations arranged and to confirm future appointments. You will not be involved in this step.

Charting and Recording the Process of Care

After the visit, you may have a chance to write a clinic note about your encounter. One method of recording the information is the SOAP (Subjective, Objective, Assessment, and Plan) format. In the subjective area, you record the things your patient told you (use quotes). Objective information includes vital signs, exam findings, and test results. Assessment is the diagnosis, often expressed as differential diagnosis with several possible causes of the patient's subjective and objective findings.

The plan includes action items such as further evaluations, medications or other treatments prescribed, follow-up visits, and instructions given to the patient or patient's caregiver *(Appendix A)*.

Many clinicians use the problem-oriented system for office record keeping. The problem-oriented system consists of a master list of patient problems, medications, surgical procedures, vaccines, and screening tests. The notes in the chart may refer to the master problem list. The problem list is updated when new problems are encountered.

Some clinicians do not use the problem-oriented system, and keep track of their patients' visits with sequential clinic notes. Clinic charts may contain clinic notes, problem lists, flow sheets, patient demographic data, lab test results, letters from consultant physicians, and records of telephone conversations.

Clinic charts are usually organized with one chart per patient or with all family members' records kept in one chart. The information in clinic charts must be kept *strictly confidential*. Do not divulge patient information gleaned from clinic charts.

Presenting Patients

When you are given opportunities to interview and examine patients on your own, it is likely that your preceptor will ask you to summarize what you learned before he or she goes in to see the patient. *Table 1* lists the steps you should follow to present the patient.

Table 1. How to Present the Patient

Keeping the delivery short and sweet is the key to a good patient presentation. Pare down all the scattered information collected during your patient interview to just the crucial, medically significant facts and organize them into a prioritized and logical order. Remember, faculty have short attention spans!

- Start with the basics: patient's name, age, sex, and race. Move on to the chief complaint.

- Follow this up with a *brief* history of the patient's present illness, being sure to include how, when, where, and, if the patient knows, why this problem started. Note the frequency and quality of discomfort and what, if anything, alleviates this problem. Be sure to include any current therapies or medications the patient is using to treat this complaint.

- Next, add any objective findings you may have noted during a physical exam (anything you can document and prove exists, such as elevated temperature and abnormal lab values).

- Finally, take a stab at what you think is wrong with the patient.

- Presenting a patient is a tough skill to master initially. It takes time and practice to know what is pertinent and what is superfluous in a patient's history. Trust your judgment. Once your preceptor has had the opportunity to assess the patient, ask about areas of your presentation that could use improvement and which areas were done well.

Writing Prescriptions

Chances are good that your preceptor will give you opportunities to write prescriptions once a course of treatment is set. **Table 2** lists the elements of proper prescription writing. **Figure 1** shows a sample prescription.

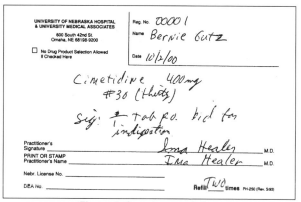

Figure 1: Sample prescription.

Table 2. How to Write a Prescription

Think of writing a prescription as writing down a recipe. Instead of writing down how to make your grandma's secret bean dip, however, you are writing down how to take the medicine that will cure the "post-bean dip blues."

- First write **Rx**.

- Then write the **name of the drug** you are prescribing—e.g., *cimetidine*.

- Now indicate **the strength** of the drug to take, indicating appropriate milligrams, grams, or other unit of measurement—e.g., 400 mg tablets.

- Indicate the **number of total pills** (or quantity if the medicine is a liquid or spray) that is to be dispensed at this time. Like writing a check, make sure you not only write the number down, but also spell out the number—e.g., #30 (thirty). This prevents someone from changing, say 30 (thirty) into 300.

- On a new line, begin the instructions for this medication by writing the word sig followed by a colon (:).

- Next, indicate **how many** to take at a given time by writing the appropriate number of dots above a corresponding number of lines—e.g., $\frac{\bullet}{|}$ = one, $\frac{\bullet\bullet}{||}$ = two, $\frac{\bullet\bullet\bullet}{|||}$ = three.

- Indicate **what** to take—e.g., tablets, drops, suppositories.

- Indicate **how** to take the medication—e.g., P.O. (orally).

- Indicate **how often** to take the medication—e.g., b.i.d. (twice daily), t.i.d. (three times per day), PRN (as needed).
  – Indicate **why** you are prescribing the medication.
  – Write the number of refills allowed.

Beyond the Clinics

If possible, observe your preceptor as she cares for patients in other venues including the hospital, nursing home, home visits, hospice, or during family conferences. Each arena of care offers unique interactions and learning experiences.

Observing other areas of your preceptor's work and private life including medical staff conferences, community outreach activities, and family activities can be rewarding and give you an idea of the life of a physician.

Your early clinical experiences can be one of the most enjoyable aspects of your medical education. These experiences provide the real world context for the basic sciences you are working so hard to master. In addition, these experiences serve to remind you of the reasons you elected to enter medicine in the first place—to care for patients and relieve suffering. Proper preparation will enhance the value of these experiences.

Appendix A: Writing the SOAP Note

Think of a SOAP note as the physician's short story. The SOAP note is a succinct and complete review of a patient encounter from start to finish. SOAP notes are most commonly written after clinical encounters to provide a written record of what ideas and information were exchanged or discovered and what the physician is going to do with that new-found information. SOAP note is an acronym for the four sections of the patient encounter report: subjective, objective, assessment, plan.

Subjective refers to what the patient tells you. The subjective portion of the SOAP note should include the reason for the visit and usually includes a chief complaint. It is helpful to state the chief complaint in the patient's own words, and quotation marks should be used liberally (e.g., "My tummy hurts."). A brief elaboration on this chief complaint is useful, and any modifying factors of the chief complaint, such as a description of the problem's onset, type of discomfort, modifying factors, duration, and what the patient has been doing for it, should be added. A sample subjective section might read:

S: Patient complains of "a tummy ache" for one day duration brought on by excessive consumption (four bowls) of "grandma's bean dip." A large and unknown quantity of Pepto Bismol has not brought relief to an abdominal discomfort described as searing and "fire"-like in nature. The patient appears to be in extreme discomfort with noticeable abdominal guarding.

The mnemonic PQRST is useful to describe a patient's symptoms:

P = Provocative or palliative—what makes this symptom better or worse?
Q = Quality—what does this pain (condition) feel like?
R = Region—where is the symptom and where does it go?
S = Severity—on a scale of 1–10, how bad is this symptom?
T = Time—when does the symptom occur, how long does it last, how long between episodes?

Objective is a documentation of all physical findings that can be *proven*. A temperature of 98.6°F can be proven as can all other vital signs (pulse, respiration rate, and blood pressure). Physical exam findings can be proven and include anything that can be palpated, measured, auscultated, or otherwise quantitated. All lab values should be included in the objective section, as well as x-ray, CT, and MRI findings. For example:

O: BP: 125/86P: 80R: 18T: 98.6

Blood work: Na (sodium): 148
Hgb (hemoglobin): 13

Positive bowel sounds in all four quadrants with noted increased borborigmy (tummy noises).

Abdominal x-ray: Air pockets and dilated bowel in all four quadrants with 18 cm distention of stomach by fundic air pocket.

The **assessment** is the clinical impression of the patient encounter; in many cases assessment is synonymous with diagnosis. The assessment should explain in one sentence your professional opinion as to what the subjective and objective information indicates about the patient's current medical condition. Keep it succinct and list a short differential diagnosis if no readily apparent assessment can be made.

A: Patient is suffering acute gastroesophageal reflux and G.I. distress due to excessive bean dip consumption.

The **plan** section is, of course, the treatment plan. Be specific but brief.

P: Patient was given 400 mg cimetidine PO b.i.d. #30 for seven days. Patient was counseled on the benefits of a balanced diet and told to return if symptoms do not improve within four days.

2. Who Pays the Bill?
An Introduction to Office Financing

William C. Minier, MD

Synopsis

Paperwork is a major part of the operation of every clinic and office; it's how the bills get paid. Because of the costs involved, health insurance companies require appropriate documentation regarding each patient visit. The information is recorded using standardized terms and numerical codes on standardized forms. Presented in narrative format, this chapter explains:

- Where to find the terminology and codes used for billing for office visits
- Types of medical insurance
- How to calculate what the patient pays and what the insurance company pays
- Governmental requirements and insurance

Introduction to Office Financing

I was making my first visit to my preceptor's office, and I was a little nervous. The busy receptionist politely asked me to have a seat. "Dr. Peterson will be with you shortly." A few minutes later, Dr. Peterson came in and introduced herself. Before we began seeing patients, she asked me back to her office and told me a little about the practice she shared with three other physicians and a physician's assistant. Then she reviewed the expectations the preceptorship coordinator had given us and asked if I had any questions. When I said no, she suggested that I just follow her for the first day and take notes. I could ask questions at the end of the day or between patients if time permitted.

Upon entering the first room, Dr. Peterson introduced me as a first-year medical student and asked the patient if I could stay in the room during the office visit. I remained quiet and observed Dr. Peterson throughout her history-taking, physical exam, and discussion with the patient. This pattern repeated throughout the day, and by the end of the afternoon, I had seen all but two of her fourteen patients. We saw patients with acute problems (e.g., colds, sore throats, back pain, stomach pain) and others with more chronic conditions, including hypertension and depression. At the end of the afternoon session, Dr. Peterson took time to review the day and answer my questions.

I asked her about the sheet she had given patients at the end of their visit while asking them to check out at the reception desk. She said that it was the office's "superbill." I asked if it was called that because it was so large. She laughed and said some patients might think so. However, it was the information the billing person needed to transfer the **CPT (Definition)** and **ICD-CM (Definition)** codes to the **HCFA 1500 (Definition)** forms. These forms were then mailed to the **PPO (Definition)** or **HMO (Definition)** so her office would be paid for their services. I stared blankly for a moment and said, "CPT, ICD-CM, PPO? What do all those letters mean? It sounds like alphabet soup." She agreed and took more time to explain.

 Definitions are supplied at the end of the chapter.

Before the insurance company pays for patient care, they need to know which services have been rendered. When insurance was less common, the doctor usually expected payment when services were provided. Under the old **fee-for-service** (FFS) *(Definition)* medical practice, with **indemnity insurance** *(Definition)*, physicians usually billed for their charges, and the insurance company paid the **usual, customary, and reasonable** (UCR) *(Definition)* charges after subtracting the **deductible** *(Definition)* and the **co-insurance** *(Definition)*. Health care was less expensive then. Insurance premiums were lower, and businesses frequently paid for part or all of the employee's (and sometimes his or her family's) health insurance premiums. As the cost of medical care began to rise, insurance companies and employers (including the federal government) wanted more information about the services for which they were paying. That is how insurance companies began using the ICD-CM coding system.

We went to Dr. Peterson's billing office where she showed me a copy of the CPT and the ICD-9-CM coding books. These books form the basis of the medical information insurance companies require prior to reimbursing covered medical services. My eyes widened at the size of the books. I asked her if I would have to learn all of that. She laughed and said no. The billing clerk would take care of the coding if we gave him accurate information about our diagnoses and procedures. She added that, after awhile, I likely would memorize some of the more common codes, such as 250.00 for NIDDM (non–insulin dependent diabetes mellitus). Basically, she explained, a physician (or nurse practitioner or physician's assistant) lists all of the diagnoses for which the patient was seen that day. If the patient just has a wart, one diagnosis is listed. If a patient has hypertension, diabetes, and elevated cholesterol (hypercholesterolemia), then all of the diagnoses associated with the reason(s) for the current visit are listed.

Then Dr. Peterson showed me one of their office's superbills and talked about how she completes the information for the billing clerk. "As you will notice," she said, "we list some of the more common diagnostic and procedural codes on our superbill. We also leave some space for times when we need to write in additional diagnostic or procedure codes." I noticed there were different codes for new and established patients and for brief, extended, or complete patient visits. I asked her how one determined whether a visit was brief, extended, or complete, and she rolled her eyes. "You don't want to know!" she said. Initially, significant variation existed among physicians in what they billed for different services. Then the **Health Care Financing Administration** (HCFA) *(Definition)*, which administers **Medicare** *(Definition)*, developed evaluation and management (E/M) guidelines. These required the physician to document the "right" amount of information under the history of present illness (HPI), the personal, family and social history (PH/FH/SH), the review of systems (ROS), and the right number of items, or "bullets," under the physical exam. However, physicians complained that they were spending more time on the documentation than they were with the patient, and HCFA revised the guidelines again. The new system is supposed to be based on physical exam findings, medical necessity, assessment (diagnoses), and the plan of treatment. Dr. Peterson said, "Just listen to the patient and do an appropriate history and physical. The billing rules will have changed again by the time you are working in an office."

She showed me a copy of the *HCFA 1500* form *(Figure 1)*. This stan-

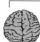

PLEASE
DO NOT
STAPLE
IN THIS
AREA

APPROVED OMB-0938-0008

CARRIER

HEALTH INSURANCE CLAIM FORM

PICA | | PICA

1. MEDICARE (Medicare #) MEDICAID (Medicaid #) CHAMPUS (Sponsor's SSN) CHAMPVA (VA File #) GROUP HEALTH PLAN (SSN or ID) FECA BLK LUNG (SSN) OTHER (ID)
[X] Medicare

1a. INSURED'S I.D. NUMBER (FOR PROGRAM IN ITEM 1)
123-45-6789A

2. PATIENT'S NAME (Last Name, First Name, Middle Initial)
Doe, Jane

3. PATIENT'S BIRTH DATE   MM DD YY   SEX   M F

4. INSURED'S NAME (Last Name, First Name, Middle Initial)
Doe, Jane

5. PATIENT'S ADDRESS (No., Street)
123 Main Street

6. PATIENT RELATIONSHIP TO INSURED
Self [X] Spouse Child Other

7. INSURED'S ADDRESS (No., Street)

CITY: Anywhere   STATE: NE

8. PATIENT STATUS
Single Married Other
Employed Full-Time Student Part-Time Student

CITY   STATE

ZIP CODE   TELEPHONE (Include Area Code)   (   )

ZIP CODE   TELEPHONE (INCLUDE AREA CODE)   (   )

9. OTHER INSURED'S NAME (Last Name, First Name, Middle Initial)

10. IS PATIENT'S CONDITION RELATED TO:

11. INSURED'S POLICY GROUP OR FECA NUMBER

a. OTHER INSURED'S POLICY OR GROUP NUMBER

a. EMPLOYMENT? (CURRENT OR PREVIOUS)   YES [X] NO

a. INSURED'S DATE OF BIRTH   MM DD YY   SEX   M F

b. OTHER INSURED'S DATE OF BIRTH   MM DD YY   SEX   M F

b. AUTO ACCIDENT?   PLACE (State)   YES [X] NO

b. EMPLOYER'S NAME OR SCHOOL NAME

c. EMPLOYER'S NAME OR SCHOOL NAME

c. OTHER ACCIDENT?   YES [X] NO

c. INSURANCE PLAN NAME OR PROGRAM NAME

d. INSURANCE PLAN NAME OR PROGRAM NAME
Medicare

10d. RESERVED FOR LOCAL USE

d. IS THERE ANOTHER HEALTH BENEFIT PLAN?
YES   NO   If yes, return to and complete item 9 a-d.

READ BACK OF FORM BEFORE COMPLETING & SIGNING THIS FORM.

12. PATIENT'S OR AUTHORIZED PERSON'S SIGNATURE I authorize the release of any medical or other information necessary to process this claim. I also request payment of government benefits either to myself or to the party who accepts assignment below.
SIGNED   DATE

13. INSURED'S OR AUTHORIZED PERSON'S SIGNATURE I authorize payment of medical benefits to the undersigned physician or supplier for services described below.
SIGNED

14. DATE OF CURRENT: ILLNESS (First symptom) OR INJURY (Accident) OR PREGNANCY(LMP)   MM DD YY

15. IF PATIENT HAS HAD SAME OR SIMILAR ILLNESS. GIVE FIRST DATE   MM DD YY

16. DATES PATIENT UNABLE TO WORK IN CURRENT OCCUPATION
FROM MM DD YY   TO MM DD YY

17. NAME OF REFERRING PHYSICIAN OR OTHER SOURCE
N/A

17a. I.D. NUMBER OF REFERRING PHYSICIAN
N/A

18. HOSPITALIZATION DATES RELATED TO CURRENT SERVICES
FROM MM DD YY   TO MM DD YY

19. RESERVED FOR LOCAL USE

20. OUTSIDE LAB?   YES NO $ CHARGES

21. DIAGNOSIS OR NATURE OF ILLNESS OR INJURY. (RELATE ITEMS 1,2,3 OR 4 TO ITEM 24E BY LINE)
1. 401.1 Hypertension
2. 250.00 Diabetes
3. 272.1 Hyperlipidemia
4.

22. MEDICAID RESUBMISSION CODE   ORIGINAL REF. NO.

23. PRIOR AUTHORIZATION NUMBER

24. A DATE(S) OF SERVICE From MM DD YY To MM DD YY	B Place of Service	C Type of Service	D PROCEDURES, SERVICES, OR SUPPLIES (Explain Unusual Circumstances) CPT/HCPCS MODIFIER	E DIAGNOSIS CODE	F $ CHARGES	G DAYS OR UNITS	H EPSDT Family Plan	I EMG	J COB	K RESERVED FOR LOCAL USE
1			99213	401.1						
2			80048	401.1						Basic Metabolic Panel
3			80061	272.1						Lipid Panel
4			81000	250.00						Urinalysis
5										
6										

25. FEDERAL TAX I.D. NUMBER   SSN EIN

26. PATIENT'S ACCOUNT NO.

27. ACCEPT ASSIGNMENT? (For govt. claims, see back)   YES NO

28. TOTAL CHARGE $

29. AMOUNT PAID $

30. BALANCE DUE $

31. SIGNATURE OF PHYSICIAN OR SUPPLIER INCLUDING DEGREES OR CREDENTIALS (I certify that the statements on the reverse apply to this bill and are made a part thereof.)
SIGNED   DATE

32. NAME AND ADDRESS OF FACILITY WHERE SERVICES WERE RENDERED (If other than home or office)

33. PHYSICIAN'S, SUPPLIER'S BILLING NAME, ADDRESS, ZIP CODE & PHONE #
PIN#   GRP#

(APPROVED BY AMA COUNCIL ON MEDICAL SERVICE 8/88)   **PLEASE PRINT OR TYPE**   FORM HCFA-1500 (12-90), FORM RRB-1500, FORM OWCP-1500

PHYSICIAN OR SUPPLIER INFORMATION

PATIENT AND INSURED INFORMATION

---

dardized form is used by federal and state governments and is accepted by most insurance companies for submitting patient services claims. The form contains demographic information (name, address, and telephone number) and identifying information about the patient's insurance policy (or policies). Having complete and accurate information (a "clean claim") is important, or payment may be denied or delayed. The billing clerk enters the services performed (CPT or procedure codes) and the diagnoses (ICD-9 codes). He also needs to indicate, for each service performed, the diagnoses for which they were done. For example, if Dr. Peterson bills for a blood glucose test, the procedure code for blood glucose must be associated with a diagnosis code supporting the ordering of that test, such as diabetes.

She also showed me the current patient charges for different levels of office visits and for some of the more common diagnostic tests. I asked Dr. Peterson how Medicare determined how much to reimburse physicians. She told me that Medicare uses a **resource-based relative value scale** (RBRVS) *(Definition)* adopted in 1992. Since 1992, the Social Security Act has required Medicare payments under the RBRVS fee schedule to be based on national, uniform **relative value units** (RVUs) *(Definition)* that are to be based on the resources used in furnishing medical services *(Brain 1)*. To determine fees, a practice typically chooses a dollar value higher than the Medicare conversion factor

1 - The payment amount for each service paid for under the physician fee schedule is the product of three factors: (1) a nationally uniform relative value for the service (2) a geographic adjustment factor (GAF) for each physician fee schedule area and (3) a nationally uniform conversion factor (CF) for the service. The CF converts the relative values into payment amounts. For each physician fee schedule service, there are three relative values: (1) an RVU for physician work (2) an RVU for practice expense and (3) an RVU for malpractice expense. For each of these components of the fee schedule, there is a geographic practice cost index (GPCI) for each fee schedule area. The GPCIs reflect the relative costs of practice expenses, malpractice insurance, and physician work in an area compared to the national average for each component.

2 - The general formula for calculating the Medicare fee schedule amount for a given service in a given fee schedule area can be expressed as:
Payment = [(RVU work times GPCI work) + (RVU practice expense times GPCI practice expense) + (RVU malpractice times GPCI malpractice)] x CF

(currently $36.1992) and multiplies that by the formula *(Brain 2)* to determine a fee. Practices usually round that figure to the nearest dollar amount, although they may set any fee higher or lower at their discretion. Medicare will still reimburse according to its own fee schedule. Dr. Peterson said that medical costs are high and can be a significant burden for patients with inadequate insurance coverage. Most of her patients have one of three major types of insurance: **commercial insurance** *(Definition)*, including FFS and managed care *(Definition)*, Medicare, or **Medicaid** *(Definition)*. There are also about 37–38 million uninsured patients, which by definition means they have a gap of greater than 365 days in their insurance coverage. "Well," I asked, "what are the differences among the different types of insurance, and which plans are the best for the patient and the physician?" She said it depended and gave me a summary of the two basic types of commercial insurance.

FFS coverage assumes the medical provider (i.e., physician, hospital) will be paid a fee for each service rendered to the patient. The patient may see any licensed provider, and the insurance claim may be filed either by the patient or by the provider of the medical service. The medical services covered and the co-insurance may vary. In addition, most policies include a deductible before insurance will begin to pay its portion. Common co-insurance ratios vary from 70/30 to 90/10, with the most common being 80/20, under which the insurance company pays 80% of the UCR charge (the prevailing cost of a medical service in a given geographic area) and the patient pays the remaining 20% *(Brain 3).*

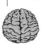
3 - Example: Your total medical expense is $5000. Your policy has a $500 deductible and the co-insurance is 80/20. You pay the first $500 as your deductible, then you pay 20% of the remaining $4500 (or $900) for a total of $1400. Your insurance company pays 80% of $4500 (or $3600).

Managed care plans generally provide comprehensive health services to their insured members with no co-insurance or deductible and with limited co-payments. The plans contract with selected hospitals, physicians, and other providers of medical services. Insured patients are expected to use contracted providers except in cases of emergency. In preferred provider organizations (PPOs) and **point-of-service** (POS) *(Definition)* plans, patients may be allowed to use noncontracted providers, but they will pay a larger portion of the fee when doing so. In health maintenance organizations (HMOs), patients are usually expected to choose one primary care physician (PCP) to manage and coordinate all of their care (i.e., a gatekeeper). Patients may be expected to request referral from their PCP before seeking nonemergent services. Most managed care plans have **quality assurance** (QA) *(Definition)* departments to ensure quality of care and **utilization review** (UR) *(Definition)* departments to monitor appropriate levels of use of services.

So, which type of plan is best for the patient and the physician? "For the patient," Dr. Peterson said, "I would recommend the plan that has the lowest premium and still protects the patient (and his family) from a catastrophic medical claim. For the physician, it would be the plan that interferes the least in his ability to care for his patients. A plan offering assistance in prevention would be an added bonus. As a physician, you will want to review all of the contracts you sign to assure you are being appropriately reimbursed for your services. I think it is fine for you to donate your services to patients in need, but you do not need to donate it to the insurance industry. And now, you and I need to perform one of the most important jobs for any physician." "What's that?" I asked. "We need to go home to our families, she replied."

I thanked Dr. Peterson and headed home, wondering how much medicine would change over the next few years.

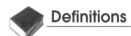

Definitions

Co-insurance: A division of responsibility for payment between the insurance company and the insured, expressed as a percent (e.g., 80/20—(insurance covers 80% of UCR, and the insured is responsible for 20% of UCR).

Commercial insurance: Commercial or private insurance falls into two broad general categories: fee-for-service (FFS) and managed care (health maintenance organizations [HMOs], preferred provider organizations [PPOs], and point-of-service [POS] plans). The distribution of health plans is approximately one-third PPO, one-third HMO, one-fourth POS, with the remainder FFS.

Current Procedural Terminology (CPT): The purpose of CPT is to provide a uniform language that accurately describes medical, surgical, and diagnostic services. The CPT book lists most procedures we perform for a patient, from a brief office visit to coronary artery bypass surgery. It also includes codes for testing, such as laboratory and radiology services.

Deductible: The portion of allowable health care expenses that an insured person must pay before insurance coverage applies. It is usually expressed as a dollar amount per calendar year; for example, $250/ calendar year means the insured must pay $250 of allowable health expenses before their insurance begins coverage by co-insurance.

Fee-for-service (FFS): A payment system where health care providers receive direct payment from the patient or the patient's health insurance company for billed charges.

Health Care Financing Administration (HCFA): The federal agency responsible for administering Medicare and for oversight of the states' administration of Medicaid, and the State Children's Health Insurance Program (SCHIP).

Health Care Financing Administration (HCFA) 1500 form: A standardized form used by federal and state governments and accepted by most insurance companies for submitting claims for services for a patient **(see Figure 1)**.

Health maintenance organization (HMO): A health plan providing a defined, comprehensive set of health services to a population within a specified geographic area for a fixed, prepaid premium (includes group, network, and staff models).

Indemnity insurance: A type of insurance plan in which the insured person may see a health care provider of his or her choice and the health care provider is reimbursed for all or part of covered services following submission of an insurance claim form (e.g., HCFA 1500 form).

International Classification of Diseases, Ninth Revision–Clinical Modification (ICD-9-CM): The ICD-9-CM is the official system of assigning codes to medical and surgical diagnoses and procedures in the United States. It is based on the World Health Organization's International Classification of Diseases (ICD).

Managed care: A system of health care characterized by comprehensive health services to insured persons using various payment and oversight methods to improve care and reduce cost. HMOs, PPOs, and POS plans are examples of this type of organization.

Medicaid: A federal government program administered by HCFA that provides medical assistance and health insurance to low-income individuals (persons eligible for Aid to Families with Dependent Children [AFDC] and Supplemental Security Income [SSI]). Services covered by Medicaid include in-patient and out-patient hospital services, laboratory and x-ray services, skilled nursing home services, physicians' services, physical therapy, hospice care, rehabilitative services, and pharmaceuticals. States may not impose restrictions or citizenship or residency requirements other than requiring that an applicant be a resident of the state. Neither the age of the applicant nor the fact that he or she works is a restriction to receiving Medicaid.

Medicare: Medicare is a federally funded system of health and hospital insurance for U.S. citizens age sixty-five years or older, for younger people receiving Social Security benefits, and for persons needing dialysis or kidney transplants for the treatment of end-stage renal disease. Coverage under Medicare is restricted to reasonable and medically necessary treatment in a hospital, skilled nursing home costs, meals, regular nursing care services, necessary special care, and home health services and hospice care for terminally ill patients. At the time of this writing, proposals are circulating in Congress to expand coverage to include prescription medications.

Point-of-service (POS) plan: POS plans combine features of both HMO and PPO plans. Members accessing care according to their HMO plan are covered according to the HMO's policies and procedures. Members accessing nonemergent care outside the network or without their primary care provider's approval pay deductible and co-insurance charges.

Preferred provider organization (PPO): A managed care plan that contracts with networks of health care providers to provide medical services according to a reduced rate. Members pay higher deductibles or co-insurance if they see noncontracted providers.

Quality assurance: A system of periodic review used by most managed care companies to ensure that quality medical care is delivered to the patients it insures. Methods used include on-site visits to physicians' offices, review of concerns voiced by insured patients, development and distribution of clinical practice guidelines (e.g., immunization schedules or asthma guidelines), and periodic review of samples of patient records.

Relative value units (RVUs): RVUs are based on calculations for physician work, practice expense, and malpractice expense. There is also a geographic practice cost index (GPCI) for each fee schedule area (to adjust for differences in cost-of-living and other variables). The Medicare fee schedule contains over 7500 codes, which correspond to the majority of the procedure codes in the CPT. The RVU is intended to compare and rate individual health care services according to the relative value of each. Specific fees are computed by multiplying the RVU by a nationally uniform conversion factor.

Resource-based relative value scale (RBRVS): This reimbursement system, designed for Medicare, bases payments on national uniform relative value units (RVUs), which are based on the resources used in furnishing a medical service (including physician work, practice expense, and malpractice expense).

Usual, customary, and reasonable charge (UCR): A reimbursement determined by the insurance company and purported to reflect the common or prevailing fee for a specific health service in a defined geographic area (may vary among insurance companies).

Utilization review: A system of oversight used by most managed care companies intended to reduce inappropriate or unnecessary medical procedures or hospitalizations. The methods used to achieve this goal include preadmission review of elective hospitalization or outpatient procedures for medical necessity, concurrent review of continued hospital stays, discharge planning to determine the level of care needed after hospitalization, and case management to assist physicians in the care of patients with complex medical or psychosocial conditions.

3. Uncertainty in Clinical Medicine

Thomas G. Tape, MD

Synopsis

Uncertainty plays a role in all medical judgments and decisions. The decision-maker may have incomplete mastery of relevant medical knowledge, medical science may not be able to provide an answer, or the correct answer may never be discoverable because of the inherent unpredictability of biologic systems. The concept of irreducible uncertainty provides a useful construct for the medical decision-maker who must make the best judgment with the currently available information.

Probabilistic methods form the basis of measuring uncertainty. Clinical indicators of disease such as symptoms, signs, and diagnostic tests are all imperfect. The probability of an indicator being present in a patient who actually has the disease defines its *sensitivity*. The probability of an indicator being absent in a patient who does not have the disease defines its *specificity*. These two measures along with disease prevalence provide the data needed to estimate the probability of disease for a patient with the clinical indicator. Clinical prediction rules, nomograms, and algorithms provide useful tools for guiding decisions when multiple clinical indicators are present.

People respond to uncertain situations with varying degrees of tolerance. Risk-averse physicians tend to order many diagnostic tests before deciding on a course of therapy. Risk-tolerant physicians may be inclined to try a therapy or adopt a wait-and-see approach if the diagnosis is uncertain. Patients' unmet expectations often arise from their failure to understand the uncertain nature of medicine or a mismatch in how the physician and the patient respond to uncertainty.

Medicine Is a Science of Uncertainty

Students of medicine often share the view of deterministic philosophers that all events are predictable and that errors simply arise from our lack of knowledge. A great deal of uncertainty in the beginning student does stem from knowledge deficit, but there are many questions medical science cannot answer. Even more difficult to comprehend is the notion that complex biologic systems are inherently unpredictable; science will never have an exact answer to some questions. This concept arose from the field of quantum mechanics and troubled a number of leading scientists, including Einstein. Nevertheless, the inability to precisely predict the behavior of complex systems of nature is now well accepted. In medicine, time pressure adds an additional dimension. Decisions often must be made quickly. The lack of time to gather more information about the patient or to search the medical literature adds to the inherent uncertainty of the underlying problem. The net result is called **irreducible uncertainty *(Definition 1)*** and must be dealt with in virtually all medical judgments and decisions.

A Clinical Example

A 25-year-old has a 2-day history of sore throat, difficulty swallowing, non-productive cough, and fever to 101°F. Physical examination discloses pharyngeal erythema, but no tonsillar exudate or cervical adenopathy. Does this patient have streptococcal pharyngitis? Should this patient be treated with antibiotics? How certain must the diagnosis be to justify treatment?

 1 - Irreducible uncertainty: Uncertainty that cannot be reduced by any activity at the moment action is required.[6]

This example is used to illustrate how to measure uncertainty.

Measuring Uncertainty

Methods for measuring uncertainty come from the fields of probability, epidemiology, and actuarial science. The most basic measure is *prevalance*, the frequency of disease. In adults presenting to primary care physicians with sore throat, the prevalence of streptococcal pharyngitis is about 10%. Thus, without any other information, one can be 90% sure the patient does not have strep throat. This patient, however, has several clinical indicators present (fever, cough, difficulty swallowing) and several indicators absent (exudate, adenopathy) that should help refine our 10% probability of strep throat. We need to know how each indicator affects the probability of disease.

The information conveyed by **clinical indicators *(Definition 2)*** is described by sensitivity and specificity. *Sensitivity* measures the proportion of patients with disease who have the clinical indicator. *Specificity* measures the proportion of patients without disease who do not have the clinical indicator. In studies of patients with sore throat, 61% of patients with streptococcal pharyngitis, and 32% of patients with other types of pharyngitis have cervical adenopathy. Thus, the sensitivity and specificity of adenopathy for strep throat are 0.61 and 0.68 (1 – 0.32), respectively. However, we do not yet have the information we need, namely the probability of strep throat in our patient who does not have adenopathy.

Bayes' theorem *(Definition 3)* provides a method to convert prevalence, sensitivity, and specificity information into probability of disease. A two-by-two table can be used to solve Bayes' theorem without resorting to complex formulas *(Table 1)*. Write whether the disease is present or absent above the columns. Write whether the clinical indicator is positive or negative to the left of the rows. The four cells of the table indicate whether the indicator is a true positive, false positive, false negative, or true negative result. Sensitivity and specificity relate to the columns of the table, and the probability of disease given the presence

2 - Clinical indicators of disease: The symptoms, signs, and diagnostic tests that are associated with a particular disease. *Symptoms* are the features of the illness described by the patient. *Signs* are clinical findings discovered by the examining clinician. *Diagnostic tests* are findings obtained by imaging procedures or laboratory analysis of clinical specimens.

3 - Bayes' theorem: A method for making probabilistic inferences developed over 200 years ago by the Reverend Thomas Bayes. In medicine, it is used to compute probability of disease from prevalence, sensitivity, and specificity. When written out in probability notation, it appears quite complex, but a mnemonic device, the two-by-two table, simplifies its application.

Table 1. 2 x 2 Table

	Disease present	Disease absent	
Indicator positive	True positives (TP)	False positives (FP)	Total positives
Indicator negative	False negatives (FN)	True negatives (TN)	Total negatives
	Total with disease	Total without disease	Grand total

Prevalence: (TP + FN) / (TP + FP + FN + TN)
Sensitivity: TP / (TP + FN)
Specificity: TN / (FP + TN)
Probability of disease when indicator positive: TP / (TP + FP)
Predictive value positive: TP / (TP + FP)
Probability of disease when indicator negative: FN / (FN + TN)
Predictive value negative: TN / (FN + TN)

Table 2. 2 x 2 Table for Streptococcal Pharyngitis

Prevalence = 10%
Sensitivity = 0.61
Specificity = 0.68
Hypothetical population of 100 patients with pharyngitis

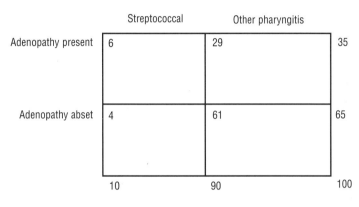

	Streptococcal	Other pharyngitis	
Adenopathy present	6	29	35
Adenopathy abset	4	61	65
	10	90	100

Probability of disease when adenopathy present (predictive value of adenopathy): 0.17
Probability of disease when adenopathy absent: 0.06
Predicitive value of no adenopathy: 0.94

or absence of the clinical indicator can be calculated from the data in the rows of the table.

Applying the data from the strep example, consider 100 patients with sore throat *(Table 2)*. Based on the prevalence of 10%, 10 would be expected to have streptococcal pharyngitis. Of those 10, the sensitivity of 0.61 implies that 6 will have adenopathy. Of the 90 with other types of pharyngitis, the specificity of 0.68 implies that 61 will not have adenopathy. The remainder of the two-by-two table can be filled in by subtraction. The probability of streptococcal pharyngitis in our patient without adenopathy is now easily calculated as 4/(4 + 61) or 0.06. Thus, the finding of no adenopathy reduces the probability of streptococcal pharyngitis from the population average of 10% to 6%.

Why bother with all these calculations if the probability of disease given no adenopathy can be looked up in a book? The answer lies in the influence of disease prevalence on predictive value of a clinical indicator. If the prevalence of streptococcal pharyngitis were 40% instead of 10%, the probability of strep given adenopathy would be 0.56 and the probability of strep given no adenopathy would be 0.28. These values are quite different from when streptococcal disease is less prevalent. Sensitivity and specificity do not vary appreciably with disease prevalence—they are properties of the clinical indicator rather than the disease prevalence. Thus, published tables of clinical indicators usually list sensitivity and specificity. If predictive values are included, remember that they apply only to the disease prevalence for which they were derived. You can use the published sensitivity and specificity values and compute predictive values for the disease prevalence that best describes your practice.

The probability of streptococcal pharyngitis given no adenopathy still does not describe our patient because it is based on only one clinical indicator. We could use published data to revise the probability estimate using each

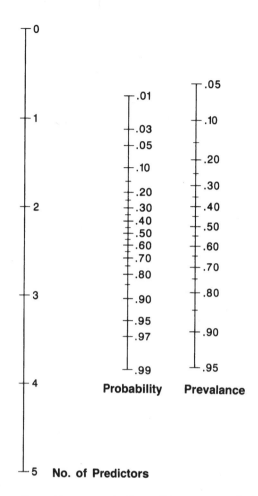

Figure 1: Nomogram for radiographic pneumonia. To use this nomogram, first determine the number of predictors present in the patient. The predictors are:
1. Temperature > 37.8°C
2. Pulse > 100 beats/min.
3. Rales
4. Decreased breath sounds
5. Absence of asthma

Place a straightedge so that it connects the number of predictors on the left line to the estimated prevalence of pneumonia on the right line. Where the straightedge crosses the center (probability) line gives the predicted probability of radiographic pneumonia. (From Heckerling PS, Tape TG, Wigton RS, et al: Clinical prediction rule for pulmonary infiltrates. Ann Intern Med 113:664–670, 1990, with permission.)

of the other indicators in turn. In practice, this tedious approach is rarely employed. For most clinical problems, a few key indicators influence the disease probability. *Clinical decision rules* show how to combine clinical indicators into an estimate of disease probability. In the strep example, adenopathy, exudate, and fever are key. If none is present, the probability of strep is 3%. If only one is present, the probability of strep is 14% and if all three are present, the probability of strep is 42%.[8]

The same information can be displayed as a *nomogram*, which is a type of graph showing how indicators relate to probability of disease. For example, the nomogram in *Figure 1* shows the probability of radiographic pneumonia as a function of five clinical indicators of pneumonia.[7] All you need to know is underlying prevalence of pneumonia in the patient population and the number of positive findings in the patient under consideration. The simple-to-use nomogram replaces a complex mathematical calculation of probability.

Clinical decision rules are often developed to provide a rapid and inexpensive means to determine whether a more expensive test or evaluation is needed. For example, the Ottawa Knee Rule[11] specifies that a knee x-ray examination is only required for acute knee injury patients with one or more of the following findings: age 55 years or older, tenderness at the head of the fibula, isolated tenderness of the patella, inability to flex to 90°, or inability to bear weight. The sensitivity of the rule is 100% and the specificity is 49%. The rule was intentionally developed to maximize sensitivity so that all patients with fractures would receive x-ray examinations.

Other types of decision rules assess prognosis. An example is the Goldman cardiac risk score, which is used to assess the risk of cardiac complications following noncardiac surgery.[5] A few elements of the clinical history and bedside examination are combined using a simple scoring system that predicts the likelihood of serious postoperative cardiac complications. This information is useful both for counseling patients about risk and for planning perioperative care.

It is important to realize that clinical decision rules have pitfalls that may lead to judgment errors. The most important caveat is that decision rules may not work well outside the patient population on which they were originally derived. For this reason, you should not apply a rule in your practice that was not validated (i.e., tested) in at least one other patient population. Another common problem results from the complex relationship of underlying disease prevalence to the calculated disease probability when applying the rule. Some rules ignore disease prevalence—for simplicity, they assume prevalence is about the same everywhere. If this assumption is false, the probability estimates will be wrong, sometimes very wrong. Decision rules that require you to estimate disease prevalence (e.g., Figure 1) are not affected by this problem. For more information on using clinical decision rules, see McGinn and colleagues, published guide.[9]

Evidence-based Medicine

A commonly asked question is: "This explicit approach to uncertainty is great in theory, but how does a busy practitioner access the information needed for clinical decision making?" Until recently, the lack of organized data on clinical findings limited the application of these methods, but collections of diagnostic strategies[2] and therapeutic trial data[3] are now available. An approach to searching for, evaluating, and incorporating clinical data into practice called *evidence-based medicine* (EBM) is rapidly gaining acceptance. EBM provides practical strategies for busy physicians to practice medicine based on the best available scientific evidence.

Table 3. Steps for Applying Evidence-based Medicine

1. Convert clinical information needs into answerable questions.

2. Track down the best evidence with which to answer them.

3. Critically appraise that evidence for its validity.

4. Apply the results of this appraisal in clinical practice.

5. Evaluate your practice of evidence-based medicine.

Adapted from Sackett DL, Straus SE, Richardson WS, et al: Evidence-Based Medicine: How to Practice and Teach EBM. Edinburgh, Churchill Livingstone, 2000.

The basic steps for applying EBM are shown in ***Table 3*** and are described in detail in Sackett and colleagues' easy-to-use handbook.[10] The first step is to frame the question in a way that is likely to be answerable from the medical literature. When searching for information to help manage a specific patient, it helps to ask the question in four parts: (1) What is the problem or disease? (2) What intervention (e.g., test or treatment) is being considered? (3) Are there alternative interventions for comparison? and (4) What are the possible clinical outcomes? The next step is to track down the evidence to answer the question. Although a literature search might seem to be the obvious next step, it is not usually the fastest or easiest way to proceed. Instead, try one of the EBM-oriented tools such as the Cochrane Library, the journal *Clinical Evidence* or the CD-ROM/Web knowledge base called *UpToDate*. The third EBM step is critical appraisal of your evidence. This means assessing the evidence for validity and applicability to your patient. For each type of clinical research study (e.g., therapy trial, diagnostic test evaluation, causation study), Sackett and colleagues have assembled a list of questions you should ask to assess whether the study findings are likely to be true. The fourth EBM step is to take the results of what you have found and use them to modify your practice of medicine. The key skill here is to decide when your patients are sufficiently like patients studied in the literature that you can reasonably apply their findings to your practice.

The last EBM step is self-assessment. You should evaluate your success in practicing your EBM skills. How often do you construct EBM questions? How often do you find answers to them? Are you able to use critically appraised evidence in your practice? EBM approaches learning and practice very differently from the traditional model of reading textbooks. Textbooks generally do a poor job of differentiating evidence from theory or opinion. Developing skills in EBM will help you better understand what is known and what is not known. EBM skills are essential to be an effective life-long learner in medicine.

Attitudes Toward Uncertainty

Physicians (and patients) respond to uncertainty with varying degrees of comfort. Those who cannot tolerate uncertainty are said to be risk-averse. Such individuals strive to maximize information before making a decision. On the other hand, risk-tolerant individuals are willing to take action in the face of considerable uncertainty. Physicians should be aware both of their own attitudes and of their patients' attitudes toward uncertainty. Consider the statement: "We don't know the cause of your fainting spells, but patients with your type of problem have a normal life expectancy." Patients who can tolerate uncertainty may appreciate the explicit discussion, whereas patients with a low tolerance for uncertainty may find the explanation completely unsatisfying. Patients may demand additional diagnostic tests in an effort to reduce the level of diagnostic uncertainty. Without an understanding of the potential for diagnostic errors, this approach may actually increase rather than decrease uncertainty. Many patients' dissatisfaction with their medical care relates to their failure to understand uncertainty or to a mismatch in tolerance for uncertainty between them and their physicians. Both patients and physicians must learn to tolerate some degree of uncertainty—it is a fact of life.

Selected Readings

1. Barton S: Clinical Evidence: A Compendium of the Best Available Evidence for Effective Health Care. London, BMJ Publishing Group, 2000.
2. Black ER, Bordley DR, Tape TG, Panzer RJ: Diagnostic Strategies for Common Medical Problems. Philadelphia, American College of Physicians, 1999.
3. Cochrane Database of Systematic Reviews. Available from BMJ Publishing Group, P.O. Box 295, London, WC1H 9TE, United Kingdom.
4. Gigerenzer G, Swijtink Z, Porter T, et al: The Empire of Chance: How Probability Changed Science and Everyday Life. Cambridge, Cambridge University Press, 1989.
5. Goldman L, Caldera DL, Mussbaum SR, et al: Multifactorial index of cardiac risk in non-cardiac surgical procedures. N Engl J Med 297:845–850, 1977.
6. Hammond KR: Human Judgment and Social Policy: Irreducible Uncertainty, Inevitable Error, Unavoidable Injustice. New York, Oxford University Press, 1996.
7. Heckerling PS, Tape TG, Wigton RS, et al: Clinical prediction rule for pulmonary infiltrates. Ann Intern Med 113:664–670, 1990.
8. Komaroff AL, Pass TM, Aronson MD, et al: The prediction of streptococcal pharyngitis in adults. J Gen Intern Med 1:1–7, 1996.
9. McGinn TG, Guyatt GH, Wyer PC, et al: Users' guides to the medical literature XXII: How to use articles about clinical decision rules. JAMA 284:79–84, 2000.
10. Sackett DL, Straus SE, Richardson WS, et al: Evidence-Based Medicine: How to Practice and Teach EBM. Edinburgh, Churchill Livingstone, 2000.
11. Stiell IG, Greenberg GH, Wells GA, et al: Prospective validation of a decision rule for the use of radiography in acute knee injuries. JAMA 275:611–615, 1996.
12. Up-To-Date in Medicine. Wellesley, MA, BDR Inc, 2000.

4. Blood-borne Pathogens, Standard Precautions, and Isolation Practices

Virginia M. Helget, RN, MSN, CIC • Mark E. Rupp, MD

Synopsis

Approximately 5–10% of patients entering hospitals in the United States will develop a **nosocomial infection** *(Definition 1)*. These infections result in thousands of deaths and cost billions of dollars each year. One of the chief goals of infection control is to prevent nosocomial infections. This is generally accomplished by interrupting the **chain of infection** *(Definition 2)*. The easiest and most frequently used mechanism is to interrupt the route of transmission (the environment). Examples of preventive measures directed at interrupting the infection chain are presented in *Table 1*.

Another major goal of infection control is to minimize the risk of health care workers (HCWs) acquiring an infection due to occupational exposure. This is largely accomplished through the use of standard precautions in the care of all patients and specific isolation precautions for the care of patients with infections that can be spread via air or contact. It also includes the use of proper protective procedures and engineering controls.

1 - Nosocomial infections: Infection that develops while the patient is in the hospital and that was not present or incubating at the time of admission to the hospital.

2 - Chain of infection: The interrelationship between a susceptible host, an infective agent, and the environment in the development of infections. When one of the trio is disrupted, infections are prevented.

Isolation Techniques

The Centers for Disease Control and Prevention (CDC) has established a guideline for isolation in hospitals. It may be adapted to fit individual facility needs. It consists of a two-tier system: standard precautions and transmission-based precautions.

Standard Precautions

Standard precautions (SPs) are used in the care of all patients. They were first described in 1985 as "universal precautions," and one may still see this terminology in some documents. SPs were developed to prevent exposure to human immunodeficiency virus (HIV) and hepatitis B virus (HBV). They have evolved over the years to include preventing exposure to all blood and body fluids and to prevent transmission of any disease by these routes *(Red Flag 1)*. To decrease confusion, the CDC renamed them "standard precautions" in 1996. It should be assumed that any patient may harbor a blood-borne pathogen, and barrier and other techniques should be used to prevent transmission. SPs apply to contact with blood, body fluids, mucous membranes, and nonintact skin *(Brain 1)*. SPs address many aspects of patient care *(Table 2)*.

1 - The greatest risk in transmitting HIV and HBV is through blood and body fluids. However, it is recognized that the same route may transmit other diseases, and it is prudent to prevent their transmission as well. Diseases that can be spread by blood and body fluids include cytomegalovirus (CMV), Epstein-Barr virus (EBV), parvovirus B19, malaria, toxoplasmosis, Rocky Mountain spotted fever, Q fever, syphilis, lyme disease, relapsing fever, bacterial diseases, and HIV 1 and 2.

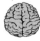

1 - It is important to protect your skin, mucous membranes, and clothing. Be cognizant of when aerosols may be generated (e.g., suctioning, centrifuging, irrigating tissues). Eye and mouth protection should be used.

Table 1. Prevention of Infectious Diseases by Category of Preventive Measure

Host	Agent	Environment (Transmission)
Appropriate exercise	Sterilization	Handwashing
Good nutrition	Disinfection	Standard precautions
Immunization and prophylaxis	Antimicrobials	Isolation techniques
		Proper disposal of waste
		Use of safety devices

Table 2. Requirements for Standard Precautions

Handwashing
- After touching blood, body fluids, secretions, excretions, and contaminated items
- Immediately after removing gloves
- Before and after patient contact
- Between dirty and clean tasks on the same patient

Gloves
- For touching blood, body fluids, secretions, excretions, and contaminated items
- For touching mucous membranes and non-intact skin

Mask, Eye Protection, Face Shield
- During procedures likely to generate splashes or sprays of blood, body fluids, secretions, excretions (e.g., suctioning, irrigating)

Gown
- During procedures likely to generate splashes or sprays of blood, body fluids, secretions, excretions (e.g., suctioning, irrigating)

Patient Care Equipment
- Soiled patient care equipment should be handled in a manner to prevent skin and mucous membrane exposures, contamination of clothing, and transfer of microorganisms to other patients and to the environment
- Reusable equipment must be cleaned and reprocessed before use in the care of another patient

Sharps
- Avoid recapping used needles
- Avoid removing used needles from disposable syringes by hand
- Avoid bending, breaking, or manipulating used needles by hand
- Place used sharps in puncture-resistant containers
- Use needleless devices, protected needles, or similar devices whenever possible

Linen and Infectious Waste
- Soiled linen should be handled in a manner to prevent skin and mucous membrane exposures and contamination of clothing and the environment
- A single bag is adequate unless it is leaking, torn, or the outside is contaminated
- Dispose of gowns, gloves, masks, and other protective equipment appropriately

Patient Resuscitation
- Use mouthpieces, resuscitation bags, or other ventilation devices to avoid mouth-to-mouth resuscitation

Patient Placement
- Patients who contaminate the environment or cannot maintain appropriate hygiene should be placed in a private room

Patient Care Areas
- Do not eat or drink in these areas
- Do not apply cosmetics (except lotion) or handle contact lenses in work areas where there is potential for exposure to blood or body fluids

Transmission-based Precautions

Transmission-based precautions are used in caring for patients with known or suspected communicable diseases. There are three categories of precautions:

1. Airborne
2. Droplet
3. Contact

Some diseases may require use of more than one category of precautions. The categories are described in **Table 3**.

Airborne precautions prevent disease spread by droplet nuclei or contaminated dust particles **(Brain 2)**. These particles may stay suspended in the air for long periods of time and can be widely dispersed. Many outbreak investigations have found air currents and building air intake locations to be involved in the spread of these diseases to remote locations in the facility. All HCWs should be immune to varicella, measles, and rubella. Vaccine should be received if immunity is uncertain.

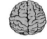
2 - Examples of diseases requiring airborne precautions are tuberculosis, measles, varicella, and disseminated zoster.

Table 3. Summary of Transmission-based Precautions

	Airborne	Droplet	Contact
Room	Private room with negative air pressure. At least 6 air exchanges per hour. All doors kept closed at all times. Patient is confined to room if possible, otherwise the patient wears a mask	Private room or patients may be cohorted. Door to the room may remain open. Patient is confined to room if possible, otherwise the patient wears a mask	Private room or cohort patients together
Respiratory protection	For entering room Respirators for tuberculosis	When within 3 ft. of patient	Consistent with standard precautions
Face shield, eye protection, mask	Consistent with standard precautions	Consistent with standard precautions	Consistent with standard precautions
Gowns	Consistent with standard precautions	Consistent with standard precautions	If contact with patient or patient environment or if environment is heavily contaminated
Gloves	Consistent with standard precautions	Consistent with standard precautions	For entering the room
Handwashing	Consistent with standard precautions	Consistent with standard precautions	Consistent with standard precautions
Equipment (e.g., stethoscopes)	Consistent with standard precautions	Consistent with standard precautions	Clean and disinfect before it is removed from the room. Use disposable items or equipment dedicated to the room if possible

Facilities that care for patients with tuberculosis (TB) are required by the Occupational Safety and Health Administration (OSHA) to have a plan for preventing transmission of TB. Deaths have occurred in HCWs due to occupationally acquired multidrug-resistant tuberculosis. It is especially important to keep a high index of suspicion to provide for early diagnosis and treatment. Patients with known or suspected TB should be placed in airborne precautions immediately. Those entering the patient room should wear respirators. HCWs are required to be fit and fitness tested for respirator use prior to wearing them. At least annual PPD skin testing of HCWs is also required.

Droplet precautions prevent diseases spread by larger particles in the air *(Brain 3)*. Droplets are generated from the source person primarily during coughing, sneezing, or talking. Because the particles are heavier, they fall out of the air more quickly. Masks need to be worn only when one is within the breathing space of the patient (about 3 ft). All HCWs should receive annual influenza vaccine to help prevent its transmission.

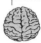

3 - Examples of diseases requiring droplet precautions are meningitis due to *Neisseria meningitidis* or *Haemophilus influenzae*, influenza, and parvovirus B19.

Contact precautions are used to prevent diseases transmitted by direct or indirect contact routes *(Brain 4)*. *Direct contact* involves skin-to-skin contact and physical transfer of microorganisms to a susceptible host from an infected or colonized person. *Indirect contact* occurs when a susceptible host encounters a contaminated intermediate object, such as a stethoscope or blood pressure cuff.

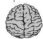

4 - Examples of diseases requiring contact precautions are vancomycin-resistant enterococci (VRE), methicillin-resistant *Staphylococcus aureus* (MRSA), *Clostridium difficile*, scabies, and shingles.

Handwashing is very effective in preventing transmission of infections. It is important to wash for 15 seconds using soap, running water, and friction, being careful to scrub around nails and between fingers. Although handwashing is the single most effective strategy to prevent infections, HCWs are known to not wash as often as indicated. Skin irritation from frequent washing and the time it takes to wash are two common reasons HCWs give for not washing as often as required. Waterless hand antiseptics have been found effective in reducing transient flora of the hands. Some products contain agents to help reduce the cracking and dryness of the skin. These waterless hand antiseptics can be used when running water is not available or to supplement routine hand washing.

Preventing Blood and Body Fluid Exposures

There are 8 million HCWs in the United States, and an estimated 800,000 needlestick or sharp-object injuries occur annually. Data suggest that at an average hospital, workers incur about 30 needlestick injuries per 100 beds per year. Therefore, HCWs are at substantial risk for HBV, hepatitis C virus (HCV), and HIV. Postexposure prophylaxis is available for preventing HIV and HBV. These infections are life-threatening and preventable.

A recent study found one-third of all graduating medical students recalled one or more exposures; less than half reported their injuries to proper authorities for follow-up. Most injuries involve various types of needles used in drawing blood or starting intravenous catheters. Injuries should be reported promptly so that postexposure prophylaxis can be initiated and eligibility for workers' benefits established. The risk of transmission for each injury varies, depending on the type of device, type of exposure (deep injury vs. superficial exposure to mucous membranes), and level of inoculum. The risk of contracting HBV, HCV, and HIV from a single percutaneous exposure is as follows:

- HBV   6–30% if unvaccinated
- HCV   0–7%
- HIV   0–0.3%

Most health care facilities are required by OSHA to have a blood-borne pathogen plan for preventing transmission to HCWs. Needleless devices, protected needles, safer passing of sharp instruments, and other devices and procedures should be used when available.

Putting It All Together

For the safety of all involved, it is important to communicate to other HCWs and professionals when a communicable condition is present or suspected. Effective techniques exist for preventing the spread of infections between patients and between patients and HCWs. These precautions involve handwashing, standard precautions and isolation, proper disposal of waste and sharps, use of immunizations and drug prophylaxis when indicated, and proper decontamination of equipment and the environment.

Preventing the spread of infection is the responsibility of each member of the health care team. It is important to be good role models for other members of the team, as well as for the patients, visitors, and family. You may be asked to reinforce the use of precautions and good aseptic practices to the family and visitors, whose cooperation and compliance in the health care setting is required.

Management

The following are key points to remember in preventing infections:

- Promptly recognize and treat communicable diseases. Communicate with other members of the team.
- Use standard precautions in the care of all patients.
- Use appropriate precautions as soon as a transmissible condition is suspected or while it is being ruled out.
- Observe facility protocols when discontinuing precautions.
- Wash your hands.

Selected Readings

1. Centers for Disease Control and Prevention, National Institute for Occupational Safety and Health (NIOSH): Preventing Needlestick Injuries in Health Care Settings. NIOSH Alert Pub. No. 2000-108, Atlanta, CDC, 1999.
2. Department of Health and Human Services, Department of Labor: Guidelines for Preventing the Transmission of *Mycobacterium tuberculosis* in Health Care Facilities. Fed Register 59:54242–54303, 1994.
3. Garner JS: Guideline for isolation precautions in hospitals. Infect Control Hosp Epidemiol 17:53–80, 1996.
4. Hospital Infection Control Practices Advisory Committee (HICPAC): Recommendations for preventing the spread of vancomycin resistance: Recommendations of the Hospital Infection Control Practices Advisory Committee (HICPAC). Am J Infect Control 23:87–94, 1995.

5. Conducting the Patient Interview

David J. Steele, PhD • William C. Minier, MD

Synopsis

The medical interview is the physician's core clinical skill. An estimated 70% of all diagnoses are made on the basis of the interview alone. The better the interview, the more accurate the diagnosis, the more likely the patient follows treatment recommendations, and the more likely both the patient and physician will be satisfied with the visit.

The medical interview is a procedure you can expect to perform about 200,000 times in your career! This chapter provides a brief overview of specific skills to enhance the quality, effectiveness, and efficiency of the interview. We begin with the generic adult interview and then offer some specific suggestions for modifying the interview for interactions with children, adolescents, and more than one person. This chapter assumes that you are the primary interviewer. It also assumes that most of your interviews in the ambulatory setting will be focused interviews designed to assess specific concerns or complaints. Full history and physical examinations, including past medical history, family and social history, and the review of systems is beyond the scope of this chapter. References to the full history and physical are provided at the end of the chapter. The topics you will need to explore for specific problems (symptoms or diseases) are highlighted in the problem-specific chapters in this book.

Getting Started

If available, review the chart to become familiar with the patient's current health problems, medications, and most recent clinic visit. Ask your preceptor if you should be aware of anything in particular in your interaction with the patient. Most clinics employ some kind of encounter form that is usually completed by a medical assistant or nurse and placed on the front of the patient's chart or on the door outside the examination room. Take a few moments to look at this form, because it typically will record the patient's name, age, vital signs, and chief complaint(s) *(Red Flag 1)*.

1 - Don't assume that the chief complaint registered on the encounter form is the only concern or the patient's most important concern. Even if a chief complaint is listed on the encounter form, it is a good idea to ask the patient directly what he/she hopes to talk about during the visit. Some patients may not disclose all of their concerns to the nursing assistant. By confirming what is on the encounter form and determining if there are other issues, you may avoid confusion and the inefficient use of time during the interview.

Introductions and Stage Setting

Always knock on the door and wait a moment before entering. When you enter, greet the patient using a polite form of address (e.g., Mr., Mrs., Ms) and the patient's full name. Introduce yourself using your full name and clearly indicate your status as a medical student or student doctor. Explain your role and make it clear that the patient's doctor will also conduct his or her own interview and examination. Finally, do what you can to arrange the environment to maximize comfort and to facilitate the face-to-face interaction. If the patient is seated on the exam table and a chair is available for both you and the patient, you may want to invite the patient to take a seat in the chair. If the patient is wearing a hospital gown that does not fully cover his or her lower body, see if a sheet is available to drape over the patient's legs. On entering the room, ask yourself, if I were in the patient's place in this interaction, what would make me more comfortable?

Example: Introductions

Jane Smith: Hi, are you Mr. Tom Doe?

Tom Doe: Hi, yes I am.

Jane Smith: I'm Jane Smith. I'm a first year medical student at State University School of Medicine. Nice to meet you. I'm working with Dr. Jones today. She has asked me to spend a few minutes reviewing your health concerns. She'll be joining us in a few minutes. Would that be okay?

Tom Doe: Sure. As long as I get to talk with her, it's fine with me.

Jane Smith: Thanks! Yes, you will get to see her too. Are you comfortable up there on the exam table or would you prefer to take this seat here while we talk?

Setting the Agenda for the Visit

Following the introductions, the most important task to accomplish in the opening 1 or 2 minutes of the visit is eliciting the patient's reasons for the visit and negotiating an agenda for the time that is available. Think of this initial part of the visit as one where you determine whether the patient has a list of concerns he or she hopes to discuss. You cannot make reasoned decisions about how to use the limited time available in the visit unless you know what is on the patient's plate. An open-ended question followed by an exhaustive "anything else?" will facilitate agenda setting and help to reduce the incidence of the frustrating, "Oh, by the way doctor, I was wondering about…," phenomenon at the end of the visit. Many interviewers err on the side of asking the patient specific questions designed to elicit the history of the present illness (HPI) immediately after hearing the first concern mentioned by the patient. The rationale given is that the patient may feel that the concern is being brushed aside. However, when the patient's initially shared concern is explicitly acknowledged, as illustrated below, it should be clear to the patient that your interest at this point is to discover all of the concerns for that day's visit and that the initial concern is not going to be ignored.

Example: Agenda Setting

Jane Smith: Now, tell me what you'd like to discuss with us today.

Tom Doe: I've been having lots of trouble with my right knee. It hurts when I put weight on it, and it feels like it catches or something when I walk. Not all the time, but enough so that I notice it.

Jane Smith: Um hum.

Tom Doe: I thought it would go away, but it hasn't so I thought I'd better check it out.

Jane Smith: I'm glad you came to see us. We'll certainly look into this for you. Now, before we address your knee pain, do you have any other problems or concerns that you'd like to discuss today?

Tom Doe: I'm not sure my blood pressure medicine is right for me. I'd like to see what my alternatives are on that.

Jane Smith: Okay, we need to check out your knee and spend some time talking about your blood pressure medications. Anything else?

Tom Doe: Nope, that's it.

Jane Smith: Alright, why don't we take these one at a time? Do you have a preference about where to start?

Tom Doe: Not really.

Jane Smith: Okay, then why don't we start with your knee problem? Tell me more about that . . ..

History of the Present Illness

After establishing the agenda for the visit, the next step is to elicit the HPI through the application of attentive listening skills and the appropriate use of both open- and closed-ended questions.

Your goal is to acquire as complete a description of the patient's symptoms as possible *(Brain 1)* and to elicit information about the patient's illness experience.

Even when you do not have the biomedical knowledge base to fully understand the patient's problem from a pathophysiologic standpoint, you can gather important data about the patient's experiences and beliefs *(Brain 2)*. The patient's beliefs and understanding affect patient behavior and response to treatment recommendations.

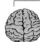

1 - Key question areas:
Location: Can you tell me where exactly it is that you feel the pain?
Quality: What does it feel like? How would you describe the pain?
Severity: How bad is this illness? What does it keep you from doing?
Timing: Do you notice your headaches coming on at any particular time of the day? Is it worse at some times than others?
Context: What were you doing when you first noticed knee pain?
Modifying factors: Is there anything you can do to make your stomachache go away? Is there anything that makes it worse?
Associated symptoms: Besides the stomachache, have you had any other symptoms that seem to go along with it?

Helping the Patient to Tell His or Her Story

Open-ended questions are valuable early in the interview and at the beginning of each new line of inquiry about a patient's problems. This type of question invites the patient to choose what he or she wants to relate and how. We are not suggesting, however, that you never use closed-ended questions. Closed-ended questions are helpful in getting specific types of information that may not have been provided in the patient's initial response. Closed-ended questions can also be helpful to patients by providing content and focus when they have difficulty relating their experiences or knowing what to tell you about their concerns. Skilled and efficient interviews use both open- and closed-ended questions in combination throughout the interview. Other techniques that can be helpful to the patient include minimal verbal responses as the use of "um hum," "yes," "go on," and echoing (repeating the last word or phrase offered by the patient). Nonverbal techniques include head nods, smiles, silence, and appropriate eye contact.

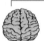

2 - Questions that can be helpful in gathering this kind of data are listed below. You do not need to ask each of these questions of every patient. Draw upon them selectively in your efforts to achieve a better understanding of your patient's story.
• What do you think causes this problem?
• Why do you think it started when it did?
• What do you think might happen if this goes untreated?
• How does this illness affect your life? Does it keep you from doing any of the things you need to do or want to do?
• Do you have any ideas about how this problem should be evaluated or treated?
• What worries you the most about this problem?
• Why did you choose to come in now for this problem?
See reference 5 for more information.

Common Questions about Conducting Interviews

What Should I Do When I Run Out of Questions or When My Mind Goes Blank?

All medical students (and experienced clinicians as well!) reach a point where they run out of questions or draw a blank because they are unsure how to understand and interpret the information presented. Sometimes, minds simply wander. A useful technique for dealing with these situations is summarization. This consists of repeating back to the patient the essence of what you have heard. This gives the patient an opportunity to check the accuracy of your understanding and a chance to correct, amend, or add new information. Summarization also gives you an opportunity to organize the information you elicited. In the process of summarizing, you may discover gaps you can ask the patient to fill in. Or, you may conclude that you have sufficient information and can move on to another line of inquiry or to the physical examination, or terminate the interview and report back to your preceptor.

Example: Summarization

Jane Smith: Okay, Mr. Doe, let me summarize my understanding of what has been going on with your knee. About a month ago you noticed that your right knee was sore the morning after you had been out jogging. You describe it as a dull ache that's there most of the time. It bothers you particularly when you climb stairs and when you push on the brakes of your car. At those times you experience sharp pains. You haven't noticed any swelling or redness. You've tried cold packs and you've taken Tylenol, but that hasn't helped. You've never had a problem with your knee before. You wonder if you might have torn the cartilage in your knee. Have I left anything out?

Tom Doe: No, I think that's about it.

Jane Smith: Oh, I also want to ask. Does resting it help? Like after a night's sleep?

Tom Doe: No, not really. It seems to stiffen up on me over night or if I've been sitting for a long time without flexing it.

Should I Take Notes?

The simple answer to this question is yes. But this yes comes with a qualification. Note-taking can interfere with the interaction, especially if you take a lot of notes.

During the course of the interview, you may need to jot down dates and other specific information that you may not readily remember. Develop your own shorthand style of note-taking so that the flow of the interaction does not have to be artificially slowed for you to write. We also recommend that you tell the patient you will be taking notes from time to time to assist you with your memory. Many patients take comfort in their physician taking notes. It assures them that they are being taken seriously and that the doctor is unlikely to forget the information they are sharing.

Common Mistakes in Medical Interviews

- Being too directive. Many interviewers get into the habit of overusing closed-ended questions. This is often done in the mistaken belief that it is more efficient to ask for specific information and yes/no responses. Being overly directive or leading is also a sign that the interviewer is pursuing his or her own agenda in the interaction. Again, seek balance. Begin with more open-ended questions and then follow up with more specific questions to fill in gaps and to get specific information. Clearly, when patients are in acute distress, flustered, or cognitively impaired, then you will need to be more directive and to use focused questions to get the information you need.
- Asking multiple questions or closing up open-ended questions by immediately appending a closed-ended question to an initial open-ended question. *Example:* Tell me about the headaches you've been having. Are they sharp or dull?
- Using medical terminology or jargon. Even simple terms such as STDs (sexually transmitted diseases) and OTCs (over-the-counter medications), to say nothing of more complicated terms such as diaphoretic, may not be readily understood by the patient. Develop

the habit of using everyday language and of translating technical terms for your patients.

Relationship-Building Skills

Unlike data-gathering or information-sharing, relationship-building is not a distinct phase of the interaction. Relationship-building is a dynamic process throughout the interaction. Listening attentively, using polite forms of address, and conveying interest in the patient's experience and concerns all contribute to the development of a therapeutic relationship *(Brain 3)*.

It is important to remember that one can show respect without necessarily liking or agreeing with choices that a patient has made. Similarly, one can empathize with another person's feelings or experience without necessarily feeling what the other person is feeling.

Tips on Interviewing More than One Person

It is not unusual for more than one person to be present in the examination room. Parents or guardians will come with their children and adolescents, spouses will accompany one another, and adult children may come with their elderly parents. A number of techniques can help reduce the complexities of interviewing more than one person.

- Greet all present and establish individual identities and the relationships between the various parties.
- Arrange seating so that you can establish comfortable nonverbal space and eye contact.
- Identify who the patient is and establish primary, but not exclusive, communication with that person.
- Clarify the reasons for the visit with all present. Establish who initiated the visit, why the other parties are present, and what each hopes to accomplish. Identify who is calling the shots and making the decisions!
- When eliciting the HPI, provide opportunities for the others in the room to add their perspectives and information if they can contribute to the story.
- If the patient is capable of interacting with you independently, you may want to negotiate some private time with the patient. The physical examination period is a good time to ask the others to excuse themselves. This can be particularly important when interacting with an adolescent patient. This helps to preserve their sense of propriety, particularly with a parent of the opposite gender, and also provides an opportunity for the adolescent to discuss issues he or she may be reluctant to bring up in front of a parent or guardian.

Interviewing Adolescents

Interviewing teenagers can be a challenge. The adolescent years are a time of growth and experimentation. Patients are coming to grips with their sexuality; peer-group acceptance is a major concern and may even be more important to the teen than acceptance by parents and

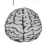

3 - A handy mnemonic for remembering specific skills that promote the development of rapport and a sound relationship is PEARLS:

P Partnership: The expressed interest in working with a patient to accomplish a desired end.

E Empathy: The capacity to understand an emotion and/or the ability to imagine what the other person might be experiencing.

A Apology: A willingness to acknowledge to the patient your role in causing the patient discomfort, distress, inconvenience, ill feelings.

R Respect: A nonjudgmental acceptance of the individuality of the patient. Treating others as you would have them treat you or someone you love.

L Legitimization: Explicitly communicating your acceptance of the patient's feelings or reactions; the expression of understanding how and why someone might react or feel as the patient does.

S Support: An explicit expression of your willingness to be available and helpful to the patient in any way that you can.

See reference 1 for more information.

family. The visit is often complicated by the fact that a parent or guardian accompanies the adolescent and feels a legitimate right to know about the teen's health status and concerns. We offer the following general recommendations:

- Remember that the adolescent is the patient and that your primary obligation is to the patient.
- Speak plainly and avoid talking down to the patient. Also recognize that efforts to gain rapport by using teen jargon can backfire.
- If the parent or guardian accompanies the patient, see page 29 for tips on interviewing more than one person. Negotiating individual time with the patient is particularly important with teens. It is the unusual adolescent who feels comfortable about discussing sexuality or the use of drugs or alcohol in front of a parent or guardian.
- If you find that the adolescent is not particularly forthcoming in response to open-ended questions, be a little more directive in your approach. You may find that the teenager opens up more as he or she becomes more comfortable with you.
- In addition to the particular concern prompting the visit, spend some time assessing psychological and behavioral risk factors *(Brain 4)*.

4 - The HEADS mnemonic can be helpful for remembering areas to explore with the adolescent.[4]

H **H**ome: "How would you say things are going at home for you?"

E **E**ducation: "How about school? Is that going well or not so well from your point of view?"

A **A**ctivities: "What kinds of things do you do for fun when you're not in school or working? Who do you do these things with? Do you have a close friend or friends? Someone you can talk to when things aren't going well?"

D **D**epression, **d**rugs: "Some kids your age start to experiment with drugs or alcohol. Is this true for you as well? Would you say you get down or feel bad a lot of the time?"

S **S**ex, **s**afety: "Do you have any questions or concerns about sex? Are you engaging in any sexual activities? Do you feel safe at home? At school? Is there any place where you don't feel particularly safe?"

Patient Education and Strategies for Maximizing Adherence

Although most students early in their careers will not have a direct role in providing a diagnosis to the patient or in establishing a treatment regimen, we provide a brief overview of techniques that are helpful in providing patient education and promoting patient adherence to treatment recommendations *(Red Flag 2)*.

2 - Provide explanation and diagnostic information as directed by your preceptor. Always remember your limitations and that the preceptor is responsible for the care of the patient.

Sharing the Diagnosis

- Explain your diagnosis in terms the patient can understand. Be clear and concise. Avoid jargon and providing too much information.
- Link your diagnostic explanation to the patient's own explanation or worries about what the problem may mean.
- Check the patient's understanding of your explanation and invite questions.

Example: Sharing the Diagnosis

Mr. Brown, based on the history you provided and on my examination, you have a condition we call costochondritis. That's a fancy name for inflammation or irritation of the point where your ribs join your breastbone. It can be very painful, but it's not a serious or dangerous condition. I know you were worried that you might be having heart problems, and I'm happy to say that's not the case. Does that make sense to you?

Communicating the Treatment Plan

- Provide a clear description of the goals of treatment and what the patient can expect.
- Provide clear, concise, and understandable instructions. Think in terms of brief chunks or sound bites. The patient needs to know:

What to do
When to do it
How often to do it
How long to do it
What to do if problems arise or if the treatment does not meet expectations
• Check for understanding.

Example: Instruction-giving to Enhance Understanding and Recall

Here's what I'd recommend for this costochondritis problem. First, I would like you to take Advil, which you can get without a prescription at the pharmacy or grocery store. I'd like you to begin by taking three pills every 4 to 6 hours. Some people take them with breakfast, lunch, dinner, and bedtime. If you experience any stomach irritation, taking them with food or milk will relieve that. As your pain begins to get better, you can start cutting back on either the number of pills, from 3 to 2 pills at a time, or the number of times a day you take them. Do you have any questions about this?

Adherence-gaining Techniques

Nonadherence with treatment recommendations is common and frustrating for the physician. It is important to recognize that you cannot force a patient to follow your advice, even when he or she has asked for it. As a physician you need to accept responsibility for providing the patient with clear explanations, good instructions, and the offer of helping the patient identify and overcome barriers to following your advice. However, beyond this effort, you are not responsible for the patient's actions or inactions. The literature on behavior-change strategies suggests that the following techniques can be helpful in promoting adherence. These techniques are predicated on the assumption that the patient has been given a clear explanation and understandable instructions.

• Ask the patient if he or she anticipates any difficulty in implementing the plan.
• Provide the patient with choices and alternatives.
• Engage in anticipatory problem solving.
• Encourage the patient to take an active role in formulating a plan for implementing the treatment.

Dealing with Difficult and Challenging Interactions

Inevitably, you will be confronted with difficult interactions. At times patients feel angry or sad or make requests that you do not feel you can meet. Sometimes bad news needs to be shared with patients or members of their families. There are no simple formulas for dealing with these situations, and a discussion of challenging interactions is beyond the scope of this chapter. See the suggested readings for more detailed consideration of the kinds of strategies than can be helpful in dealing with difficult interactions.

Selected Readings

1. Clark W, et al: Faculty development course materials. McLean, VA, American Academy on Physician and Patient. Available at www.physicianpatient.org.
2. Cole SA, Bird JB: The Medical Interview: The Three-Function Approach. St. Louis, Mosby, 2000.
3. Coulehan JL, Block MR: The Medical Interview: A Primer for Students of the Art, 3rd ed. Philadelphia, F.A. Davis,1997.
4. Goldenring JM, Cohen E: Getting into adolescent heads. Contemp Pediatr 5:75–90, 1988.
5. Kleinman A: Patients and Healers in the Context of Culture: An Exploration of the Borderland between Anthropology, Medicine, and Psychiatry. Berkeley, CA, University of California Press, 1980.

6. Telephone Triage

John J. Vann, MD • Jeffrey D. Harrison, MD

Synopsis

A substantial portion of any medical practice involves phone management. Frequently, patients, parents, spouses, or professional caregivers will call requesting advice. These calls will include questions regarding the treatment of specific problems, requests for prescriptions, advice regarding the need to be seen, and in many cases reassurance that everything is okay.

The purpose of this chapter is not to define all phone triage scenarios, but rather to provide a framework from which to assess the broad range of calls that a clinician could receive.

The other chapters in this book provide specific questions and red flags that need be addressed for a given problem. Detailed texts and computerized algorithms exist for professional phone triage services, but one overriding rule of thumb remains true in all cases: when in doubt, the patient should be seen.

Differential Diagnosis

When triaging phone calls, there are three assessment options to consider:

1. Immediate evaluation by a health care provider
2. Medical evaluation is indicated soon, but not emergently
3. Medical evaluation is not indicated; home or self-care is appropriate

The conditions requiring immediate evaluation are those that are potentially life threatening or functionally disabling. The red flags noted in other sections of this book will guide the need for immediate evaluation *(Table 1) (Red Flag 1).*

 1 - The following complaints could indicate life-threatening problems: chest pain, shortness of breath, difficulty breathing, severe headache, mental status change, acute neurologic deficit, penetrating injury, new-onset seizure, infant with high fever, vomiting or diarrhea for more than 24 hours, or suicidal

Other conditions will not warrant immediate evaluation but will require greater care than can be provided by the patient or home caregiver. These individuals should be seen, but how soon should be mandated by the severity of the problem, the potential for the problem to worsen, and the timing of the call.

Finally, some conditions can be managed with phone advice alone. The level of comfort that the caller and student have with the condition will aid in this determination. The option of being seen immediately should be offered, particularly if the condition worsens or changes *(Table 2).*

History

In the typical in-clinic encounter, approximately 85% of the diagnosis comes from the history; in the phone encounter 100% of the diagnosis comes from the history. The same general format should be used as in any patient encounter. It is important to document accurately and completely this history and what the caller was instructed to do.

Table 1. Selected Potentially Life-threatening Problems

Complaint	Possible Cause
Chest pain	MI, aortic dissection, pneumothorax, pneumonia
Short of breath, difficulty breathing	MI, PE, asthma attack, pneumonia, pneumothorax, COPD
Severe headache ("worst ever")	Meningitis, subarachnoid bleed, tumor
Mental status change	Stroke, infection (CNS, pneumonia, sepsis) electrolyte imbalance, hypoxia, drug overdose
Acute neurologic deficit	Stroke, TIA, intercranial bleeding (epidural or subdural hematoma)
Penetrating injuries	Occult bleeding, neurovascular injuries, pneumothorax
New-onset seizure	CNS infection, tumor, drug withdrawal
Infants or elders with high fever (> 102.5°F); 0–6 weeks (T > 100.5°F rectal)	Systemic infection
Persistent vomiting/diarrhea (> 24 hours)	Gastroenteritis
Suicidal or homicidal ideations	Depression, psychosis

MI = myocardial infarction; PE = pulmonary embolism; COPD = chronic obstructive pulmonary disease; CNS = central nervous system; TIA = transient ischemic attack

Table 2. Examples of Conditions to Be Managed Over the Phone

Condition	Possible Advice
Over-the-counter medication (OTC) dosage	Offer correct dose
Upper respiratory infection	Push fluids, OTC cough and cold medication
Superficial abrasion or laceration	Clean wound, sterile dressing, tetanus status, signs and symptoms of infection
Sunburn	OTC analgesia, cool compress
Insect bite (mosquito, chigger)	Calamine topical, OTC antihistamine

In the typical office encounter, the background and identification of the patient is given when he or she registers. In the phone encounter the following information needs to be obtained as the call begins *(Figure 1)*:

- Who the patient is
- Age (date of birth will aid in referencing who the patient is in the case of common names)
- Gender
- Usual physician
- Who the caller is
    Patient—first-hand information
    Someone calling for the patient
    Health care professional (nurse, EMT) *(Table 3)*

The first step in the evaluation is to obtain the reason for the call. This will serve as a guide to ask the appropriate questions regarding the history of the present illness (HPI). Important factors to elicit regarding the problem include:

- Duration
- Location

- Severity
- Context ("I get chest pain when I lie down")
- Quality
- Modifying factors
- Associated signs and symptoms
- Timing

```
Date: _____        Time:_____

Name of Patient: _____
Phone: _____

Name of Caller: _____
Relationship: _____

Age: ____    Sex: _____    D/O/B: _____    Physician: _____

Presenting Problem/Symptoms: _____
_____
_____
_____

Pertinent Past History: _____

Current Medication: _____
Allergies: _____

Social History: _____ Family History: _____

Review of Systems: _____
_____

Assessment: _____

Recommendations/Actions:_____
_____

Does caller agree?_____

Told to call back or be seen if problem worsens?_____

Other comments:_____

Signature:_____
```

Figure 1: Sample triage documentation form.

You must then obtain a pertinent past medical history (PMH) because this information will not be available unless asked and can have a strong influence on the advice given. An example would be an insulin-dependent diabetic with vomiting and diarrhea. This is a patient at risk for diabetic ketoacidosis (DKA) and should probably be seen expeditiously. Pertinent inquiries include:

- Previous illnesses
- Current illnesses
- Medications
- Allergies
- Recent surgery or procedures

A targeted social and family history (SH, FH) that relates to the reason for the call or could affect the outcome should be obtained. An example would be a patient with chest pain who had a parent who died prematurely from a heart attack; this situation would suggest the need for more immediate evaluation. Inquiries to consider include:

- Living arrangements (who is available to take care of the patient?)
- Transportation availability (could the patient get to care if needed?)
- Patient's functional status (ability to initiate self care)
- Family members with associated illness

A review of systems (ROS) pertinent to the reason for the call should also be obtained.

Table 3. Caller Experience

Caller	Considerations
New parents	Will have many questions and may have minimal prior experiences with common problems; often seeking reassurance that a condition is normal
Patients with chronic condition (asthma)	Will often have good insight into their status; past experience of the caller may be valuable to the student
Health care professionals (LPN at nursing home)	Will generally know the patient. Reasonable to ask what **they** think needs to be done.
Patients with newly diagnosed chronic illness (diabetes)	Patient and family inundated with large volume of information. Many questions and concerns without prior experience

Physical Examination

Although the phone encounter does not allow the student to examine the patient, there are still objective findings that can be used to formulate an assessment.

- How does the caller sound? Is the patient short of breath, confused or calm?
- Can the caller describe what he sees? Can the caller describe the rash, swelling, breathing pattern, or other pertinent information?

The student needs to develop a picture in his or her mind of what the patient looks like to aid in making an assessment and plan.

Testing

Although formal testing is not available during a phone encounter, important additional information often can be obtained. For example, an individual with diabetes can provide home glucose monitoring, a parent can take a child's temperature, or an asthmatic can provide peak flow measurements.

Putting It All Together

Phone management entails the determination of illness without the benefit of seeing the patient. Based on the phone encounter you must decide if the patient needs to be seen immediately, at a later time, or not at all.

An accurate initial assessment may be difficult to obtain. You should not always feel that an immediate answer is necessary. Consulting a text, physician, or other health professional and returning the call is acceptable in cases where a life-threatening condition is not involved. If the assessment suggests a life-threatening condition, then calling 911 immediately is appropriate *(Brain 1).*

In cases where the assessment is not felt to be life-threatening, arrangements need to be made for follow-up in a reasonable time frame. This evaluation will be determined by timing and severity of the condition. The comfort of the caller with waiting will also guide the timing of the follow-up encounter. Remember, when in doubt it is safer to have the patient seen.

Home care or self-care is a reasonable decision in many cases. In many professional phone triage centers, this recommendation is the single most common one offered. The option of calling back or being seen if the condition changes should always be given to the caller.

A separate call type that deserves mention involves the request for prescription refills. Most practices will have specific policies regarding refills, and you should familiarize yourself with those policies. As a student, you will not have authority to call in prescriptions or refills; however, it is important that a consistent message be given to the patient. If you are unsure whether or not a prescription will be called in, you should tell that to the caller rather than suggest what may be decided by the physician. You will need to obtain the medication they request, the dosage taken, and the pharmacy they use. In cases where the patient is unsure of the medication or dosage, the pharmacy can be an excellent source of information. Be alert to the drug-seeking patient who requests opioid analgesics and other drugs of abuse (e.g., Ritalin).

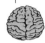

1 - If the caller is not the patient, he or she should hang up and call 911. In many emergency medical systems (EMS), this allows the operator to have the caller's address automatically. If the patient is the caller, then the risk of being unable to complete the 911 call exists. In these cases you should place the call, keeping the caller on another line if possible, or call back quickly to ensure that help is on the way.

Management

You will need to develop a framework of phone assessment and treatment, just as you would for a routine office visit. A thorough history is the single most important component of the phone encounter. With experience and practice you can become skilled at providing accurate assessments and plans based on a phone encounter. Liberally consult written resources, your preceptor, and other consultants until you have gained confidence. Remember: when in doubt, have the patient seen.

Selected Readings

1. Schmitt Barton D: Pediatric Telephone Protocols: A Quick Reference. Littleton, CO, Decision Press, 1993.
2. Wheeler SQ, Windt JH: Telephone Triage: Theory, Practice and Protocol Development. Florence, KY, International Thompson Publishing, 1995.

7. Health Care Maintenance Examination for Infants and Children

Kristine L.S.P. McVea, MD, MPH

Synopsis

Congenital abnormalities may become manifest only after several weeks or months of life. One purpose of the health care maintenance (HCM) examination of children is to screen for these physical and developmental abnormalities. Fortunately, most children enjoy good health, so another important function of this visit is to provide preventive services and counseling to prevent accidents and disease. Anticipatory guidance of parents regarding normal development, nutrition, discipline, and safety is an important component of these preventive services.

Setting the Stage for the Physical Examination

You will not be able to do an adequate physical exam if the child is upset and crying. Here are a few tips to set the stage for a quiet, happy patient:

- Try your best not to disturb or awaken sleeping children until you have completed all of the auscultatory parts of your exam.
- Perform as much of the exam as possible with the child in the parent's arms or on the parent's lap.
- Older infants and preschool children are often anxious about being examined by a person in a white coat, so consider removing it before entering the room.
- Distract bored or unhappy children with a small stuffed animal or squeaky toy (wash between patients!).
- For fussy, crying infants, encourage mom to breast-feed during the exam or have a parent offer the child a bottle or pacifier.
- Avoid aggressive body language: sit at a lower level than the patient whenever possible, avoid prolonged eye contact, use a soft voice, smile and coo at infants.

Most importantly, *take your time!* Rushing or pushing children only makes both you and the child nervous and distressed. Avoid physically restraining children whenever possible; it traumatizes them and only makes them more resistant the next time they come to the clinic. It is better to take a few minutes longer to coax the child through the exam than to hurry him through using force and making him upset.

Another important point is to get parents on your side by providing positive reinforcement and making the whole experience as pleasant as possible for the child. Too often you will hear parents say, "Get up on that table or I am going to slap your face!" or "If you don't stop crying, the doctor is going to give you a shot!" That only increases the child's anxiety and makes the experience worse. When parents make negative, threatening comments, you can use the situation as an opportunity for teaching better parenting skills if you approach the situation in a sensitive way. Do not directly criticize parents, or you will put them on the defensive. Rather, start with an objective, nonjudgmental statement: "David seems to be very frightened by his visit to the doctor today. He is crying as if he thinks I am going to hurt him." Get the parent to be your partner in making the child feel more secure by asking for input: "What kinds of things do you think we could do to help him calm down and feel less afraid?" You may have to suggest things to some parents; sitting on the parent's lap, talking in a soothing voice, rubbing the child's back, or holding the child's hand might all be options. Next, ask the parent to do the specific nurturing behavior: "Why don't we have David sit on your lap, and you can hold the stethoscope to his chest for me. If you could tell him, 'You are doing just fine' a few times in a soothing voice, I think that would help, too." Finally, be sure to praise the parents for the good job they did: "David seems a lot calmer now, Mr. Jones. Thank you for your help."

Praising children often during the exam is also important. The more they are praised for cooperating with the easy parts of the exam, the more confident they will be and the more likely they will be to participate in the more threatening parts. For example, listen to the heart initially for 1 second, then praise the child. Listen again for 2 seconds, and praise the child. Listen again for 3 seconds; praise the child. Then praise the child again after listening to each of the cardiac listening areas. After all that praise, listening to the lungs will be a snap.

Vital Signs

For HCM exams of children, growth measurements are probably the single most important part of the visit. Growth should be measured in a consistent manner at every HCM visit and plotted on an age- and gender-appropriate growth chart *(Red Flag 1)*.

1 - Deviations from the following should prompt an evaluation by the physician, beginning with a *detailed* diet history: frequency of feedings, amount of formula, how formula is prepared, length of nursing sessions, and other foods and liquids that are consumed.
- Infants should regain their birth weight by 2 weeks of age.
- Children should maintain their growth curve and should not cross 2 percentile lines on the curve.

Weight should be recorded on naked infants (no diapers, no nothing!) and on children who have removed their shoes, coats, sweaters, and any other heavy articles of clothing. Although parents often want to know their child's weight in pounds, it is often more convenient to record kilograms in the medical record because drug dosages and other calculations are based on the metric system. Clearly label the units used on chart.

Length in children younger than about 18 months of age should be measured in the supine position on a hard board. The head should be stabilized and the body and legs stretched out straight in order to get an accurate measurement. Length should be measured from the crown of the head to the heel. For older children who are able to stand up straight, height should be measured in stocking feet. The child should stand up as tall as possible with the chin maintained in the horizontal position. A ruler or stadiometer should be used to mark the height of the crown of the head. Again, label the units (i.e., inches or centimeters) clearly in the chart.

Head circumference is measured using a tape placed over the midforehead, extending around the most prominent part of the occiput. Errors in measurement are common, so recheck any suspicious readings.

2 - Systolic blood pressure or dystolic blood pressure > 95% for age and sex measured on three separate occasions = hypertension.

Blood pressure should be measured on all children older than 3 years of age. Normal values vary by age *(Table 1) (Red Flag 2)*.

Physical Examination of Infants and Young Children

Certain elements of the physical exam are more frightening or unpleasant for children. The following sequence will help minimize their anxiety. Undress the child as you go.

Table 1. Blood Pressure Levels for the 90th and 95th Percentiles of Blood Pressure for Boys Aged 3–17 Years by Percentiles of Height

Age (yr)	Blood Pressure Percentile*	Systolic Blood Pressure by Percentile of Height (mmHg)†							Diastolic Blood Pressure by Percentile of Height (mmHg)†						
		5%	10%	25%	50%	75%	90%	95%	5%	10%	25%	50%	75%	90%	95%
3	95th	104	105	107	109	111	112	113	63	63	64	65	66	67	67
4	95th	106	107	109	111	113	114	115	66	67	67	68	69	70	71
5	95th	108	109	110	112	114	115	116	69	70	70	71	72	73	74
6	95th	109	110	112	114	115	117	117	72	72	73	74	75	76	76
7	95th	110	111	113	115	116	118	119	74	74	75	76	77	78	78
8	95th	111	112	114	116	118	119	120	75	76	76	77	78	79	80
9	95th	113	114	116	117	119	121	121	76	77	78	79	80	80	81
10	95th	114	115	117	119	121	122	123	77	78	79	80	80	81	82
11	95th	116	117	119	121	123	124	125	78	79	79	80	81	82	83
12	95th	119	120	121	123	125	126	127	79	79	80	81	82	83	83
13	95th	121	122	124	126	128	129	130	79	80	81	82	83	83	84
14	95th	124	125	127	128	130	132	132	80	81	81	82	83	84	85
15	95th	127	128	129	131	133	134	135	81	82	83	83	84	85	86
16	95th	129	130	132	134	136	137	138	83	83	84	85	86	87	87
17	95th	132	133	135	136	138	140	140	85	85	86	87	88	89	89

Blood Pressure Levels for the 90th and 95th Percentiles of Blood Pressure for Girls Aged 3–17 Years by Percentiles of Height

Age (yr)	Blood Pressure Percentile*	Systolic Blood Pressure by Percentile of Height (mmHg)†							Diastolic Blood Pressure by Percentile of Height (mmHg)†						
		5%	10%	25%	50%	75%	90%	95%	5%	10%	25%	50%	75%	90%	95%
3	95th	104	104	105	107	108	109	110	65	65	65	66	67	67	68
4	95th	105	106	107	108	109	111	111	67	67	68	69	69	70	71
5	95th	107	107	108	110	111	112	113	69	70	70	71	72	72	73
6	95th	108	109	110	111	112	114	114	71	71	72	73	73	74	75
7	95th	110	110	112	113	114	115	116	73	73	73	74	75	76	76
8	95th	112	112	113	115	116	117	118	74	74	75	75	76	77	78
9	95th	114	114	115	117	118	119	120	75	76	76	77	78	78	79
10	95th	116	116	117	119	120	121	122	77	77	77	78	79	80	80
11	95th	118	118	119	121	122	123	124	78	78	79	79	80	81	81
12	95th	120	120	121	123	124	125	126	79	79	80	80	81	82	82
13	95th	121	122	123	125	126	127	128	80	80	81	82	82	83	84
14	95th	123	124	125	126	128	129	130	81	81	82	83	83	84	85
15	95th	124	125	126	128	129	130	131	82	82	83	83	84	85	86
16	95th	125	126	127	128	130	131	132	83	83	83	84	85	86	86
17	95th	126	126	127	129	130	131	132	83	83	83	84	85	86	86

* Blood pressure percentile was determined by a single measurement.
† Height percentile was determined by standard growth curves.

From National High Blood Pressure Education Program Working Group on Hypertension Control in Children and Adolescents: Update on the 1987 task force report on high blood pressure in children and adolescents: A working group report from the National High Blood Pressure Education Program. Pediatrics 98:649–655, 1996, with permission.

- Observe the whole child. Is this a normal-looking, healthy child?
- Face
    1. Normal features
    2. Facial rashes (these are almost universal in newborns)
- Heart
- Lungs
- Chest wall, breast buds
- Abdomen
- Pulses: femoral and radial (checking for coarctation of the aorta)
- Hip exam *(Brain 1)*
- Umbilicus *(Red Flag 3)*
- Genital exam: check males for undescended testes. Pull back foreskin on uncircumcised males.
- Anus: in infants check for diaper dermatitis, normal placement
- Lower and upper extremities for bony deformities and tone
- The rest of the skin
- Inguinal and axillary lymph nodes
- Spine: check infants for spina bifida occulta and bony deformities. Older children beginning about age 10 years should be checked for scoliosis *(Brain 2)*.
- Head, including fontaneles (should be open until about 9–12 months of age)
- Neck: check for masses, thyromegaly, tracheal deviation, adenopathy
- Eyes
    1. Red reflex in infants. Note that you should not try to pry infants' eyes open. Cradle the child in one arm and gently bounce the infant's head up and down. Use your other hand to look through the ophthalmoscope.
    2. Check children over 3 months of age for **strabismus** *(Definition 1) (Red Flag 4)*. Ensure that their red reflexes are symmetric and that they have a normal cover–uncover test *(Brain 3)*.
    3. Pupils
    4. Extraocular muscles. Use a toy to attract the child's attention to perform this.
- Mouth
    1. Check infants for cleft palate, including palpation of the soft palate.
    2. In infants, note the presence of thrush, a white exudate that can not be scraped off the tongue or buccal mucosa.
    3. Note the presence of erupting teeth, dental hygiene, caries.
    4. Check the posterior pharynx. It is difficult to check without a tongue blade, but rarely worth the trauma it causes.
- Ears
    1. Formation of external ears in infants, presence of preauricular pits.
    2. External auditory canal. Note presence of cerumen impaction *(Brain 4)*.
    3. Tympanic membrane. Use pneumatic otoscopy (a "puffer") to evaluate for middle ear effusion if there is a history of ear complaints or a recent otitis media.
- Neurologic exam
    1. Infants younger than 6 months of age may still exhibit the following primitive reflexes:
        Moro reflex *(Brain 5)*
        Tonic neck reflex *(Brain 6)*
    2. Tone, strength, and the presence of any abnormal posturing should be noted in infants.

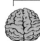

1 - This exam should be performed at every HCM visit up to 1 year of age to check for developmental hip dislocation. Two tests are used: The **Ortolani test** is performed with the child supine. The examiner faces the child's feet and grasps the knees. With the hip in flexion, gently adduct then abduct the hip. In an abnormal test, a palpable jerk and an audible "click" or "clunk" is heard as the femur slips back into the acetabulum. The **Barlow test** involves placing gentle pressure over the knee with the hip in flexion and adduction. A click is heard and palpated in an abnormal test as the unstable hip shifts.

3 - The umbilical cord should separate by 1 month of age. Some infants are left with umbilical granulomas that need cauterization. Small (< 3 cm) umbilical hernias are common, especially in black infants, and usually close spontaneously by school age.

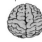

2 - The **forward bend test** is performed with the naked back exposed and the patient bending forward from the waist. An asymmetric rib hump is seen on the concave side of a spinal curvature. This is a subtle finding, and the examiner must look closely to see it.

1 - **Strabismus:** Misalignment of the eyes.

4 - Strabismus can lead to vision loss (amblyopia).

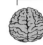

3 - The **cover–uncover test** requires the child to fixate at both distance and near vision. To perform the test, have the patient look at an object (toy or eye chart) 10 feet away. Note the position of the light reflex, and then obscure the vision in the patient's left eye with your right hand. In an abnormal test, the uncovered eye will move to fixation. Uncover the eye, allowing the patient to fixate with both eyes, then repeat the procedure with the other eye. Next, look for more subtle movements by alternately covering the eyes (like a windshield wiper) and watching for fixation movement as the eye is uncovered.

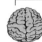

4 - Dark brown or black cerumen should be removed by the use of irrigation in the clinic or by daily use of hydrogen peroxide combined with water rinses for several weeks. Soft, yellow wax may be removed carefully under direct otoscopic visualization with a curette. Older children may be able to cooperate with cerumen removal by lying down on the table, but young children need to be restrained and have their heads stabilized against the examination table to prevent injury.

Development

Apart from the growth parameters, development is the most important portion of the HCM exam for preschool children. A variety of methods are available for screening children for developmental delays. Some practices have parents complete a developmental screening form. Others have prompts printed on age-specific encounter forms that list the appropriate milestones for that age. Some clinics perform a full Denver Developmental Screening Test on all 1-year-olds. *Table 2* lists age-appropriate milestones achieved by 90% of children at specified ages.

Immunizations

These recommendations change frequently as new vaccines are developed. For the most recent immunization schedule, check the following Web sites:

- American Academy of Pediatrics: www.aap.org/family/parents/immunize.htm (see also policies section for additional information).
- Centers for Disease Control National Immunization Program: www.cdc.gov/nip *(Red Flag 5)*.

Anticipatory Guidance

Advice to the parent (and child when appropriate) regarding normal development, parenting, and safety issues should be provided at each visit. The topics covered will vary depending on the population of children and the individual family. *Table 3* covers recommended screening tests and appropriate ages to address them. Here are some general categories to cover:

1. **General baby care**—Cord care, bathing, skin care, clothing, comforting crying babies, diaper rash
2. **Injury prevention**—Car seats/seat belts, air bags, supine sleep positioning, rolling/falls, childproofing home, no infant walkers, poisoning/Ipecac, smoke detectors, gun safety, bike helmets, water safety/drowning, stranger danger, violence prevention, burns, pedestrian hazards
3. **Nutrition**—Breast-feeding support; formula preparation; introducing solids; weaning; healthy diet; iron-rich foods; limiting juice; sweets; hot dogs, peanuts, and popcorn as choking hazards; normal decrease in toddler appetite
4. **Dental health**—Teething, brushing teeth, baby bottle tooth decay, fluoride supplementation, regular dental check-ups
5. **Development**—Normal developmental stages, appropriate toys, sleeping through the night, limiting computer/TV time, reading, toilet training, bed-wetting, tantrums, preschool, school readiness
6. **Parenting**—Discipline, time out, sibling rivalry, intentional injury prevention, choosing childcare, bonding, divorce, parental smoking/drug or alcohol use, talking with teachers, latchkey kids, sexual education, communication skills
7. **Illness**—Immunization schedule/side effects, smoke-free environment, thermometer use, when/how to seek care for illness episodes, handwashing

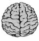

5 - The Moro reflex is elicited when holding the infant in a supine position. When the infant's head is briefly allowed to fall backward, the infant first flings his or her arms out (abducts and extends the arms and opens the hands), then the infant grasps toward the examiner (by adducting and flexing the arms). This reflex should be symmetric and present in all newborns.

6 - To elicit the tonic neck reflex, the infant should be placed supine on the table. The head should be turned gently but quickly to one side. The child should assume a "fencing position" with the ipsilateral arm extended, and the contralateral arm positioned with the elbow flexed and the hand extended upward.

5 - Children with sickle-cell disease, anatomic or functional asplenia, HIV infection, immune deficiency, treatment with immunosuppressive therapy or radiation therapy (including chemotherapy, corticosteroids), transplantation, cardiac disease, pulmonary disease (including asthma), cerebrospinal fluid (CSF) leaks, renal insufficiency, or diabetes mellitus are considered high risk and require influenza and additional pneumococcal immunizations. Check the American Academy of Pediatrics *Red Book* or one of the immunization Websites for more information.

Table 2. Developmental Milestones

Age	Personal-Social	Fine-motor	Language	Gross Motor
2 months	Smiles	Follows to midline	Says "ooh" / "ahh"	Lifts head
4 months	Regards own hand	Follows past midline, grasps rattle, claps hands together	Laughs	Lifts head up 90°, sits with head steady
6 months	Works for toy out of reach	Follows 180°, reaches	Squeals, turns to rattling sound	Pulls to sit without head lag, rolls over, bears weight on legs, lifts chest up with arm support
12 months	Feeds self, plays pat-a-cake	Grasps raisin with thumb and finger, bangs 2 cubes	Says "dada" / "mama" but not specific to parent, jabbers, combines syllables	Gets to sitting, sits without support, pulls to stand, stands holding on, stands 2 seconds
18 months	Plays ball with examiner, waves bye-bye, drinks from cup, helps in house	Scribbles	Says "dada" / "mama" to specific parent, says 3 other words	Walks well, stoops and recovers, walks backward
2 years	Removes garment, uses spoon/fork		Knows 6+ words, combines words	Runs, walks up steps, kicks ball forward
3 years	Puts on clothing, brushes teeth with help, washes and dries hands		Knows 6 body parts, speech is half understandable, has 100-word vocabulary	Jumps up, throws ball overhand
4 years	Puts on T-shirt	Copies vertical line and letter O, able to wiggle thumb	Knows use of 3 objects; counts 1 block; uses 2 objects, 1 color, 2 adjectives, 2 actions	Balances on each foot 2 seconds, does broad jump
5 years	Prepares cereal, brushes teeth without help, plays board/card games, dresses without help	Copies+, draws person with 3 parts	Speech all understandable; knows 4 colors; 4 prepositions, and 4 actions	Balances on each foot for 3–4 seconds, hops

Source: Denver II DA Form 5694 ©1990 W.K. Frankenburg and J.B. Dodds

Table 3. Screening Tests

Recommended Test	Age	Red Flags
Hearing testing	Newborns,* preschool	> 15 dB at 500–2000 Hz
Visual acuity	Yearly, beginning at 3 years	< 20/40 in either eye
Hematocrit or hemoglobin	9 months**	Hct < 33% Hgb < 10.5 gm%
Urinalysis	5 years	≥ 1+ proteinuria, hematuria, or glucosuria, leukocyte esterase +
Lead screening	Yearly, ages 1–6 years. History in all patients, blood lead levels in high-risk populations†	≥ 10 mg/dL
Tuberculin test	High risk: annually‡ Low risk: periodically (age 1, 4–6 years)	> 10 mm induration
Cholesterol	> 2 years in high-risk individuals§	> 170 mg/dL total cholesterol; LDL > 110

The child fails this developmental screen if they are unable to do *one* of these tasks by the age indicated.
* Using either evoked otoacoustic emissions (EOAE) or auditory brainstem response (ABR)
** May also screen older, preschool children who are recent immigrants from undeveloped countries or low socioeconomic status
†Universal blood lead screeing in **communities** at high risk include areas with > 27% of housing built before 1950 or with high rates of exposed children. **Individuals** at risk include children living/visiting/receiving childcare in houses (1) built before 1950, (2) built before 1978 and recently remodeled, or children who (3) have siblings with lead poisoning.
‡ Immigrants from countries with high TB prevalence, medically underserved low-income populations, residents of long-term care facilities, close contacts of persons with TB.
§ If parents or grandparents developed coronary artery disease, peripheral vascular disease, cerebral vascular disease *or* sudden cardiac death before 55 years of age or if parent has cholesterol level > 240 mg/dL.
Hct = hematocrit, Hgb = hemoglobin, LDL = low-density lipoprotein; TB = tuberculosis.

8. **Exercise**—Fitness, limiting sedentary activities, age/developmentally appropriate activities, competition/team sports, protective equipment
9. **Social**—Normal social development, playmate interaction, bullies, friends, peer pressure, tobacco/drug/alcohol use prevention

Selected Readings

1. Johns Hopkins Hospital: Harriet Lane Handbook, 15h ed. St. Louis, Mosby, 2000.
2. National High Blood Pressure Education Program Working Group on Hypertension Control in Children and Adolescents: Update on the 1987 task force report on high blood pressure in children and adolescents: A working group report from the National High Blood Pressure Education Program. Pediatrics 98:649–655, 1996.
3. Schor EL (ed): Caring for Your School-age Child: Ages 5 to 12. Elk Grove Village, IL, American Academy of Pediatrics, 1999.
4. Shelov SP, Hannemann RE (eds): Caring for Your Baby and Young Child: Birth to Age 5. Elk Grove Village, IL, American Academy of Pediatrics, 1998.

Web Sites

American Academy of Pediatrics: www.aap.org. See the series of materials in The Injury Prevention Program (TIPP).

8. The Health Care Maintenance Visit for Adolescents

Kristine L.S.P. McVea, MD, MPH

Synopsis

Adolescence is a time of increasing independence and experimentation with health risk behaviors. The purpose of the adolescent preventive services visit is to help the patient establish a healthy lifestyle and to provide parents with advice about their child's health needs. The emphasis of these visits should be on health promotion, health guidance, and interventions that target social problems such as alcohol use and unintended pregnancies. There should be less emphasis on the diagnosis of biomedical problems and the physical examination. The American Medical Association's Guide for Adolescent Preventive Services (GAPS) describes the following components of a health maintenance visit for adolescents.

Visit Orientation

Beyond age 11 years (depending on the maturity of the child), adolescents should be interviewed privately, without a parent present. This gives you time alone with the adolescent to discuss sensitive issues. Parents should also have the opportunity to meet with the physician privately, both to address their questions and for you to provide anticipatory guidance regarding their child's physical, emotional, and social development. Set the stage for this early in the interview. Although your role is to help enhance communication between the child and parent, encouraging adolescents to discuss sensitive topics with other responsible adults is a healthy thing. In order to have a frank discussion with your adolescent patients, you must assure them that you will maintain confidentiality *(Brain 1)*. Make sure both the parent and the child understand these ground rules before proceeding *(Red Flag 1)*.

Medical History

This is often done most efficiently before the parent leaves the room. Include:

- Current health problems
- Past health problems, hospitalizations, surgeries
- Medication allergies
- Medications
- Immunization record
- Family history, including risk of coronary artery disease, hypertension, diabetes, peripheral vascular disease, cancer, psychiatric disease, and substance abuse
- Social history: family composition, school and grade level

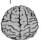 **1** - Office policies should ensure confidentiality. Billing sheets or bills for services that will be seen by parents should not mention "genital warts," for example, unless the patient agrees to reveal that information to them.

 1 - If the patient reveals information about potentially *life-threatening* behavior (e.g., suicidal or homicidal ideation, IV drug addiction), you must let him or her know that you cannot maintain confidentiality. Other information may be revealed by the adolescent that falls into a gray area (e.g., pregnancy, alcohol abuse, abusive relationship) of serious things that parents should know about, but may not constitute an immediate threat to the patient's life. In these instances, you should encourage the patient to share (with your help) this information with his or her parents. If the patient refuses, you must balance the benefit of having an ongoing therapeutic relationship with the patient against the cost of keeping the parents in the dark. I recommend arranging short follow-up intervals with these teens, and letting them know you will continue to maintain confidentiality as long as they act responsibly and keep their appointments.

Adolescent Interview

Use a conversational style and open-ended questions to explore the following topic areas:

- Physical maturation (secondary sex characteristics, menarche, regularity of menses, understanding of pubertal changes)
- Safety (driving while impaired; seat belts; motorcycle, bicycle, and all-terrain vehicle (ATV) helmets; smoke detectors; fighting; gang membership; weapons; safe storage and removal of firearms)
- Diet (junk food, fat and cholesterol intake, vegetables and fruits, dieting, bulimia, anorexia, calcium intake in females)
- Exercise (team sports, injury prevention)
- Sexual behavior (onset of sexual activity, birth control, sexually transmitted disease (STD) symptoms, HIV risk, condom knowledge/use, abstinence counseling, sexual coercion, sexual orientation, exchange of sex for money or drugs, past STD and pregnancy history)
- Tobacco, alcohol and drugs (experimentation; regular use; addiction; all forms of tobacco, including bidis, cigars, and chewing tobacco; binge and daily drinking; glue/inhalant sniffing; marijuana; anabolic steroids; diet pills; over-the-counter or prescription drugs for nonmedical purposes; IV drug use)
- Depression (mood, school performance, family dysfunction, suicidal ideation, psychiatric history, past suicide attempts)
- Abuse (emotional, physical, sexual abuse, partner abuse)
- School (truancy, grades, learning disabilities, attention deficit disorder, future plans, employment)
- Peers (best friend, peer pressure, tobacco, drug, or alcohol use)
- Family (relationships, source of conflict, discipline, parental alcohol or drug abuse, divorce)
- Dreams for the future

As you work through these areas use praise to reinforce healthy lifestyle choices. If you identify problems, provide guidance and explore potential solutions with the patient. Do not hesitate to address difficult issues, such as multiple sexual partners, but avoid lecturing or being judgmental. Frame your approach in terms of helping the patient be as healthy as possible; that is your job. To do that, you need to be critical of the unhealthy *behaviors*, but at the same time be unconditionally supportive of the *person*. (For example, do not say, "You are too fat," but instead, "I would like to help you achieve a healthier weight"). Tailoring your prevention message to the adolescent's particular social circumstances and life goals will help motivate him or her to make difficult lifestyle changes. (For example, "You told me that music is a very important part of your life. I am concerned that your smoking may not only cause health problems, but may also harm your singing voice").

Providing information alone may not be sufficient, because many patients know they need to make changes but do not know how. Suggest specific, concrete things the patient can do, and negotiate a plan that the adolescent understands and can agree to. ("If your boyfriend doesn't want to use condoms, you could tell him, 'Having safe sex is best for both of us'"). Remember, lifestyle changes are never easy to make, so be patient. Focus on a few key areas and arrange follow-up visits to monitor the patient's progress and to set new goals.

Physical Examination *(Brain 2)*

GAPS recommends an annual preventive services visit. However, a complete physical examination is only recommended during three of those visits (during early adolescence [11–14 years], middle adolescence [15–17 years], and late adolescence [18–21 years]) unless warranted by clinical signs or symptoms. Most of the visits should be devoted to health guidance (see below), and the medical interview is given priority. Here are the elements of the physical exam to cover:

- Height, weight, body mass index (weight/height^2) and growth curve *(Red Flag 2)*
- Blood pressure

- General appearance, hygiene
- Head and scalp (seborrhea)
- Facial skin (acne, facial hair)
- Eyes
- Ears
- Mouth (dentition, oral hygiene, posterior pharynx)
- Neck (masses, adenopathy, thyromegaly)
- Heart
- Lungs
- Breasts *(Brain 3)*
  1. For girls, note the Tanner stage for breast development *(Table 1) (Red Flag 3)*
  2. For older girls, begin teaching breast self-examination (BSE)
- Abdomen
- Male genitalia
  1. Tanner stage *(Table 2) (Red Flag 4)*
  2. Visual inspection for genital warts if sexually active
  3. Testes (masses, descended)
  4. Teach testicular self-exam (TSE)
  5. Inguinal hernia
- Female genitalia
  1. Tanner stage *(Table 3)*
  2. Vaginal discharge
  3. If the girl is sexually active, discuss performing a Pap smear with gonorrhea and chlamydia screening (even if asymptomatic). It is probably best to perform this at the same visit if feasible.   Also complete a bimanual exam *(Brain 4)*.
- Femoral pulses and inguinal lymph nodes
- Knee, ankle, and shoulder exam. Note joint laxity, instability, or previous injury. This is especially important in student athletes.
- Spine for scoliosis
- Skin (tattoos, piercings, nevi, sun exposure, athlete's foot, tinea)

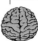
2 - Children may have been taught not to allow inappropriate genital touching by strangers, and they need to be reassured that medical exams by physicians are acceptable. ("I am going to check your private parts today, but it is okay because I am a student doctor and your mom [or the nurse] is here with you"). When examining the genitalia of an adolescent of the opposite sex, have a chaperone present.

2 - Adolescents with weight loss > 10% of previous weight or BMI < 5% of normal for age should be assessed for organic disease and eating disorders. Adolescents with BMI > 95% are overweight, and those at the 85–94% are at risk for becoming overweight. (See Chapter 44 for more information.)

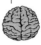
3 - It is extremely common for boys to develop either unilateral or bilateral gynecomastia during adolescence. Take this opportunity to reassure the boy that this is normal, common, and will go away in time. Unilateral breast development is also common among girls at the onset of puberty.

3 - Therlarche (breast development) before age 7 in white girls or age 6 years in black girls *or* after 13 years of age is out of the range of normal. Additional endocrinologic evaluation is needed. The average age of menarche is 12.8 years.

4 - Boys who develop sexual characteristics before 9 years of age and those who do not develop these characteristics by 13.5 years of age are out of the range of normal. They need additional endocrinologic evaluation.

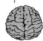
4- When performing the exam, take time to explain the procedure in detail first, and answer the patient's questions. Use the smallest adult-size speculum possible for the exam, and warn the patient before each step. The procedure will be extremely uncomfortable if the patient has tense vaginal muscles. To help with relaxation, initially insert one finger into the vagina and apply gentle downward pressure before slowly guiding the speculum over the top of your finger.

Table 1. Breast Development

Tanner Stage	Description	Normal Age (Years)
I	No breast buds	
II	Breast bud and papilla are elevated	7–13
III	Further enlargement of breast and areola	10–13
IV	Areola and papilla form a second mound above the level of the rest of the breast	11.5–13.5
V	Mature breast with projection of papilla only, recession of areola to the mound of breast tissue	12–18

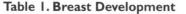

From Wilson JD, Foster DW, Kronenberg HM, Larsen PR (eds): Williams' Textbook of Endocrinology, 9th ed. Orlando, FL, W.B. Saunders, 1998. Adapted from Marshall WAA, Tanner JM: Variations in pattern of pubertal changes in girls. Arch Dis Child 44:2291–2303, 1969; and Roche AF, Wellens R, Attie KM, et al: The timing of sexual maturation in a group of U.S. white youths. J Pediatr Endocrinol Metab 8:11–18, 1995.

Table 2. Male Genital Development

Tanner Stage	Genital	Normal Age	Pubic Hair	Normal Age (Years)
I	Preadolescent		Vellus growth only	
II	Scrotum and testes enlarged, and thickening and reddening of scrotal skin	10.5–12.5	Sparse growth of long, slightly pigmented, downy hair at base of penis	12–13
III	Enlargement of penis in length with some increase in breadth. Further growth of testes and scrotum	12.5–13.5	Hair is darker, coarser, curlier and spread sparsely over junction of pubes	13–14
IV	Penis is further enlarged in length and breadth, with development of glans. Testes and scrotum further enlarged. Darkening of scrotal skin	13.5–15	Hair adult in type, but area covered is smaller, no spread to thighs	14–15
V	Adult in size and shape	15	Adult in quantity and type, spread to medial surface of thighs.	15–16

From Wilson JD, Foster DW, Kronenberg HM, Larsen PR (eds): Williams' Textbook of Endocrinology, 9th ed. Orlando, FL, W.B. Saunders, 1998. Adapted from Marshall WAA, Tanner JM: Variations in pattern of pubertal changes in boys. Arch Dis Child 45:13–23, 1970.

Table 3. Female Pubic Hair Development

Tanner Stage	Pubic Hair	Normal Age (Years)
I	Vellus hair only	
II	Sparse growth of long, slightly pigmented, downy hair	8.5–12
III	Hair is darker, coarser, curlier, and spreads to the pubic junction	9–13
IV	Hair adult in type, but area covered is smaller, no spread to thighs	11.5–13
V	Adult in quantity and type, spread to medial surface of thighs; inverse triangle distribution	13+

*Black girls enter puberty approximately 1–1.5 years earlier than white girls and begin menses 8.5 months earlier.
From Wilson JD, Foster DW, Kronenberg HM, Larsen PR (eds): Williams' Textbook of Endocrinology, 9th ed. Orlando, FL, W.B. Saunders, 1998. Adapted from Marshall WAA, Tanner JM: Variations in pattern of pubertal changes in girls. Arch Dis Child 44:2291–2303, 1969; and Roche AF, Wellens R, Attie KM, et al: The timing of sexual maturation in a group of U.S. white youths. J Pediatr Endocrinol Metab 8:11–18, 1995.

Screening Tests / Immunizations

See *Tables 4* and *5*.

Parent Interview

During a private interview, allow the parent time to address any specific concerns. Use time to discuss the following health guidance issues:

- Normal adolescent development in terms of physical, social, sexual, and emotional development
- Parenting concerns (communication skills, discipline strategies, family time, discussion of health-related behaviors, increased independence and privacy)
- Modeling healthy behaviors (diet, exercise, tobacco/alcohol/drug use, safety)
- Safety (new drivers, weapons inaccessible, smoke detectors)
- Social development (monitoring social activities for alcohol, tobacco, and drug use or sexual activity)

Table 4. Screening Tests

Preventive Service	Selected Patients	Red Flags
Serum cholesterol (non-fasting)	> 19 years or if parent has cholesterol level > 240 mg/dL or family history is unknown or patient has cardiovascular disease risk factors (smoking, HTN, DM, obesity)	> 170 mg/dL total cholesterol
Fasting lipoprotein analysis	Elevated serum cholesterol screening test or if parents or grandparents developed coronary artery disease, peripheral vascular disease, or sudden cardiac death < 55 years of age	LDL > 110 mg/dL
STD screening	All sexually active adolescents *Gonorrhea*—cervical culture or immunologic test of cervical fluid (females), urine leukocyte esterase (males) *Chlamydia*—immunologic test of cervical fluid (females), urine leukocyte esterase (males) *Human papilloma virus*—visual inspection *Syphilis*—VDRL or RPR if high risk (previous STD or > 1 partner past 6 months *HIV*—if high risk (IV drug use, hx STD, > 1 partner past 6 months, exchanged sex for drugs or money, male engaged in sex with other males, sexual partner of person at risk for HIV)	
Tuberculin test (PPD)	High risk (exposed to active TB, lived in homeless shelter, have been incarcerated, immigrants from high prevalence area low income, work in health care setting)	> 10 mm induration
Pap smear	Females > 18 years or sexually active	

HTN = hypertension, DM = diabetes mellitus, LDL = low-density lipoprotein cholesterol, STD = sexually transmitted disease, VDRL = Venereal Disease Research Laboratory test for syphilis, RPR = rapid plasmin reagin, HIV = human immunodeficiency virus, hx = history of, PPD = purified protein derivative, TB = tuberculosis.

Table 5. Immunizations

Immunization	Selected Patients
MMR #2	If not given at school entry
Hepatitis B series	Hep B #2 should be administered at least 1 month after the first dose. Hep B #3 should be administered at least 4 months after the first dose and > 2 months after the second dose.
Tetanus-diphtheria booster	Recommended at age 11–12 if > 5 years have elapsed since last dose of DT or DTP. Boosters recommended every 10 years.
Varicella	Previous immunity based on clinical judgment/history. 1 dose anytime after 1 year of age, 2 doses at least 4 weeks apart for children ≥ 13 years old

MMR = measles-mumps-rubella, DT = diphtheria-tetanus, DTP = diphtheria-tetanus-pertussis.

Follow-up

End your visit by creating a follow-up plan with both patient and parents present. You may need to schedule additional appointments with the adolescent only or with both the parent and adolescent to further address issues that surfaced during the initial visit.

Suggested Reading

Elster AB, Kuznets NJ: Guidelines for Adolescent Preventive Services. Baltimore, Williams & Wilkins, 1994.

9. Health Care Maintenance for Adults

Jim Medder, MD, MPH

Synopsis

Health promotion and disease prevention activities have been shown to reduce the number of premature deaths and morbidity from disease and injury *(Definition 1)*. Ten diseases or conditions account for 80% of all deaths in the U.S. each year, and over half of these deaths may be attributable to lifestyle choices and other preventable causes. In general, younger individuals are more likely to suffer death or disability from injuries, whereas older individuals are more likely to suffer from chronic diseases.

1 - Health promotion: Strategies related to individual behaviors or lifestyle that maintain or enhance well being or health (e.g., good nutrition, adequate physical activity).

Primary disease prevention: Prevent disease or condition from developing by removal or modification of risk factors or causes of disease or injury (e.g., immunizations, counseling a patient not to start smoking).

Secondary disease prevention: Screening tests for early detection of asymptomatic disease or measures to prevent recurrence (e.g., mammography screening, aspirin therapy after myocardial infarction).

Risk Assessment

Preventive services should be individualized for each person based on the presence or absence of risk factors, including age and gender. Risk factors are found in several parts of the patient's history:

- Past medical history (e.g., personal history of skin cancer or heart attack)
- Family history (e.g., family history of breast cancer or premature coronary artery disease)
- Social and personal history (e.g., tobacco use or multiple sexual partners without condom use)

Because risks may change over time, a periodic update or review of risk factors should be performed. In addition to risk assessment, ages or dates of previous screening tests and immunizations should be elicited.

Behavior Change Counseling

Because behavior change is difficult and long-term success rates are low, clinicians and patients often become frustrated and may give up trying to change or stop unhealthy behaviors. A different way of defining success involves the application of the Five Stage Process of Readiness for Change model *(Table 1)* in which success involves moving the patient from one stage of readiness for change to the next stage. For example, reframing success as having a patient who is unwilling to quit smoking to start thinking about cessation helps allay frustration. Good interviewing and counseling techniques and appropriate follow-up are especially important in motivating patients to change long-standing habits. The U.S. Preventive Services Task Force developed the following principles for patient education and counseling:

- Develop a therapeutic alliance
- Counsel all patients
- Ensure that patients understand the relationship between behavior and health
- Work with patients to assess barriers to behavior change
- Gain commitment from patients to change
- Involve patients in selecting risk factors to change
- Use a combination of strategies
- Design a behavior-modification plan
- Monitor progress through follow-up contact
- Involve office staff

Table 1. Five Stage Process of Readiness for Change

Stage	Definition	Goal
Precontemplation	Not thinking about change and may not be aware of need for change, (e.g., "I really don't want to quit—smoking relieves my stress.")	Help the individual to become aware of reasons supporting change and encourage him/her to think about the possibility of future change (e.g., "I understand you are under a lot of stress—I think we could find a way to help you deal with this stress more effectively and safely than smoking.")
Contemplation	Thinking about the need for change and may have attempted to make this change in the past. Currently, has not made a committed decision to change in the near future and doesn't have a plan for change (e.g., "I know I should stop smoking, but I don't know if I can.")	Help move the individual toward a committed decision to change (e.g., "Let's discuss the barriers to quitting that you see and maybe together we can find ways to get around those barriers.")
Preparation	Has made a committed decision for change but lacks a concrete realistic plan for change that takes barriers and resources to change into account; plans to start within a month (e.g., "I want to quit soon, but I don't know how I should go about it.")	Help the individual to develop such a plan, including a specific, time-limited first step (e.g., "What do you think about cutting back to half a pack per day and setting a quit date for 2 weeks from now?")
Action	Has initiated plan for change within months (e.g., "I stopped smoking about 4 months ago.")	Provide follow-up contact that will help motivate and support the individual (e.g., "Four months is really good; you should be very proud.")
Maintenance	Is successfully continuing the process of change beyond 6 months (e.g., "I've not smoked a cigarette in the past year.")	Provide follow-up contact for reassurance and support (e.g., "That's really great—by not smoking you're decreasing your risk for heart and lung problems.")
Relapse	Has relapsed (e.g., "I was doing really good until I went out for a drink with friends. Everyone was smoking, and I borrowed a couple of cigarettes from my friend.")	Help the patient evaluate the experience in a way that will facilitate future change. Be supportive and reframe the experience to help the individual quickly get back into preparation/contemplation (e.g., "Just because you smoked a couple of cigarettes doesn't mean that you've failed—it's just a temporary lapse. You did so well for so long—you can do it again.")

From Prochaska JO, Diclemente CC, Velicer WF, et al: Predicting change in smoking status for self-changes. Addictive Behavior 10:395–406, 1985, with permission.

Recording Preventive Services

A health care maintenance flow sheet on the front of the patient's chart is an excellent method of keeping track of preventive services. The dates and results of counseling, screening tests, and immunizations are recorded in one place and can quickly be reviewed when the patient presents for acute or chronic care visits to determine what preventive services are due *(Figure 1)*.

Adult Preventive Care Flow Sheet

Name

D.O.B.

No.

PUT PREVENTION INTO PRACTICE

ALLERGIES:

Health Counseling

(Circle if appropriate)										
1. Alcohol and Drugs	Date									
2. Aspirin	Type(s)									
3. Dental and Oral Health	Date									
4. Hormone Replacement Therapy	Type(s)									
5. Domestic Violence										
6. Family Planning	Date									
7. Folate	Type(s)									
8. Injuries (e.g. seat belts, falls)										
9. Nutrition	Date									
10. Occupational Health	Type(s)									
11. Osteoporosis										
12. Physical Activity	Date									
13. Polypharmacy	Type(s)									
14. Self-Exams (skin, breast, testicular)										
15. STDs/HIV Infection	Date									
16. Tobacco	Type(s)									
17. _____										
18. _____										

Screening and Tests

Suggested Examinations and Tests:*

BLOOD PRESSURE	DEPRESSION	HEIGHT/WEIGHT	PROSTATE EXAM/PSA	TUBERCULIN SKIN TESTING
BREAST EXAM	DIGITAL RECTAL EXAM	MAMMOGRAPHY	SIGMOIDOSCOPY	URINALYSIS
CHOLESTEROL	FECAL OCCULT BLOOD	ORAL CAVITY EXAM	SKIN EXAM	VISION
COGNITIVE AND FUNCTIONAL IMPAIRMENT	GLAUCOMA	PAP SMEAR/PELVIC EXAM	TESTICULAR EXAM	
	HEARING	PLASMA GLUCOSE	THYROID FUNCTION/EXAM	

* Specific preventive protocols should be tailored to the patient's risk factors and based on discussion between the patient and provider

Examinations and Tests	Schedule										
		Date									
		Result									
		Date									
		Result									
		Date									
		Result									
		Date									
		Result									
		Date									
		Result									
		Date									
		Result									

Immunizations

Immunization/Frequency

Influenza	Date						
≥ 65 YRS. OR IMMUNOCOMPROMISED YEARLY	Manuf. & Lot No.						

Pneumococcal	Date				Tetanus and Diphtheria	Date	
≥ 65 YRS. OR IMMUNOCOMPROMISED ONE DOSE	Manuf. & Lot No.				ALL ADULTS EVERY 10 YEARS	Manuf. & Lot No.	

Varicella	Date				Rubella	Date	
NON-IMMUNE ADULTS TWO DOSES DELIVERED 4-8 WEEKS APART IF IMMUNIZED AFTER AGE 13 YEARS	Manuf. & Lot No.				WOMEN OF CHILDBEARING AGE AND HEALTH CARE WORKERS WITHOUT EVIDENCE OF IMMUNITY OR PRIOR IMMUNIZATION ONE DOSE	Manuf. & Lot No.	

Hepatitis B	Date			
ADULTS AT INCREASED RISK 3 OR 4 DOSE SERIES	Manuf. & Lot No.			

Other Immunizations

Date	
Manuf. & Lot No.	
Date	
Manuf. & Lot No.	
Date	
Manuf. & Lot No.	
Date	
Manuf. & Lot No.	
Date	
Manuf. & Lot No.	
Date	
Manuf. & Lot No.	

Figure 1: Adult preventive care flow sheet.

Recommendations

These recommendations are for patients 18 years and older. Periodic health examinations (visits specifically for prevention) should be scheduled at appropriate intervals throughout life based on age and gender. Younger adults should be seen every 1–3 years, whereas those 65 years and older should be seen annually. Preventive services also can be performed while a patient is being seen for medical care of unrelated problems (e.g., a 30-year-old male presents with acute sinusitis, and the clinician recommends tobacco cessation, lipid screening, and a tetanus booster). This latter approach is necessary because many patients do not visit physicians except when they are acutely sick or injured.

Preventive services may be categorized as:

- Screening to detect diseases or conditions in asymptomatic individuals
- Counseling for behavior or lifestyle change
- Immunizations to prevent infectious diseases
- Chemoprophylaxis or drug therapy to prevent disease or its recurrence

Screening

The following lists areas to be screened and the relevant populations who should be screened:

- Problem drinking: All users of alcohol *(Brain 1)*
- Symptoms and signs of drug abuse: All persons (see Chapter 59)
- Polypharmacy: Persons 65 years and older *(Brain 2)*
- Domestic and neighborhood violence: All persons. Sample screening questions include: "Do you feel safe at home?" or "Is anyone ever violent when you have arguments?" (see Chapters 31 and 46).
- Cognitive and functional impairment: Persons age ≥ 65 years (screening tools include the Mini Mental Status Exam and activities of daily living) (see Chapter 42)
- Depressive symptoms and suicide ideation: All persons (depression is prevalent throughout the population), especially those at a higher risk, including young adults, women, the elderly, and those with a history of the following: prior episode of depression, family history of depressive disorder, prior suicide attempt, chronic or serious medical condition, lack of social support or living alone, stressful life events (e.g., recent divorce, separation, bereavement, or unemployment), sexual abuse, current substance abuse, and women in postpartum period. Persons with sleep disorders, chronic pain, or multiple unexplained somatic complaints should also be evaluated for depression (see Chapter 14 for symptoms and more detailed information).
- Blood pressure: All persons at each visit (at least every 2 years if < 140/85 and annually if diastolic is 85–89)
- Height, weight, **body mass index** *(Definition 2)*: All persons at each visit
- Vision (Snellen chart): Persons age ≥ 65 years
- Hearing: Persons age ≥ 65 or those regularly exposed to excessive noise *(Brain 3)*
- Skin exam: Family or personal history of skin cancer, history of increased exposure to sunlight, or presence of precursor lesions (e.g., dysplastic or certain congenital nevi) *(Red Flag 1)*

1 - All users of alcohol should be asked the type of alcohol used, number of drinks per occasion, number of drinks per week, and screening questions, such as the CAGE questionnaire. Men who have more than 4 drinks per occasion or 14 per week or women who have more than 3 drinks per occasion or 7 drinks per week may have an alcohol problem. Positive responses to the CAGE questionnaire may also indicate risk of alcohol abuse. See Chapter 59 for more detailed information.

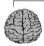

2 - An increased risk of side effects and drug–drug interactions may result in falls or other injuries when patients, especially the elderly, take multiple medications.

2 - Body mass index (BMI) = weight in kilograms divided by height in meters squared (kg/m²). **Overweight** is defined as BMI of 25–29.9, whereas obesity is BMI ≥ 30.

3 - Patients should be asked about symptoms of trouble hearing and examined for impaired hearing with otoscopy and audiometry if symptoms are present.

1 - Warning signs of skin cancer (ABCDs):
- Asymmetry
- Border irregularity
- Color variation
- Diameter > 6 mm

- Oral cavity exam: Persons exposed to tobacco or excessive amounts of alcohol or those with symptoms or lesions suspicious of cancer detected through self-examination
- Thyroid exam for thyroid nodules: History of upper-body irradiation in infancy or childhood
- Symptoms and signs of thyroid dysfunction: Older persons, postpartum women, or persons with Down syndrome *(Brain 4)*
- Symptoms and signs of peripheral arterial disease: Older persons, smokers, or persons with history of diabetes mellitus
- Testicular exam and teach/encourage periodic testicular self exam: Men age 15–35 years, especially if have history of cryptorchidism, orchiopexy, or testicular atrophy
- Pap test: Every 1–3 years for women who have been sexually active and have a cervix (pelvic exam is done at the same time as Pap test) *(Red Flag 2)*
- Breast exam and teach/encourage monthly breast self-exam: Women age 20–39 every 3 years and women age 40–69 every 1–2 years
- Mammography: Women age 40–69 every 1–2 years *(Brain 5, Red Flag 3)*
- Dipstick urinalysis (screening for asymptomatic bacteriuria): Women age ≥ 65 or women with diabetes mellitus
- Fasting lipids: Men age 35–65 years and women age 45–65 years *(Brain 6, Brain 7);*
- Fasting blood sugar: Persons age ≥ 45 every 3 years (specific diabetes mellitus preventive medicine flow sheets are available) *(Red Flag 4)* (see Chapter 27)
- Fecal occult blood test (FOBT): Persons age ≥ 50 annually *(Brain 8)*
- Sigmoidoscopy: Persons ≥ 50 years every 5 years *(Red Flag 5)*
- Syphilis: Persons who seek treatment for other sexually transmitted diseases (STDs), exchange sex for money or drugs, have multiple or new sex partners, or are sexual contacts of persons with syphilis
- Chlamydia and gonorrhea: High-risk women (those who are younger than age 25, exchange sex for money or drugs, have multiple or new sex partners, have history of STD, are sexual contacts of persons with chlamydia or gonorrhea, and do not consistently use barrier protection)
- Human immunodeficiency virus (HIV): Persons treated for another STD; persons who exchange sex for money or drugs; those who have multiple sexual partners; past or present illegal injected drug users; persons whose past or present sexual partners are/were HIV-infected, illegal injected drug users, or bisexual; those with long-term residence or birth in an area with high prevalence of HIV infection; persons who received blood transfusion between 1978 and 1985; men who have sex with other men after 1975
- Hepatitis B and C: Persons with more than one sex partner in past 6 months, persons with recent STD, men who have sex with other men, household contacts and sex partners of hepatitis B or C carriers, illegal injected drug users who share needles and their sexual partners, health care workers, institutionalized persons and those who work with them, hemodialysis patients, hemophiliacs and other recipients of certain blood products, and international travelers to high-risk areas
- Bone mineral content (e.g., dual energy x-ray absorptiometry [DEXA]): Perimenopausal women not taking estrogen or at increased risk for osteoporosis, such as women with a history of bilateral oophorectomy before menopause; early menopause; slender build;

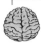

4 - Symptoms and signs of hypothyroidism or hyperthyroidism may be subtle and nonspecific (e.g., fatigue, weight change); one should have a low threshold for diagnostic testing with TSH.

2 - Women at high risk (history of genital warts, other STDs, multiple sexual partners, or abnormal Pap test) should be screened more often. If previous Pap tests have consistently been normal and the patient is at low risk, Pap tests may be discontinued after age 65.

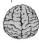

5 - Screening women age 40–49 with mammography is controversial because of conflicting results in studies of this age group. A recent NCI and NIH Consensus Panel has recommended screening women at average risk every 1–2 years in this age group. A rule of thumb is to screen every 2 years for age 40–49 and annually beginning at age 50. Individualized screening is recommended for women age > 70 because of lack of research studies in this age group.

3 - Women at higher risk (primarily women with a mother or sister who had premenopausal breast cancer or a personal history of breast or gynecologic cancer) should have earlier and more frequent mammography screening.

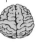

6 - The National Cholesterol Education Program recommends screening at least every 5 years starting at age 20 with a fasting lipid profile. Screening between ages 65 and 75 should be individualized for each patient.

7 - Coronary artery disease (CAD) risk factors:
- Men ≥ 45 years
- Women > 55 years or premature menopause without estrogen-replacement therapy
- Family history of premature CAD defined as myocardial infarction or unexplained sudden death before:
  Age 55 in father or brothers
  Age 65 in mother or sisters
- Current tobacco use
- Hypertension (> 140/90 or on antihypertensive medication)
- Low HDL cholesterol (< 35)
- Diabetes mellitus
- Sedentary lifestyle
- Obesity

HDL ≥ 60 is a negative risk factor (i.e., it is protective against CAD).

sedentary lifestyle; excessive alcohol use; low dietary calcium intake during adolescence; or caucasian or Asian women
- Tuberculosis (TB) skin test (PPD): Persons with close contact to someone with TB; persons with certain underlying medical disorders; members of medically underserved, low-income population, including homeless; illegal injected drug users; residents of long-term care facility; or immigrants or refugees within 5 years from country in which TB is common *(Brain 9)*
- Hemoglobin electrophoresis (screening for thalassemia, sickle cell trait and disease, and other hemoglobinopathies): Young adults of Caribbean, Latin American, Asian, Mediterranean, or African descent who want to have children
- Ophthalmology consult for eye exam and glaucoma testing: History of diabetes mellitus, African Americans age > 40 years, caucasians age > 65, family history of glaucoma, or history of severe myopia

Counseling

Substance Use
- Tobacco cessation and use of nicotine replacement therapy: All tobacco users
- Moderation in alcohol use: All alcohol users (Moderation is a maximum of two drinks per day for men and one drink per day for women.) (see Chapter 59)
- Avoid illegal injected drug use and sharing of needles and syringes; referral to drug treatment program: Users of illegal injected drugs

Diet and Exercise
- Limit fat and cholesterol; emphasize grains, fruits, and vegetables; eat a variety of foods; moderate sugar and salt/sodium use; and maintain caloric balance/ideal weight: All persons (see Chapter 44)
- Maintain adequate calcium intake: Women
- Regular physical activity: All persons

Injury Prevention
- Lap-shoulder belts: All persons
- Helmets while riding motorcycle, bicycle, or all-terrain vehicle: Persons at risk
- Avoid alcohol and other drug use while driving, swimming, boating, bicycling, hunting, or operating dangerous machinery: All alcohol/drug users
- Smoke detector in home; test periodically: All persons
- Safe storage of firearms in home with gun and ammunition locked up separately and kept out of reach of children: Persons with firearms in the home
- Hot water heater temperature set to 120°F: Persons with children or adults age ≥ 65 in the home
- Cardiopulmonary resuscitation (CPR) training for household members: Persons with children or adults age ≥ 65 in the home
- Occupational/environmental exposures and hazards: All persons *(Brain 10)* (see Chapter 45)
- Fall prevention: Persons age ≥ 75 or persons age ≥ 70 who have risk factors for falls *(Brain 11)* (see Chapter 33)

4 - High-risk groups for diabetes mellitus should be screened more often and at a younger age than the general population. Risk factors include overweight (BMI ≥ 25 kg/m²), parent or sibling with diabetes, members of a high-risk ethnic population (e.g., African-American, Hispanic American, Native American, Asian American, Pacific Islander), delivered a baby weighing > 9 lb or have been diagnosed with gestational diabetes mellitus, hypertensive (≥ 140/90), HDL cholesterol level ≤ 35 mg/dl and/or a triglyceride level ≥ 250 mg/dl, and previous fasting blood glucose ≥ 110 and < 126 mg/dl.

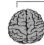

8 - Although it is tempting to test the patient's stool for occult blood during the digital rectal exam, this approach is problematic when screening asymptomatic individuals. Without proper preparation of the patient, false-positive and false-negative tests are more likely. Patients should be instructed to avoid aspirin, nonsteroidal anti-inflammatory drugs (NSAIDs), and other drugs that may cause bleeding (e.g., warfarin) for 7 days prior to testing. Three days prior to testing they should avoid vitamin C in excess of 250 mg per day (supplements and dietary sources), red meat, and raw fruits and vegetables. Because colorectal cancers do not bleed continuously and uniformly, the patient is also instructed to test two different areas of three consecutive bowel movements.

5 - Those at higher risk for colorectal cancer than the general population should be screened earlier and more frequently, often using colonoscopy. High-risk persons include those with history of colorectal cancer or polyps; women with history of breast, ovarian, or endometrial cancer; history of inflammatory bowel disease; first-degree relative with colorectal cancer or polyps, especially at young age; or family history of familial adenomatous polyposis, hereditary nonpolyposis colorectal cancer, or cancer family syndrome.

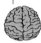

9 - Underlying medical conditions at high risk for TB include history of HIV, diabetes mellitus, end-stage renal disease, hematologic and reticuloendothelial diseases, intestinal bypass or gastrectomy, chronic malabsorption syndromes, silicosis, cancers of the upper GI tract or oropharynx, prolonged steroid use or immunosuppressive therapy, and being 10% or more below desirable body weight.

Sexual Behavior

- STD prevention, including avoiding high-risk behavior and using condoms or female barrier contraceptive with spermicide: Persons at risk (see Chapters 40 and 56)
- Contraception counseling to prevent unintended pregnancy: Men and women capable of having children (see Chapter 17)

Dental Health

- Regular visits to dentist, daily flossing, and brushing after meals with soft- or medium-bristled toothbrush and fluoride toothpaste: All persons

Miscellaneous

- Counsel about the known risks and uncertain benefits of screening for prostate cancer: Men age 50–65 **(Brain 12)**
- Discuss advanced directives, including living will and durable power of attorney: Persons age ≥ 65 or persons with terminal condition
- Ultraviolet exposure skin protection: Family or personal history of skin cancer; presence of nevi; immunosuppression; increased sun exposure; or light skin, eye, and hair color **(Brain 13)**

Immunization

- Tetanus-diphtheria (Td) boosters: All persons every 10 years
- Rubella vaccine: Women considering pregnancy who are not immune by history or serology and health care providers
- Pneumococcal vaccine: Persons age ≥ 65; persons with chronic illness, including cardiovascular disease, respiratory disease, diabetes mellitus, alcoholism, cirrhosis, or cerebrospinal fluid leaks; immunocompromised individuals with splenic dysfunction (e.g., sickle cell anemia), anatomic asplenia, Hodgkin's or non-Hodgkin's lymphoma, multiple myeloma, chronic renal failure, nephrotic syndrome, organ transplantation, or other conditions associated with immunosuppression; persons with HIV infection; or residents of special environments with increased risk (e.g., certain Native American populations)
- Influenza vaccine each fall: Persons age ≥ 50; residents of chronic care facilities; history of chronic cardiopulmonary disorders, metabolic disorders (including diabetes mellitus), hemoglobinopathies, immunosuppression (including HIV and cancer), or renal dysfunction; health care workers
- Hepatitis B vaccine: Persons up to age 24 without reliable history of hepatitis B infection or previous immunizations and those persons at high risk for hepatitis B infection
- Hepatitis A vaccine: Persons who live in or travel to area where disease is endemic or where periodic outbreaks occur, men who have sex with men, illegal injected drug users, institutionalized persons or workers, or military personnel
- Varicella vaccine: Healthy persons who are not immune, especially health care workers, family contacts of immunocompromised persons, or those who live/work in day care, institution, or college settings

Chemoprophylaxis

- Multivitamin with 0.4–0.8 mg folic acid: Women planning or capable of pregnancy who have not had a previous pregnancy with a neural tube defect **(Red Flag 6)**

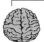

10 - Ask about work, home, travel, and recreational or hobby exposures to physical trauma or injury, chemicals, dust, noise, or other hazards and the use of protective measures or equipment (e.g., respirators) and monitoring techniques (e.g., work site measurements of air or water quality).

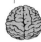

11 - Safety measures for the home include good lighting in hallways and stairwells, removal of objects on floors that predispose to falls, and the use of handrails and traction strips in stairways and bathtubs. Risk factors for falls include decreased visual acuity, decreased physical activity, impaired cognitive function, and polypharmacy with medication side effects that decrease alertness (see Chapter 33).

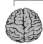

12 - Older men, African-American men, and men with a family history of prostate cancer are at higher risk. Routine screening of men for prostate cancer with prostatic specific antigen (PSA) and digital rectal (prostate) exam is controversial. The American Cancer Society and several other organizations recommend annual PSA screening in men age 50 years and older with a life expectancy > 10 years and digital rectal exams beginning at age 40. However, other organizations, such as the U.S. Preventive Services Task Force, do not recommend screening with PSA because research has not proven that screening decreases mortality and treatment for prostate cancer has significant side effects. Currently, several randomized clinical trials are underway in the U.S. and Europe that may resolve this controversy.

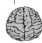

13 - Advise patients to avoid excess exposure and midday sun (between 10:00 A.M. and 3:00 P.M.), use protective clothing, including long sleeve shirt and wide brim hat, and apply sunscreen with an SPF ≥ 15.

6 - Folate should be taken at least 1 month prior to conception through the first trimester. Women who have had a prior pregnancy with neural tube defect should consult their physician about the desirability of using a higher dose of folate (4.0 mg) to prevent recurrence of neural tube defects.

- Counsel about the benefits and risks of postmenopausal hormone replacement therapy: All peri- and postmenopausal women (see Chapter 43) *(Brain 14) (Red Flag 7)*
- Discuss potential benefits and risks of routine aspirin prophylaxis (75–325 mg daily): Men age 40–84 with coronary artery disease risk factors or persons with history of myocardial infarction, transient ischemic attack, or ischemic stroke *(Red Flag 8)*

Selected Readings

1. Executive Summary of the Third Report of the National Cholesterol Education Program (NCEP) Expert Panel on Detection, Evaluation, and Treatment of High Blood Cholesterol in Adults (Adult Treatment Panel III). Bethesda, MD, National Heart, Lung, and Blood Institute, 2001.
2. National Vital Statistics Reports, Vol. 47, no. 19. Hyattsville, MD, National Center for Health Statistics, 1999.
3. Office of Disease Prevention and Health Promotion: Put Prevention into Practice: Clinician's Handbook of Preventive Services, 2nd ed. McLean, VA, International Medical Publshing, Inc, 1998.
4. Prochaska JO, Diclemente CC, Velicer WF, et al: Predicting change in smoking status for self-changes. Addictive Behavior 10:395–406, 1985.
5. Report of the Expert Committee on the Diagnosis and Classification of Diabetes Mellitus. Diabetes Care 25:S5–S20, 2002.
6. U.S. Preventive Services Task Force: Guide to Clinical Preventive Services, 2nd ed. Washington, DC, U.S. Department of Health and Human Services, 1996.

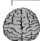

14 - Estrogen helps to protect postmenopausal women from cardiovascular disease, fractures due to osteoporosis, and menopausal symptoms, such as hot flashes and mood swings. For women with a uterus, progesterone supplementation should also be given to reduce the risk of endometrial cancer from unopposed estrogen.

7 - Contraindications to hormonal replacement therapy (HRT) include history of undiagnosed vaginal bleeding, active liver disease, thromboembolic disorder, or hormone-dependent cancer, such as breast or endometrial cancer.

8 - Precautions and contraindications to aspirin chemoprophylaxis include aspirin allergy, poorly controlled hypertension or other risk factors for hemorrhagic stroke, liver disease, kidney disease, history of gastrointestinal (GI) bleeding or peptic ulcer disease, or bleeding disorder.

10. Complementary and Alternative Medicine

Laeth Nasir, MBBS

Synopsis

The use of alternative medicine by the public has increased dramatically over the past several years *(Brain 1)*. Alternative medical practices have always been surrounded by a great deal of controversy, to the extent that even what constitutes "alternative" or "complementary" medicine is a matter of debate. Eisenberg et al. suggest the following definition of alternative medical therapies: "those interventions that are not taught in medical schools and are not generally available in U.S. hospitals."[2] Complementary and alternative medicine (CAM) therapies range from relatively uncontroversial practices, such as relaxation, meditation, and massage, to interventions such as high-dose vitamin therapy, herbal supplements, or unusual diets, that have unknown effects and may interfere with orthodox medical treatments.

 1 - An estimated 40% of people in United States have used an alternative therapy in the past year.

Physicians should concern themselves with the use of alternative therapies by their patients for a number of reasons. Adverse effects of an alternative therapy may be the cause of a patient's presenting symptoms. Therapies that are utilized without the physician's knowledge may interfere with conventional medical treatment. Inappropriate use of alternative therapies may prevent patients from seeking more effective care in a timely fashion. Also, unconventional health beliefs may affect the acceptance or use of conventional medical therapies unrelated to their presenting complaint (e.g., the avoidance of immunizations). In addition, the use of certain alternative therapies may be safe and efficacious for the prevention or treatment of some conditions.

Types of Alternative Therapies

Thousands of forms of alternative therapies exist, ranging from generations-old ethnic folk remedies to modern, quasiscientific therapies carried out by a single or handful of practitioners in a particular region. Because of this, it is unrealistic to expect the primary care physician to have a working knowledge of many of these therapies. Often, the physician will be called on to judge the merits of a particular therapy without access to scientific studies or even unbiased opinion. This chapter reviews a number of the more common types of therapies used by patients. Keep in mind that many individuals use a number of therapies simultaneously.

Relaxation Techniques, Meditation, and Prayer

Practices include biofeedback, progressive muscle relaxation, and various types of meditation.

Philosophy

Most forms of meditation have their basis in Far Eastern traditional practices or religion. It is thought that repeatedly "stilling the mind" in meditation and withdrawing attention from the material world allow the individual to attain enlightenment by perception of the true nature of the universe. Biofeedback and progressive muscle relaxation are Westernized forms of these practices that have been largely accepted into mainstream medical practice. Prayer, both personal and intercessory, is practiced universally.

Typical Practice

These therapies are most often practiced on a regular basis, often daily or even more frequently.

Benefits

These therapies, particularly meditation, are often efficacious in reducing anxiety and may have positive effects on a number of physiologic parameters, such as a reduction in blood pressure. In addition, some studies suggest that regular spiritual practice has benefits on overall health. In general, these techniques are extremely safe. However, there have been anecdotal reports of worsening symptoms in persons with psychiatric disorders who have attempted certain types of intensive meditation practices.

Herbal Therapies, Vitamins, and Nutraceuticals

Patients often use herbs, vitamins, or nutraceuticals to treat a symptom or to prevent illness in much the same fashion as over-the-counter or prescribed pharmaceuticals. Herbs may be taken individually or in combination with other herbs, vitamins, or nutraceuticals.

Philosophy

The use of herbal substances is common to virtually all healing traditions, including conventional medicine, where a significant proportion of medications are derived from plant products.

Typical Practice

Herbs are usually purchased through a retailer such as a health food store or pharmacy, but may be obtained elsewhere or even gathered by the patient.

Benefits

Many herbs have been shown to be relatively safe and beneficial for a wide spectrum of disorders. For example, *Ginkgo biloba* has been shown to be useful in the treatment of dementia, and ginger is effective in the treatment of nausea and vomiting.

The quality of herbal therapies available in the United States varies a great deal because of the lack of external oversight of the industry. Although most of the popular herbs are probably safe, few scientific studies exist regarding many of them. Little is known about herb–herb or herb–drug interactions. In addition, the mutagenic or carcinogenic potential of many herbal substances remains unknown, particularly in long-term use *(Red Flag 1)*.

Nutraceutical is a catchall term applied to a number of substances—often hormones, minerals, or proteins—said to enhance the functions of specific biochemical pathways in order to prevent or treat illness *(Red Flag 2)*. Many individuals take vitamin supplements to treat or prevent disease. A growing body of evidence suggests that modest vita-

1 - It has been reported that some herbs imported into the United States have high levels of pesticide residues, heavy metals, or other contaminants. Poisoning has been reported from the deliberate admixture of medications with the herbs, as well as the ingestion of inaccurately identified herbs.

2 - Some nutraceuticals such as L-tryptophan have resulted in death due to impurities in manufacturing processes. Other nutraceuticals pose a theoretical hazard because of their source (e.g., some types of melatonin are obtained from animal brain tissue).

min supplementation is beneficial for the prevention of a number of degenerative disorders. Women of childbearing age in the U.S. are advised to supplement their diets with folate in order to reduce the incidence of neural tube defects in their offspring *(Red Flag 3)*.

Massage, Chiropractic, and Other Manipulative Therapies

Every culture has a form of therapeutic massage. In general, massage is used to help resolve myofascial complaints and promote feelings of well being. Types of massage vary in style and intensity. The use of massage is extremely safe for virtually any individual when carried out by a professional therapist. The major drawback of massage is its relatively high cost *(Red Flag 4)*.

Philosophy
Chiropractic and osteopathic practices differ somewhat in philosophy and style, but in general, they both hold that many illnesses are due to subtle malalignment in the axial or appendicular skeleton.

Typical Practice
Manipulative techniques that briefly move joints beyond their normal physiologic range are used to treat a variety of disorders.

Benefits
Most commonly, manipulative therapies attempt to resolve problems of myofascial spasm or restriction. However, treatment of other illnesses or the prevention of disease is sometimes the focus of this type of treatment *(Red Flag 5)*.

Homeopathy

Homeopathy is a system of medicine developed in the 19th century by a German physician, Samuel Hahnemann, and was practiced extensively in Europe and the U.S. until the practice began to decline in the 1930s. This therapy is currently enjoying resurgence in popularity.

Philosophy
In classical homeopathy, unlike orthodox medicine, the practitioner does not attempt to diagnose a particular illness. Instead, he or she takes an extremely detailed history of the patient's physical and emotional symptoms, then selects a substance having the potential to *exactly reproduce* the patient's symptoms if administered in an undiluted state. This substance is then serially diluted to the extent that little or none of the original material is present in the diluent, and it is this "remedy" that is administered to the patient. Practitioners of homeopathy claim that the process of dilution creates a substance that has a specific healing effect. A number of theories have been advanced to explain the possible mechanism of action of homeopathic preparations including a "memory" effect of water, low-intensity microwave radiation that has an effect on biologic systems through resonance with these systems, and highly complex nonlinear systems such as those envisioned by chaos theory.

Benefits
Homeopathy is most commonly used for chronic medical conditions such as migraine headaches, irritable bowel syndrome, and hay fever. Because of the extremely dilute nature of these remedies, the homeopathic treatment itself is safe.

3 - Some individuals ingest doses of vitamins that are high enough to cause acute or chronic toxicity. "Megavitamin" therapy may also interfere with the absorption of medications or other nutrients, resulting in illness or deficiency states.

4 - Some styles of vigorous massage (such as Rolfing) have been rarely implicated in patient injury or death.

5 - Too frequent or vigorous manipulation may result in excessive joint mobility and, less commonly, fractures, stroke, or spinal cord compression. These complications are rarely a problem when a practitioner with adequate training is performing the treatment.

Acupuncture

In this therapy, thin needles are inserted into various locations in the body in order to prevent or treat illness or to provide surgical analgesia.

Philosophy

Acupuncture is a component of ancient traditional Chinese medical practice and is sometimes used in concert with other elements of Chinese medicine, such as spiritual practice, herbal therapy, exercise, and dietary modification. Briefly, traditional Chinese medical theories see human beings as animated through a universal force called *qi* (pronounced "chee"), which runs through the body in a stereotyped fashion in channels called meridians. To be in perfect health, an individual's flow of qi must be in balance. If the qi becomes unbalanced, illness results. Chinese medical treatments are aimed at recalibrating the flow of qi. In the case of acupuncture, it is thought that needles placed and manipulated at certain points along the meridians will serve to modulate qi.

Typical Practice

For chronic medical conditions, a series of treatments are commonly performed at intervals.

Benefits

Acupuncture is often used for conditions such as acute or chronic pain, nausea, narcotic detoxification, and anxiety or depression and to assist the recovery of neurologic function after a stroke. The effects of acupuncture are thought to be mediated through the release of endorphins and other neurotransmitters in the central and peripheral nervous systems *(Red Flag 6)*.

6 - Although acupuncture is an extremely safe treatment modality when carried out by a qualified practitioner, complications can occur. Bleeding and bruising, infection, injury to vital body organs, and even death have been reported.

Patient History of Alternative Medicine Use

Because many patients seen in a general outpatient practice use one or more alternative therapies, it is important to quiz patients about their use of various therapies. Taking a history on the use of unconventional therapies can be difficult. Patients often avoid telling their physicians about the therapies that they are using for fear that they will be ridiculed or dismissed. Sometimes patients will test a physician's reaction to the use of alternative therapies by casually reporting the use of an innocuous vitamin or herb. Responding to the bait with friendly interest or nonjudgmental concern, the physician is often rewarded by fuller disclosure on future visits. To get complete information from a patient, the physician should directly, but cautiously, ask patients about alternative therapy use:

- "What herbs or vitamins do you take?" *(Brain 2)*
- "What do you take them for?" *(Brain 3)*
- "Do you know what substances the tablets you take contain?" *(Brain 4)*
- "Are you using any other therapies for this problem?"
- "Is anyone else helping you with this problem?" *(Brain 5)*

It may be useful to cautiously explore patients attitudes toward orthodox medicine.

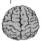

2 - Asking all patients specific questions about their use of vitamins, herbs, and nutraceuticals is important. A significant minority of patients will fail to report herb or vitamin use with less direct questioning.

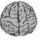

3 - The answer to this question often will give the clinician some insight into the patient's health beliefs.

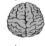

4 - Frequently, nutraceuticals, vitamins, or herbal supplements are complex mixtures. Examining the container itself for a detailed list of ingredients is often useful (keeping in mind that the label may not be accurate).

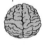

5 - Identifying other practitioners that the patient is in contact with may be important.

Physical Examination

The use of alternative therapies seldom results in specific physical changes; however, a number of folk or ethnic remedies leave physical marks that may be mistaken for signs of illness or abuse by the unwary practitioner. Individuals from the Middle and Far East may consult practitioners who treat illness by cauterizing parts of the body with red-hot irons (*maqua*), resulting in burn scars. A number of massage techniques used widely in the Far East (known as *gua sha* in China) may result in local petechiae or bruising. Cupping (the practice of applying containers to the skin after evacuating air by means of a flame) is practiced in many parts of the world and may result in discrete round bruises at the site of the treatment.

Putting It All Together

Many patients use alternative therapies, and the use of these therapies in the United States is likely to grow. Ideally, the health care provider should identify patients who use these therapies, accurately identify the therapies themselves, assess whether the therapy is causing or is likely to result in adverse effects, and ascertain whether or not the therapy is appropriate for the condition for which it is being used. In addition, the patient should be screened for atypical and potentially hazardous health care beliefs, such as the avoidance of immunizations. Finally, the physician should assess whether there is scientific evidence to suggest that the practice is efficacious. This information can be shared with the patient. Obviously, the extent to which a patient will follow his or her health care provider's recommendations on any topic will depend largely on the relationship between patient and provider. Sensitivity to the patient's beliefs and needs, as well as good negotiating skills, is usually required for the provider to have an impact on patient actions.

Management

Most patients who use alternative therapies are eager to collaborate with their physician in developing a plan to evaluate and test alternative treatments for their problems. In general, keeping two commonsense guidelines in mind will result in a good outcome for all concerned. First, the physician should not feel obligated to condone the use of any alternative treatment unless he or she is reasonably certain that the symptoms the patient is seeking relief from are not due to a condition (e.g., cancer or infection) requiring intervention with a proven treatment modality. Second, the physician should be in a position to make a rough assessment of the risk/benefit ratio of the treatment and communicate this to the patient *(Red Flag 7)*.

 7 - For all alternative therapies, a number of questions should be asked. (1) Has an adequate medical work-up of the symptom or symptoms been carried out? (2) Is the therapy reasonably safe, and is it being used for an appropriate indication? (3) Is it interfering or does it have potential to interfere with orthodox medical treatments that are being used simultaneously?

Selected Readings

1. Eisenberg DM: Advising patients who seek alternative medical therapies [see comments]. Ann Intern Med 127:61–9, 1997.
2. Eisenberg DM, Davis RB, Ettner SL, et al: Trends in alternative medicine use in the United States, 1990–1997: Results of a follow-up national survey. JAMA 280:1569–1575, 1998.
3. Fugh-Berman A: Alternative Medicine—What Works: A Comprehensive, Easy-to-Read Review of the Scientific Evidence, Pro and Con. Tucson, AZ, Odonian Press, 1996.
4. Helms J: Acupuncture Energetics: A Clinical Approach for Physicians. Berkeley, CA, Medical Acupuncture Publishers; 1995.
5. Lewith GT, Kenyon JN, Lewis PJ: Complementary Medicine: An Integrated Approach. Oxford, Oxford University Press, 1996.

11. Abdominal Pain in Children

David R. Mack, MD

Synopsis

Abdominal pain is a common affliction of children and adolescents. The pain may be acute in onset or, as occurs in up to 20% of school-aged children, recurrent in nature. **Recurrent** or **chronic abdominal pain** is a definition *(Definition 1)* and not a diagnosis. Using current methodologies, a discrete organic cause can be identified in one-third of children with recurrent abdominal pain, whereas no known structural, inflammatory, or biochemical cause can be identified to explain the recurrent pain in the remaining two-thirds of children. These latter children are classified as having nonorganic or functional recurrent abdominal pain, and, in the long-term, about half will have resolution of their pain. In the setting of acute abdominal pain, the history, physical examination, and testing are directed toward identifying surgical or medical emergencies where immediate action is indicated. History and physical examination for patients with recurrent abdominal pain are directed toward making a definitive diagnosis so that appropriate directed testing is undertaken or referral considered for those without the typical signs or symptoms of functional abdominal pain. Empirical pharmacologic therapies are generally not indicated for recurrent abdominal pain; rather education, reassurance, and ongoing support during office follow-up visits for these children and their families are important to ensure that growth and development remain normal and other insidious signs and symptoms are not present.

1 - Recurrent abdominal pain of childhood: Paroxysmal abdominal pain in children between the ages of 4 and 16 years that occurs at least once per month for at least 3 consecutive months and that is severe enough to disrupt normal activities.

Differential Diagnosis

Acute Abdominal Pain

- Acute appendicitis
- Hernias, torsion *(Brain 1)*
- Intussusception *(Red Flag 1)*
- Volvulus
- Urinary tract infection
- Food poisoning, gastroenteritis
- Extra-abdominal etiologies (referred pain)—pneumonia, intracranial
- Other (inflammation of solid organs, hollow organs, or blood vessels)

Recurrent Abdominal Pain

- Urinary tract infection
- **Constipation** *(Definition 2)*
- **Functional** *(Definition 3)*
- Carbohydrate intolerance *(Brain 2)*
- Gastrointestinal inflammation (infectious and noninfectious)

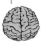

1 - The blood supply to organs may be impaired (i.e., ischemia) by a number of mechanisms— telescoping of the intestines (intussusception), twisting or rotation of hollow organs such as the intestines (volvulus), or solid organs such as the testes (testicular torsion), or following protrusion of intestines through the wall of a body cavity (incarcerated hernia). In all cases, there is marked pain, and this is an emergency situation requiring rapid restoration of blood flow.

1 - Intussusception is characterized by the sudden onset of severe abdominal pain in infants typically aged 6–24 months (variable). It may occur in a previously well child or during intercurrent GI infection.
There may be relief between peristaltic waves. Pallor and vomiting will be noted before and after attacks; lethargy ("knocked-out look") also may be evident. Later abdominal distention, bile-stained vomitus, or currant-jelly stool may occur. Look for a sausage-shaped mass in the upper abdomen and Dance's sign.

- Choledochal cyst *(Red Flag 2)*
- Other (e.g., gynecologic, renal, gall bladder, liver, tumors, psychiatric, poisoning, metabolic)

History

Acute Abdominal Pain

Have the patient or the parent describe the pain ("Tell me about your pain. What symptoms are you experiencing?") Record the following:

- Location, radiation, onset, and length of time of pain
- Fever
- Reduced appetite, lethargy
- Vomiting and characteristics of vomitus
- Diarrhea and characteristics of fecal discharge
- Dysuria, hematuria, urinary frequency
- Menstrual history if age and gender appropriate
- Prescription and nonprescription drugs, supplements, preparations *(Brain 3)*

Recurrent Abdominal Pain

Ask the patient or parent about:

- Pain that awakens the child from sleep
- Pain localized well away from the umbilicus
- Pain referred to back, shoulder, flank or groin
- Exacerbating features (e.g., foods, positioning)
- Relieving maneuvers (medications, positioning, foods)

Note any other symptoms the patient is experiencing, especially:

- Fever
- Weight changes and growth
- Emesis
- Urinary symptoms (dysuria, hematuria, frequency, dribbling)
- Stool characteristics (e.g., frequency, character, color)
- Appetite, energy, mood
- Dysmenorrhea
- Headache, syncope, dizziness, weakness, confusion
- Joint pain
- School performance, substance abuse, peer relationships, self and peer activities

Record the family history. "Tell me about your family."

- Intestinal diseases (e.g., inflammatory bowel disease, peptic ulcer disease, irritable bowel disease, pancreatitis)
- History of migraines (e.g., association with abdominal migraine in children)
- Family dynamics, disorders, and how family members deal with the pain

Physical Examination

Acute Abdominal Pain

The following elements should be checked in the physical exam:

- General observation: positioning of the patient (fetal positioning, motionless, stooped gait) and alertness *(Brain 4)*

2 - Constipation: A condition in which bowel contents are hard in consistency, difficult to pass, infrequent and often incompletely evacuated.

3 - Functional abdominal pain: There are three forms classified by anatomic location: (1) The most common form is periumbilical in location. (2) In the epigastric form, the pain is in the upper abdomen and is accompanied with early satiety, bloating, belching, nausea or vomiting and may also be referred to as nonulcer *dyspepsia.* (3) In the infraumbilical form, pain is felt across the lower abdomen and is accompanied by cramping, abdominal distention, or bloating and altered stool consistency or frequency. This latter form is equivalent to irritable bowel syndrome in adults.

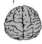

2 - Primary lactose intolerance rarely affects children under the age of 2 years, but does increase in prevalence with increasing age. All ethnic groups are variably affected (e.g., caucasians 15%; Mexican Americans 75%; African Americans 75%; Asians 90%).

2 - A choledochal cyst is a dilation of the common bile duct that children are born with. It presents with pain, yellowish staining of the skin, and sclera of the eyes (i.e., jaundice), and sometimes a mass is felt in the upper abdomen. Although uncommon, it is a very serious condition because dilation of the common bile duct does not allow for normal bile, which can lead to liver dysfunction and pancreatitis.

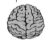

3 - Many drugs are associated with hepatitis and pancreatitis. Excess vitamins may also cause disease (e.g., excess vitamin C predisposes to urolithiasis).

- Vital signs, including temperature, height and weight
- Growth *(Brain 5)*
- Oropharynx, tympanic membranes, sinuses
- Skin pallor or jaundice, temperature, rashes
- Extremities—**clubbing** *(Definition 4)*
- Node tenderness, size, and location
- Oral: check odors, hydration, ulceration
- Check breath sounds, air entry, accessory muscle usage
- Abdominal inspection (include inguinal areas, genitalia) for distention and masses, movement with respiration *(Brain 6)*, peristalsis, **Cullen's** and **Grey Turner's sign** *(Definition 5)*
- Auscultation *(Brain 7)*
- Palpation (e.g., soft, tender, signs of **peritoneal irritation** [*Definition 6*]), masses, organomegaly, **McBurney's point** *(Definition 7)*
- **Psoas sign** *(Definition 8)*, **Dance's sign** *(Definition 9)*, **Carnett's sign** *(Definition 10)*

Recurrent Abdominal Pain

This exam should include:

- General observations: note positioning and general habitus
- Growth parameters and vitals *(Brain 8)*
- Skin: look for discoloration or pallor, rashes, striae, scars, dilated vessels, edema, petechiae
- Oral *(Brain 9)*
- Sinuses
- Eyes: check for jaundice, inflammation
- Hair texture and nails: check for signs of malnutrition
- Extremities: check for clubbing, arthritis, sacral abnormalities, leg-length discrepancy, reflexes
- Lymph nodes
- Abdomen: check for distention, masses, organomegaly, tenderness, fluid
- Perianal (e.g., tags, fissures, fistulas, abscess, warts, trauma) *(Brain 10)*
- Rectal: record stool volume and consistency, rectal vault size, presence of blood

Testing

Acute Abdominal Pain

Usually a complete blood count (CBC), urinalysis will suffice. Various other blood tests may be of benefit depending on clinical suspicion (e.g., amylase/lipase if pancreatitis suspected, pregnancy test).

Plain radiographs of the abdomen are rarely beneficial with acute abdominal pain. Computed tomography (CT) is the best test for pancreatitis and may be required for appendicitis. Other tests may include air or barium enemas, barium upper gastrointestinal (GI) with small bowel series, and ultrasound.

Recurrent Abdominal Pain

An initial screen for all patients with recurrent abdominal pain should include a CBC and an erythrocyte sedimentation rate (ESR). Anemia

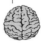
4 - Patients with peritoneal irritation, such as in appendicitis, will walk with a stooped gait and will find movement increases pain, whereas lying in a fetal position with legs drawn is more comfortable.

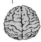
5 - Patients with low height-to-weight ratios other signs of calorie deprivation such as hair, nail, or skin changes may have more chronic underlying disorder now manifesting with acute abdominal pain.

4 - Clubbing: Normally, the depth of the index finger at the base of the nail is less than its depth at the distal interphalangeal joint. A depth at the base of the nail equal to that at the distal interphalangeal joint is above normal and indicates clubbing. Clubbing may be familial but is also associated with chronic GI, pulmonary, cardiac, hepatic, endocrine, infectious, and neoplastic conditions.

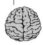
6 - Respirations are abdominal in the pediatric patient. If the abdominal wall fails to move during respiration, an acute condition requiring surgery is likely at hand.

5 - Cullen's and Grey Turner's signs: Bluish discoloration around the umbilicus (Cullen) and flanks (Grey Turner) that occurs in acute hemorrhagic pancreatitis.

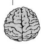
7 - The absence of peristaltic sounds is significant and evidence of ileus.

6 - Signs of peritoneal irritation: Patients with inflammation of the peritoneum experience greatest relief from pain by lying supine, motionless with knees flexed. There is tenderness when abdominal pressure from touching the abdomen is suddenly released (rebound tenderness) both over and away from the site of the inflamed organ causing the peritoneal irritation. There may also be muscular resistance to palpation of the abdominal wall (guarding) and may progress from voluntary process to one independent of will (involuntary guarding) to the point of boardlike abdominal rigidity.

7 - McBurney's point: Used to locate the appendix, this is the point on the anterior abdominal wall lying 11/2–2 inches above the anterior superior spine of the ileum. The appendix is below the straight line that joins this point and the umbilicus.

or elevated ESR with recurrent abdominal pain necessitates further investigation. Other useful screening procedures include a urinalysis and culture, because one of the most common causes of recurrent abdominal pain is urinary tract infection. Fecal examination for ova and parasites may also be of benefit because parasites such as *Giardia lamblia* are common and may manifest only with vague abdominal pain.

A lactose breath hydrogen test is another simple noninvasive test that is definitive for lactose intolerance. Empirical diagnosis can be difficult in children. Management is lactose avoidance or lactose supplementation (don't forget calcium supplements to meet recommended requirements).

A barium upper GI exam is one of the most common radiologic procedures performed. The best use of a barium upper GI is in combination with a small bowel series for evaluation of anatomic alterations. These tests are not reliable for evaluating suspected mucosal lesions in children.

Other diagnostic tests should be individualized and may include various blood tests and imaging tests (e.g., barium, ultrasound, CT, magnetic resonance imaging [MRI]).

Endoscopic (esophagogastroduodenoscopy, colonoscopy) procedures have generally replaced barium examinations for evaluation of intestinal mucosal diseases (e.g., inflammatory lesions).

The primary care physician can have a major role at well-child visits to help prevent the development of fear and anxiety for parents and children with recurrent abdominal pain that can lead to excessive consultations and testing. The primary care physician can discuss parenting styles, the importance of open family communication, and having a loving environment for healthy child development.

Putting It All Together

Acute onset of abdominal pain can be disconcerting to those involved and requires careful evaluation to ensure that the cause is not a surgical emergency. Although older children may present with typical signs and symptoms, younger patients may have less typical presentations. For children in whom there continues to be a diagnostic dilemma despite consultation with surgical colleagues, a period of hospital observation may be indicated *(Consultation and Referral 1)*.

Recurrent abdominal pain is a broad descriptive term used to define a heterogenous group of patients in whom over 100 causes of pain have been identified. Functional disorders are most common, and the diagnosis of functional recurrent abdominal pain should not be one of exclusion. Improved diagnostic techniques have identified an organic basis for recurrent abdominal pain in about one-third of patients. Thus, the primary care physician has a significant role in advocating a referral when the history, physical examination (including evaluation of growth parameters), or screening tests suggest problems, even though other symptoms may be minimal *(Consultation and Referral 2)*.

8 - Psoas sign: The test is performed by having the patient lie on his or her left side. The examiner slowly extends the right thigh, stretching the iliopsoas muscle. The sign is positive if extension produces pain.

9 - Dance's sign: A slight retraction in the neighborhood of the right iliac fossa.

10 - Carnett's sign: Palpation of the abdomen when the child is asked to raise his head. This maneuver increases superficial muscle tenderness so it can be distinguished from intra-abdominal tenderness.

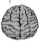

8 - Children with functional recurrent abdominal pain have normal growth parameters, appear healthy on physical exam, have normal lab tests, and are older than 4 years of age.

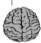

9 - The mouth is the first part of the intestinal tract. A careful inspection may provide clues to intestinal tract diseases. For example, small ulcers with surrounding erythema (aphthous stomatitis) occur in chronic intestinal inflammation (e.g., Crohn's disease). Tumors of the nervous system visible on the tongue (mucosal neuromas) may be a clue to abnormal intestinal nerves leading to chronic constipation (e.g., multiple endocrine neoplasia type IIb). Brownish discoloration of the lips may be a clue that growths from the lining of the intestinal tract (i.e., polyps) are present in the intestinal tract (e.g., Peutz-Jeghers syndrome). Fungal infections (e.g., candidiasis [caused by *Candida albicans*]) of the mouth may indicate a serious immune disorder in older children.

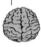

10 - The anal verge and rectum are the last parts of the intestinal tract, and, similar to the mouth, a careful inspection may yield important clues. For example, skin outgrowths (tags) and cracks of the lining of the anus (fissures) may indicate that large, hard stools have been passed by the patient. They may also suggest chronic mucosal inflammation when combined with the presence of passage from the inside of the intestine to the skin (fistula) or abscesses by the anus. A diagnosis of internal hemorrhoids is unlikely because these are extremely unusual in children. One should have a high index of suspicion for child abuse when there is any sign of trauma or a sexually transmitted disease such as perianal warts.

1 - Referral should be considered in patients with severe acute onset pain, bilious vomiting, hematochezia, or an increasing symptomatology complex.

Management

Follow-up should be arranged for patients with acute abdominal pain if their symptoms do not disappear in 48 hours or if their symptoms worsen over the next 24-hour period. Some children will need to be hospitalized for observation, and this should be done in consultation with other specialists as indicated.

Functional abdominal pain often affects the entire family, so therapy must be directed at the family as a unit. Successful therapy depends on education, reassurance and ongoing support. The goals are to reduce tension and stress while promoting normal school attendance and activities. When speaking with families, the physician may wish to compare abdominal pain with headaches because most family members will understand that the pain associated with headaches is real, but rarely from a serious underlying problem. Medications, including sedatives, anticholinergics, and antispasmodics, are not efficacious. The role of increased dietary fiber is controversial. Hospitalization is rarely required for functional abdominal pain, but referral should be considered in any child who has a history, physical examination, or screening tests that raise the suspicion of organic disease. Defined causes of recurrent abdominal pain will lead to specific interventions that can be administered in collaboration with the consultant.

2 - Referral should be considered for children with chronic pain and children who are outside the compatible age range for functional pain. These children may have characteristics of pain, evidence on the physical examination suggesting organic disease, or an abnormal screening laboratory evaluation. Additionally, evidence of psychologically stressful stimuli or environmental reinforcement of pain behavior may be lacking.

Selected Readings

1. Boyle JT: Recurrent abdominal pain: An update. Pediatr Rev 18:310–320, 1997.
2. Drumm B, Rhoads JM, Stringer DA, et al: Peptic ulcer disease in children: Etiology, clinical findings, and clinical course. Pediatrics 82:410–414, 1988.
3. Hyams JS, Burke G, Davis PM, et al: Abdominal pain and irritable bowel syndrome in adolescents: A community-based study. J Pediatr 129:220–226, 1996.
4. Mahajan L, Wyllie R: Chronic abdominal pain of childhood and adolescence. In Wyllie R, Hyams JS (eds): Pediatric Gastrointestinal Disease, 2nd ed. Philadelphia, W.B. Saunders,1999, pp 3–13.
5. National Digestive Diseases Information Clearinghouse: www. niddk.nih.gov /health/digest/pubs/lactose/lactose.htm.
6. Pena BM, Taylor GA, Lund DP, et al: Effect of computed tomography on patient management and costs in children with suspected appendicitis. Pediatrics 104:440–446, 1999.
7. Scholer SJ, Pituch K, Orr DP, et al: Clinical outcome of children with acute abdominal pain. Pediatrics 98:680–685, 1996.

12. Allergic Diseases

Russell J. Hopp, DO

Synopsis

The concept of an allergic disease, as commonly understood by the lay public, includes a wide variety of untoward systemic and local reactions. For the purpose of this discussion, this chapter will focus entirely on those disease entities that have known (or suspected) immunoglobulin E (IgE)–mediated associations. The major allergic diseases (IgE-mediated) include allergic rhinitis, eczema, food allergy, hives (on occasion), asthma, and anaphylaxis. Each entity will be discussed separately, although an individual may present with more than one allergic disease.

Allergic Rhinitis

Synopsis

Allergic rhinitis is a common medical problem, affecting nearly 15% of the American population. It usually starts in childhood and often continues into adulthood. Allergens include indoor exposures, such as pets or house-dust mites, and outdoor allergens, such as pollens. Symptoms of allergic rhinitis include itching, sneezing, rhinitis, and nasal congestion.

Differential Diagnosis

- **Chronic sinusitis *(Definition 1)***
- **Viral rhinitis *(Definition 2)***
- **Adenoid hypertrophy *(Definition 3)***
- Nonallergic rhinitis with eosinophils
- Vasomotor rhinitis
- Anatomic obstruction

History

"What bothers you the most about your nose?" The following are significant:

- Itchy—often present chronically in IgE-mediated rhinitis
- Congested—suggests a chronic process, assists in therapy decisions
- Runny—same significance as congested
- Sneezing—usually a signal of IgE mediation
- Snoring—helps with differential, because adenoid hypertrophy and severe allergic rhinitis are commonly associated with snoring
- Several (or all) of the above symptoms—suggests severity

"What times of the year do you have these problems?"

- Seasonal—suggests an outdoor allergen is the cause
- Year around—suggests an indoor allergen is the cause
- Year round with seasonal exacerbations—suggest both indoor and outdoor allergens are responsible for the symptoms

1 - Chronic sinusitis: An infection of the sinuses, usually bacterial, that has been continuously present ≥ 6 weeks.

2 - Viral rhinitis: A viral rhinosinusitis, usually caused by a rhinovirus and usually lasting ≤ 10 days.

3 - Adenoid hypertrophy: Anatomically enlarged adenoids, obstructing the posterior nasal vault, and leading to clinical symptoms.

"What medications have you taken to help your nasal problems? Have they helped?"
- Antihistamines—helps with differential diagnosis and treatment plans
- Decongestants—helps with differential diagnosis and treatment plans
- Combinations of both—helps with differential diagnosis and treatment plans
- Nasal sprays (which types?)—helps with differential diagnosis and treatment plans

"Do you have other problems at the same time as your nasal symptoms?"
- Itchy, burning, or watery eyes—additional IgE-mediated target organ
- Cough—additional IgE-mediated target organ (lungs)
- Wheezing—additional IgE-mediated target organs (lungs)
- Hives—additional IgE-mediated target organs (skin)
- Eczema—often a precursor in young children of allergic rhinitis

"What is the usual color of your nasal or posterior nasal drainage?"
- Clear—usually associated with noninfectious rhinitis
- Green, yellow, or white—often associated with infectious rhinitis

Physical Examination

- Ears, looking for serous otitis media or eustachian tube dysfunction
- Face, for nasal crease, allergic shiners, lower eyelid creases
- Nose, for turbinate size, color, and secretions
- Throat, for tonsil size, posterior nasal drainage, and lymphatic studding on posterior pharyngeal wall
- Lungs, for wheezing, prolonged expiratory phase
- Skin, for eczema, hives

Testing

The diagnosis is primarily based on the history and physical examination. A nasal smear for eosinophils (> 10% of total cells) might provide supportive evidence. Skin testing is available by referral to an allergy specialist. A total serum IgE is rarely helpful.

Putting It All Together

Allergic rhinitis has historically been viewed as an insignificant illness by the medical community and lay public. This is partly explained by the commonness of upper respiratory tract symptoms in the general population, especially in children. Also, the symptoms are not life-threatening and virtually never require hospitalization. This characterization is changing, however, as the evidence of allergic rhinitis as a risk factor for the development of associated diseases, especially asthma, mounts. Additionally, its complexity as a disease entity and its impact on the patient's quality of life are becoming better appreciated. Its economic impact on the patient and on society for over-the-counter (OTC) medications, prescription costs, and lost days of work and school is tremendous.

Management *(Consultation and Referral 1)*

Avoiding allergens is the first step in a progressive treatment strategy for allergic rhinitis. The identification and subsequent avoidance of

1 - Consider referral for allergic rhinitis when:
- Symptoms last for more than 4 months each year
- Daily medication is required
- Symptoms of wheezing or asthma begin
- Frequent sinusitis or otitis media is present

indoor and outdoor allergens will help prevent allergic reactions. Regardless of any pharmacologic therapy that is introduced, consistent environment control is paramount *(Brain 1)*.

In mild seasonal allergic rhinitis with only occasional symptoms, the administration of rapid-onset, oral, nonsedating H1-antihistamines when symptomatic or the administration of **cromoglycate** *(Definition 4)* to eyes, nose, or both is recommended.

In moderate seasonal disease with prominent nasal symptoms, the daily administration of an intranasal steroid, begun early in the season, is reasonable. An oral (or possibly topical) antihistamine is added as necessary for additional nasal symptoms. Topical cromoglycate for eye symptoms can be helpful. Long-term requirement for intranasal steroids strongly suggests the necessity of allergy immunotherapy *(Brain 2)*.

The treatment of perennial allergic rhinitis includes the regular use on intranasal steroids, or cromoglycate for very young children. Oral antihistamines, with or without decongestants, can be added as needed.

Food Allergy

Synopsis

IgE-mediated food allergy can cause a variety of local and systemic clinical responses. This is due to the fact that mast calls and basophils, containing specific IgE antibodies to the specific food, are widely distributed throughout the body.

The foods most responsible for allergic reactions in infants include cow's milk, eggs, peanuts, and soy. These same foods, along with wheat, tree nuts, fish, and shellfish, can be responsible for allergic reactions in children. In adults, peanuts, tree nuts, fish, and shellfish are common sources of food allergies.

History

Food allergy can cause lip or tongue swelling, abdominal cramping, abdominal pain or diarrhea, hives, wheezing, or anaphylaxis. Rhinitis can occur with other symptoms, but chronic rhinitis is generally not caused by food ingestion. Food allergies occasionally can be a cause of chronic hives or, more often, eczema, but most often the symptoms of food allergy are of sudden onset.

Physical Examination

Because food allergy manifests as an IgE-mediated response, many target organs can be affected. The physical examination findings are variable and could include hives, wheezing, and angioedema. No particular physical finding is diagnostic of a food allergy.

Testing

Allergy skin testing is the gold standard for identifying food allergy. There are, however, many false positives, especially in individuals with other allergies. False negatives are exceedingly rare. Single-blind or double-blind food challenges should only be done by allergists.

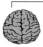

1 - Common allergens causing allergic rhinitis and ways to control them include:
- House-dust mites: Cover mattress and pillow, and wash bedding in hot water
- Pets: Remove from house
- Pollens: Run air conditioning, and change furnace filters regularly
- Molds: No vaporizers in bedroom

4 - Cromoglycate: Sodium cromolyn is a mast cell stabilizer. It is available in ophthalmic, nasal, and pulmonary formulations.

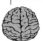

2 - The role of allergen immunotherapy is to alter the immunologic reactivity so that natural re-exposure to the offending allergen results in a lessened allergic response. Allergy immunotherapy reduces the associated inflammatory response (late-phase reaction) and the need for medication. Although immunotherapy should be initiated by an allergy specialist, it can be administered by any physician who understands how to recognize and treat anaphylaxis.

Management

Avoidance of the food causing the local or systemic allergic reactions is the *only* appropriate therapy for food allergy. Injectable epinephrine and oral antihistamines should be provided for school and home and for eating at restaurants to treat unintentional exposure. A Medi-Alert bracelet or necklace is also advisable. Food allergies can last a lifetime, and severe allergies always warrant co-management with an allergist if one is readily available.

Hives (Urticaria)

Synopsis

Hives can be localized or widespread, associated with other allergic diseases, or independent of other allergic diseases. Hives are itchy, although burning or tingling sensations can be felt. Hives are due to the local release of histamine from mast cells into the skin, causing a typical wheal and flare reaction. IgE reactions cause a minority of chronic hives. Mast cells and basophils have receptors, other than IgE receptors on their surfaces. Opioid receptors, for example, can be activated by any opioid medications, causing histamine and other mediator release. Hives can be acute or chronic, with 6 weeks being the usual dividing line for classification. Chronic hives are often difficult to manage and often do not have an obvious cause. Infection-triggered acute hives are not uncommon, especially in children, but chronic hives are rarely triggered by a chronic or occult infection.

Differential Diagnosis

- Erythema multiforme
- Vasculitis

Testing

Under most circumstances, laboratory testing has a limited role in acute hives. Individuals with seasonal allergic rhinitis or pet allergies can have hives when exposed to the relevant allergen, and the temporal association often becomes clear. Chronic hives can be a frustrating entity, and referral to an allergist for appropriate testing and laboratory screening is valuable.

Management

When acute hives appear as the sole clinical presentation, antihistamines are generally the most reasonable therapy. Continuous, long-acting, and nonsedating antihistamines are preferred. They should be continued for a week or two beyond the last hive outcropping. Intermittent antihistamine therapy often will be suboptimal. With severe acute hives, oral corticosteroids can be added. Chronic hives are difficult to manage. Continuous antihistamines are the cornerstone of therapy.

Anaphylaxis

Synopsis

There are probably few emergencies more critical than systemic anaphylaxis. In many cases the accidental or inappropriate exposure to an allergen, usually by the oral or intravenous route, triggers an explosive release of histamine and other mediators from systemic basophils and tissue mast cells. These chemicals can cause severe edema, bronchospasm, circulatory collapse, hives, flushing, and laryngospasm. Any or all of these reactions can occur. Food, antibiotics, latex, insect stings, and radiocontrast dyes are common agents. Some individuals have exercise-related anaphylaxis. On occasion, no cause can be determined.

History

The sudden, often dramatic, onset of localized or systemic symptoms should be considered as a possible anaphylactic reaction. The symptoms often include bronchospasm, circulatory collapse (variably), hives, flushing, and laryngospasm.

Physical Examination

The sudden set of multiple (usually) allergic symptoms can include:

- Wheezing
- Hypotension or shock
- Hives or diffuse, localized erythema
- Laryngeal stridor
- Angioedema

Differential Diagnosis

- **Vasovagal attacks** *(Definition 5)*
- Carcinoid syndrome
- Postmenopausal flushing
- Alcohol ingestion
- Panic attacks
- Vocal cord dysfunction

5 - Vasovagal: A collection of systemic symptoms mediated by the vagal nerve. Paleness; cold clammy skin; and fainting are all common. Vasovagal symptoms are often triggered by fear.

Testing

Referral to an allergist is the recommended starting point to evaluate the possible causes of an anaphylactic event. If an obvious cause is evident (e.g., peanut ingestion), strict avoidance will be necessary for life.

Management

The treatment for anaphylaxis is epinephrine (adrenaline) by injection. Antihistamines, although helpful, are always second-line therapy. Immediate transfer to an emergency room for prolonged observation is necessary. For prophylaxis, injectable epinephrine and oral antihistamines should be available at school and home and for eating at restaurants. A Medi-Alert bracelet or necklace is also advisable.

Selected Readings

1. Joint Task Force on Practice Parameters, American Academy of Allergy, Asthma and Immunology, American College of Allergy, Asthma and Immunology, and the Joint Council of Allergy, Asthma and Immunology: The diagnosis and management of anaphylaxis. J Allergy Clin Immunol 101:S465–S528, 1998.
2. Juhlin L, Landor M: Drug therapy for chronic urticaria. Clin Rev Allergy 10:349–369, 1992.
3. Kaplan AP: Urticaria: The relationship of duration of lesion to pathogenesis. Allergy Proc 11:15–18, 1990.
4. Kay AB: Allergy and allergic diseases: First of two parts. N Engl J Med 344:30–37, 2001.
5. Kay AB: Allergy and allergic diseases: Second of two parts. N Engl J Med 344:109–113, 2001.
6. Naclerio RM. Allergic rhinitis. N Engl J Med 325:860–869, 1991.
7. Sampson HA: Food allergy, part 1: Immunopathogenesis and clinical disorders. J Allergy Clin Immunol 103:717–728, 1999.
8. Sampson HA: Food allergy, part 2: Diagnosis and management. J Allergy Clin Immunol 103:981–989, 1999.

13. Ankle Injuries

Christopher C. Madden, MD

Synopsis

The ankle is one of the most commonly injured joints in the body, and the ankle **sprain** is the most common injury in sports *(Definition 1)*. Any activity involving running and jumping places the athlete at risk for ankle injury. Although most ankle injuries are lateral ankle sprains, it is important to recognize fracture or dislocations, syndesmosis sprains, peroneal tendon subluxation, and midfoot sprains. A pertinent history and thorough physical examination will allow confident diagnosis and treatment of most ankle injuries. Imaging, although often normal in the acute setting, can be useful if used appropriately. Most ankle injuries do well with conservative treatment, and many athletes return to sport between 1 and 6 weeks, depending on the severity of injury.
Appropriate diagnosis and treatment of ankle sprains can prevent long-term complications such as pain, laxity, impingement, and degenerative arthritis. Twenty to forty percent of patients complain of residual symptoms after ankle sprains. If symptoms persist beyond 2–3 months, consultation with an orthopedist or other sports medicine physician is appropriate.

Differential Diagnosis

* Ligamentous injuries *(Brain 1)*
  Lateral ankle sprain *(Definition 2)*
  Medial ankle sprain *(Definition 3)*
  Syndesmosis sprain *(Definition 4)*
  Midfoot sprain *(Definition 5)*
* Fracture (bone vs. cartilage) *(Definition 6)*
* Tendon injuries (e.g., Achilles, peroneal, posterior tibial, flexor hallucis, tibialis anterior)
  Tendinopathy (chronic/overuse) *(Definition 7)*
  Tendon strain or rupture (acute)

History

* "Tell me about the injury."
* "What happened exactly?" (Identify mechanism of injury to localize anatomic structure injured.)
* "When did the injury occur? Did your pain start right away or slowly?" Determine if the injury was acute (e.g., sprain or strain) or chronic (e.g., tendinopathy).
* "When and where did you notice swelling or bruising?" This will help localize the injury.

1 - Sprain: Disruption (tear) of ligamentous fibers.
Strain: Disruption of tendon or muscle fibers.

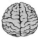

1 - Grading of ankle sprains:
* Grade I (ligaments minimally torn): Minimal swelling, pain, no ligamentous laxity with firm endpoint (attempted stretch of ligament results in abrupt stop at ligament end point)
* Grade II (ligament or ligaments partially torn): Mild-moderate swelling or ecchymosis, pain, mild-moderate ligamentous laxity with soft end point (attempted stretch of ligament results in nonabrupt or "soft" stop at ligament end point)
* Grade III (ligament or ligaments completely torn): Severe swelling or ecchymosis, pain, severe ligamentous laxity with no end point

2 - Lateral ankle sprain: Injury to anterior talofibular (ATF), calcaneolfibular (CF), or posterior talofibular (PTF) ligaments. The ATF ligament is most commonly injured.

3 - Medial ankle sprain: Injury to the deltoid ligament.

4 - Syndesmosis sprain: Injury to the structures at the distal tibia-fibula joint. These include anterior and posterior ligaments and the interosseous membrane. This injury is also referred to as a high ankle sprain.

5 - Midfoot sprain: Injury to any of the smaller intertarsal ligaments of the midfoot. The midfoot includes the navicular, cuboid, and cuneiform bones.

- "Where exactly is most of your pain, and what increases the pain?" Localize the injury to specific anatomic structures if possible.
- "Were you able to walk on the injured ankle?" If no, suspect fracture or severe sprain. "Did you return to activity and when?" This helps predict severity of injury.
- "Did you hear a pop?" This often indicates ligamentous rupture or fracture.
- "Do you have any numbness or tingling?" This could indicate neurological injury *(Red Flag 1)*
- "Have you noted any losses in motion or strength?" Find out if other structures are involved.
- "How has the injury been treated so far?" Determine if the patient has taken any anti-inflammatory medicine; used crutches, rest, or ice; or seen a rehabilitation specialist.
- "Have you injured the area previously? Does your ankle 'twist or roll' easily?" Determine if this is a chronic problem such as instability, predisposing to acute injury.

Physical Examination

The main goal of the physical exam is to anatomically localize the injury and to rule out injuries associated with significant potential morbidity. Exam of the injured ankle should always be compared with the uninjured side *(Brain 2)*. In addition, examination of the foot should routinely accompany the ankle exam. Brief palpation of foot structures can screen for associated injuries (e.g., midfoot sprain) and will help determine the need for a more complete foot exam *(Red Flag 2)*. A complete ankle exam should be conducted as follows:

1. **Inspection.** Check for:

- Localized swelling
- Deformity (fracture/dislocatioin)
- Ecchymosis or abrasions

2. **Palpation.** Locate anatomic structures injured:

- Bones (proximal fibula, distal malleoli, base of fifth metatarsal, navicular)
- Ligaments (lateral–anterior talofibular (ATF), calcaneal fibular (CF), posterior talofibular (PTF), medial–deltoid, high–syndesmosis, midfoot)
- Tendons
- Other soft tissues (joint capsule, retrocalcaneal bursa)
- Note crepitation (gross: fracture; fine: tendinopathy) and tendon thickening (Achilles)
- Foot structures (bones and ligaments of midfoot and forefoot)
- **Range of motion:** Active and passive *(Definition 8)*
- Plantar flexion (35–40°), dorsiflexion (15–20°), inversion, and eversion (inversion:eversion ratio ~ 2:1)

3. **Strength testing.** Note areas of weakness and pain with manual muscle testing (e.g., for pain with resisted ankle eversion, think peroneal muscle strain)

- Plantar flexors, dorsiflexors, inverters, everters, foot intrinsics (look for areas of specific injury)

6 - Chondral or osteochondral lesion: Cartilage can be fractured alone (chondral) or in combination with bone (osteochondral). When present, chondral lesions usually affect the talar dome (top of talus).

7 - Tendinopathy: General tendon pathology involving inflammation or degeneration. Degenerative change, rather than inflammatory change, may be present at the onset of tendon symptoms. The term more appropriately describes tendon pathology, especially at the patellar tendon and rotator cuff tendons, compared to the terms *tendinitis* and *tendinosis*, which mean inflammation in a tendon and degeneration in a tendon, respectively. Both may be present during the acute presentation.

1 - Suspect **fracture** if the patient is unable to take any steps on the injured ankle, or if she describes hearing a loud crack or pop. Suspect **neurologic injury** if the patient reports numbness or tingling in the affected ankle.

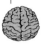

2 - Starting the examination with the uninjured ankle will allow the patient to relax and build trust in the physician, making the exam of the injured ankle less difficult. Findings on the injured side should always be compared to the noninjured side. Everyone's "normal" may be different—the patient's baseline can be established using the noninjured extremity.

2 - The examination should be used to localize the patient's injury to specific anatomic structures. The examiner should focus on ruling out injuries associated with significant morbidity (see Red Flag 1).

8 - Active range of motion: Patient voluntarily moves the ankle using his or her muscles.

Passive range of motion: Examiner moves the ankle through its motion while the patient attempts to relax. Significant muscle guarding may indicate pain associated with a fracture or severe sprain. Passive motion places a stretch on potentially injured ligaments and tendons, often resulting in pain over the injured structures.

4. **Neurovascular** assessment

- Sensory exam (ankle injuries often associated with stretch neuropraxia)
- **Proprioception** *(Definition 9)*. Proprioception can be grossly tested by having patients stand on their injured ankle (if able) and closing their eyes. This maneuver should be repeated standing on the uninjured side. If the patient wobbles more or greater muscle work (observe foot muscles contracting or "shivering") is noted while standing on the injured side, proprioception is likely decreased.
- Dorsalis pedis and posterior tibial pulse
- Deep tendon reflexes

5. **Specific tests** (test specific anatomic structures; all tests are compared to opposite uninjured side)

- **Anterior drawer test** (ATF ligament). Assess for laxity (increased anterior translation), grinding or clunking (degenerative joint disease [DJD], osteochondral lesion, fracture), and soft end point (significantly torn ligaments). In 10–15° of ankle plantar flexion, stabilize the patient's distal tibia with one hand while cupping the heel with the your dominant hand. Have the patient relax and apply an anterior force to the hindfoot, assessing anterior translation (forward movement of the talus) and any grinding *(Figure 1)*.
- **Talar tilt test** (ATF and CF ligaments). Assess for laxity (increased tilt) and soft end point. Test the ankle in both 0° (CF and ATF) and 20–30° (ATF > CF) plantar flexion. Hand position is the same as in the anterior drawer test. Apply an inversion stress to the ankle, assessing for increased tilt and soft end point. This is a more difficult and less reliable test than the anterior drawer test *(Figure 2)*.
- **Syndesmosis squeeze test** (syndesmosis ligaments and interosseous membrane). Assess for pain over the syndesmosis. The syndesmosis is made up of three ligaments and the interosseous membrane. The test is performed by grasping the tibia and fibula just above the midcalf and squeezing them toward each other. A positive test results in pain over the syndesmosis *(Figure 3)*. A syndesmosis, or high ankle sprain, is diagnosed clinically by tenderness over the tibiofibular ligaments combined with a positive syndesmosis squeeze or positive external rotation stress test. Fracture and tibia-fibula joint instability should be ruled out by x-rays.
- **Thompson test** (Achilles tendon rupture). Assess for absence of plantar flexion. Lay the patient in the prone position with feet hanging over the end of the table. Squeeze the calf and observe for passive plantar flexion. Absence of plantar flexion is a positive Thompson test and indicates a completely torn Achilles tendon *(Figure 4)*.

Testing

Primary care physicians may follow the Ottawa Ankle Rules when considering plain x-rays in the evaluation of acute ankle and foot pain *(Red Flag 3)*. The rules help determine when to order an x-ray to rule out a fracture. They are only valid in patients older than 18 years of age, and they should be used to assess only acute ankle injuries presenting within 10 days of injury. Sensitivity is 100% for detecting fractures of the ankle, and specificity is 90% for the ankle.

9 - Proprioception: The ankle's ability to tell the brain where it is in space ("position sense"). Proprioceptors are located in the soft tissues of the ankle and their function is lost with each subsequent injury.

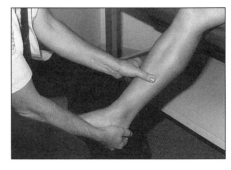

Figure 1: Anterior drawer test.
(From Brown DE: Ankle and leg injuries. In Mellion MB, Walsh MW, Shelton GL (eds): The Team Physician's Handbook, 2nd ed. Philadelphia, Hanley & Belfus, 1997, pp 579–592, with permission.)

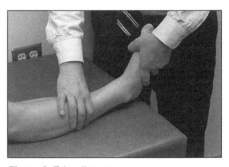

Figure 2: Talar tilt test.
(From Brown DE: Ankle and leg injuries. In Mellion MB, Walsh MW, Shelton GL (eds): The Team Physician's Handbook, 2nd ed. Philadelphia, Hanley & Belfus, 1997, pp 579–592, with permission.)

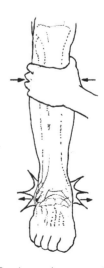

Figure 3: Syndesmosis squeeze test.
(Adapted from Ward DW: Syndesmotic ankle sprain in a recreational hockey player. J Manipulative Physiol Ther 17:385–394, 1994.)

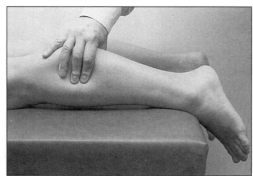

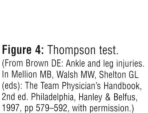

Figure 4: Thompson test. (From Brown DE: Ankle and leg injuries. In Mellion MB, Walsh MW, Shelton GL (eds): The Team Physician's Handbook, 2nd ed. Philadelphia, Hanley & Belfus, 1997, pp 579–592, with permission.)

3 - Ottawa Ankle Rules to rule out fracture (not including foot):
An ankle x-ray series is necessary if there is malleolar pain and any of the following:
- Bony tenderness involving the distal 6 cm of the posterior edge or tips of either the medial or lateral malleolus
- Inability to bear weight (cannot take four steps) immediately or in the office

Plain radiographs, using anteroposterior (AP), lateral, and mortise views, are the most practical and cost-effective means to assess the injured ankle. Other forms of imaging, including computer tomography (CT), magnetic resonance imaging (MRI), stress radiography, bone scanning, and arthrography, are available for a more detailed assessment of complex injuries but often are most appropriately left in the hands of the specialist.

Putting It All Together

Most patients presenting with acute ankle pain will have a lateral ankle sprain. A good history will uncover the mechanism (e.g., inversion) and circumstances surrounding the injury. Physical examination will localize the injury to specific anatomic structures (e.g., lateral ligaments: ATF and CF) and will rule out other significant injury. The Ottawa Ankle Rules can help ascertain when x-rays are indicated.

Management

After serious causes of ankle pain are ruled out, most ankle injuries, particularly sprains, can be treated conservatively following acute and rehabilitation phase principles.

Ankle sprains usually improve with conservative treatment, and athletes commonly return to sport between 1 and 6 weeks, depending on the severity of injury. Psychosocial issues related to decreasing a patient's normal physical activity (e.g., runner who must suddenly stop running) or removing a competitive athlete from sport must be addressed. Frustration can lead to poor compliance with proper treatment. Conditioning should be maintained with nonimpact activities such as pool-running or stationary bicycling. Often a practical question to ask the patient is: "Is our management plan realistic for you?" If the answer is no, develop another approach that will satisfy both the patient and the physician.

Acute phase management focuses mainly on pain control, reduction of swelling, maintenance of range of motion, and protection from further injury. The mnemonic PRICES can be used to remember acute phase management *(Treatment 1).* Range of motion can be maintained by having the patient "write" the alphabet in the air with his feet.

The rehabilitation phase begins as soon as pain will allow it. Range of motion and strength are top priorities. Conditioning can be maintained with pool-running or exercise bicycling early on. Walking, jogging, and sport-specific activities are added as pain allows. Proprioception retraining can be performed by having the patient stand on the affected ankle and balancing for increasing periods of time. Inadequately rehabilitated proprioception can lead to recurrent ankle sprains, resulting in ankle instability. The ankle should be functionally supported using taping or bracing, and anything beyond a grade I injury should be functionally supported with bracing or taping for at least 6 weeks. An Air Cast ankle stirrup can be used in more severe sprains. Although most patients successfully return to activity or sport between 1 and 6 weeks, there is no specific time that ensures ideal return. Overall, readiness for return to activity or sport is best predicted successfully if these criteria are met:

- Full ankle range of motion
- Near normal strength (~80%)
- Pain-free activities and exam (including stress tests)

Frequent patient follow-up is recommended. For minor injuries, the athlete may be reassessed in 2 weeks and at appropriate time intervals thereafter. More worrisome injuries can be reassessed at the end of the first week. If symptoms are worsening despite appropriate treatment or do not completely resolve by 2–3 months, referral to a specialist is recommended *(Consultation and Referral 1).*

Selected Readings

1. Bull RC: Handbook of Sports Injuries. New York, McGraw-Hill, 1999.
2. Fallat L, Grimm DJ, Saracco JA: Sprained ankle syndrome: Prevalence and analysis of 639 acute injuries. J Foot Ankle Surg 37:280–285, 1998.
3. Mellion MB, Walsh MW, Madden C, Putukian M (eds): The Team Physician's Handbook, 3rd ed. Philadelphia, Hanley & Belfus, Inc, 2001.
4. Sallis RE, Massimino F: ACSM's Essentials of Sports Medicine. St. Louis, Mosby, 1996.
5. Trojian TH, McKeag DB: Ankle sprains: Expedient assessment and management. Physician Sports Med 26:29–40, 1998.

1 - PRICES treatment for acute phase injury:

P Protection: Use crutches until patient can walk pain-free without limp.

R Rest: *absolute rest:* means complete rest from activity until pain-free; *relative rest:* indicated participation in pain-free activities only (e.g, "If it hurts, don't do it").

I Ice : Apply 20–30 minutes three times daily (practical tip: advise icing during meals—often the only time younger patients take time) and after activity, to decrease pain and swelling.

C Compression: Use of an Ace wrap decreases swelling, but does not provide support.

E Elevation: Keep leg above level of heart while sitting: this uses gravity to decrease swelling.

S Support: Use functional taping or bracing with minor injuries to allow more timely return to sport; this provides some protection and support.

1 - Referral to a primary care sports medicine physician or an orthopedist is recommended with worsening symptoms despite proper treatment or symptoms lasting longer than 2–3 months.

14. Anxiety and Depression

Jeffrey L. Susman, MD

Synopsis

Although anxiety and depression are extremely common conditions, they often present occultly or with somatic (bodily) signs and symptoms. Screening tools, such as the PRIME-MD **(Figure 1)**, can be used to help identify individuals suffering from anxiety and depression problems. Many common medical problems are associated with depression and anxiety. A thorough history and physical examination are important to appropriately detect treatable, underlying causes of mood disorders. It is imperative to uncover patients with suicidal intent, comorbid psychiatric conditions such as substance abuse, and relevant social issues. Patients with less severe cases often respond to counseling alone, whereas more severe problems are usually treated with a combination of counseling and medication. Referral, consultation, or hospitalization is indicated in patients who are actively suicidal, are refractory to treatment, or have complicated comorbidities.

Differential Diagnosis

- **Stress, life events, usual swings in mood.** Every individual reacts to the daily ups and downs of living. People often talk about being "stressed out" or "in a funk." Most individuals recover quickly from these temporary problems. It is important to distinguish between transient, minimally impairing mood changes and those that are clinically important **(Brain 1)**.
- **Medical conditions and medication use.** A wide variety of medical problems are associated with depression and anxiety. Examples of common problems linked with depression include cancer, endocrine problems such as hypothyroidism, and infections such as hepatitis and human immunodeficiency virus (HIV). Medications, including steroids, hormones, and antihypertensives, are commonly associated with depression. Anxiety symptoms can be associated with thyroid disease and hormone-producing tumors. In addition, medical diseases can cause symptoms that mimic mood disturbance. For example, a patient with advanced arthritis might exhibit less interest in activities that exacerbate pain, have substantial fatigue, and have a change in appetite related to medication.
- **Substance abuse.** Abuse of many substances, including alcohol, cocaine, and even the use of over-the-counter (OTC) remedies (such as decongestants or ephedra, a commonly used botanical), can cause depression or anxiety symptoms.
- **Other mental health problems.** Many other mental health problems are associated with depression and anxiety. For example, a patient with **obsessive-compulsive disorder (Definition 1)** or **social phobia (Definition 2)** may develop depression related to their primary mental health disorder. Bipolar disorder (manic depression) is associated with alternating periods of depression and mania (expansive,

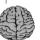

1 - *Anxiety* and *Depression* are lay terms that are not very specific in meaning. Anxiety and depression are not the variations in mood that all of us feel from time to time, related to life events and countless other factors. Serious anxiety and depression problems are persistent and significantly impair function. To help standardize the diagnosis of psychiatric disorders, the *Diagnostic and Statistical Manual of Mental Disorders* (DSM) was developed. This classification scheme provides standard criteria for each psychiatric disorder. A primary care version, the DSM-IV-PC, begins with common symptoms and outlines, in algorithm form, the appropriate diagnosis.

1 - Obsessive-compulsive disorder: Disorder made up of obsessions (recurrent thoughts and impulses) and compulsions (rituals or mental routines) that significantly impair a person's life.

2 - Social phobia (social anxiety disorder): "Marked and persistent fear of one or more social or performance situations in which the person is exposed to unfamiliar people or to possible scrutiny by others."[1]

Brief Patient Health Questionnaire

This questionnaire is an important part of providing you with the best health care possible. Your answers will help in understanding problems that you may have.

Name_____ Age_____ Sex: ☐ Female ☐ Male Today's Date _____

1. Over the <u>last 2 weeks</u>, how often have you been bothered by any of the following problems?

	Not at all	Several days	More than half the days	Nearly every day
a. Little interest or pleasure in doing things.....................	☐	☐	☐	☐
b. Feeling down, depressed, or hopeless	☐	☐	☐	☐
c. Trouble falling or staying asleep, or sleeping too much	☐	☐	☐	☐
d. Feeling tired or having little energy	☐	☐	☐	☐
e. Poor appetite or overeating	☐	☐	☐	☐
f. Feeling bad about yourself — or that you are a failure or have let yourself or your family down	☐	☐	☐	☐
g. Trouble concentrating on things, such as reading the newspaper or watching television	☐	☐	☐	☐
h. Moving or speaking so slowly that other people could have noticed? Or the opposite — being so fidgety or restless that you have been moving around a lot more than usual	☐	☐	☐	☐
i. Thoughts that you would be better off dead or of hurting yourself in some way	☐	☐	☐	☐

2. Questions about anxiety.

	NO	YES
a. In the <u>last 4 weeks</u>, have you had an anxiety attack—suddenly feeling fear or panic?...	☐	☐

If you checked "NO", go to question #3,

b. Has this ever happened before?	☐	☐
c. Do some of these attacks come <u>suddenly out of the blue</u> — that is, in situations where you don't expect to be nervous or uncomfortable?..	☐	☐
d. Do these attacks bother you a lot or are you worried about having another attack?	☐	☐
e. During your last bad anxiety attack, did you have symptoms like shortness of breath, sweating, your heart racing or pounding, dizziness or faintness, tingling or numbness, or nausea or upset stomach?	☐	☐

3. If you checked off <u>any</u> problems on this questionnaire so far, how <u>difficult</u> have these problems made it for you to do your work, take care of things at home, or get along with other people?

Not difficult at all	Somewhat difficult	Very difficult	Extremely difficult
☐	☐	☐	☐

Figure 1: PRIME-MD patient health questionnaire. Major depressive disorder is possible if 1a or 1b and five or more of 1a–i are checked as "more than half of the days." 1i should be counted if checked at all. Other depressive illness suggested if 1a or b and 2–4 of 1a–i are checked. Panic syndrome suggested when 1a–e are marked "yes."
(From Spitzer RL, Kroenke K, Williams JBW, et al: Validation and utility of a self-report version of PRIME-MD: The PHQ Primary Care Study. JAMA 282:1737–1744, 1999, with permission.)

irritable, or elevated mood) *(Brain 2)*.

- **Grief and bereavement.** Most individuals will feel depressed after the loss of a loved one. Although these symptoms can be severe initially, most individuals will improve by 2 months.

History

For All Patients with Anxiety or Depression *(Brain 3)*

- "Tell me how you are doing? What is your life like? What symptoms are you experiencing? What do you think is going on?"
- "Tell me about your medical history. Do any members of your family have a mental health problem?" Uncover history that may be relevant to diagnosing other medical or mental health problems that may be contributing to the patient's symptoms.
- "Tell me about the medications you take. Do you take any other supplements, vitamins, or nonprescription medications? Do you use alcohol? Do you use any other drugs?" It is important to inquire about substance use, OTC medications, supplements, and vitamins.

For Depression

"Tell me about your life and how things are going. How do you see the future? Do you feel down, blue, or depressed?" Assess the patient's mood. The mnemonic SIG-E-CAPS is helpful to assess for the signs and symptoms of major depressive disorder *(Brain 4)*:

S Sleep: "How have you been sleeping recently?" Many patients will wake up early in the mornings (early morning awakening) or sleep restlessly.

I Interest: "How has your interest in your work, family, hobbies been? What do you do to have a good time?" Solicit input from family, friends, and coworkers when possible.

G Guilt: "How do you feel about yourself and life in general? Do you feel guilty or at fault for anything?"

E Energy: "Do you feel tired or fatigued?"

C Concentration: "How has your work [or school or housework] been going? Do you find you forget things or have a hard time getting things done?"

A Appetite: "How has your appetite been? Are you as hungry as you used to be?"

P Psychomotor disturbance: "Describe your day. How has your ability to get up and go been?" Does the patient exhibit psychomotor retardation or agitation? *(Brain 5)*

S Suicide: "Have you ever felt you would be better off dead? Ever had thoughts of harming yourself?" *(Red Flag 1)*

Anxiety

For patients with anxiety, worries, fears, or recurrent and persistent thoughts or behaviors that are troublesome:

- "Tell me about your problems. Do you have times when you are fearful, worried, or have repeated thoughts or behaviors that interrupt

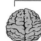

2 - Bipolar disorder is characterized by alternating periods of depression and mania. Mania consists of elevated, expansive, or irritable mood; increased energy levels; and decreased need for sleep. Patients often engage in compulsive or capricious behavior (e.g., spending large sums of money, engaging in risky sexual behaviors). They may have inflated self-esteem and are often distractible and jump from one subject to another (flight of ideas).

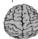

3 - Many patients will not present with a problem or symptoms directly suggestive of depression or anxiety. Indeed, somatic (bodily) symptoms such as back pain, headache, or stomachache are the most common presenting symptoms of depression. Likewise, patients with anxiety often emphasize the physical aspects of their illness. The use of a screening instrument (e.g., the PRIME-MD Patient Health Questionnaire, Zung Self-Rating Depression Scale, or Beck Inventory) can uncover patients with significant depression and anxiety problems (see Figure 1).

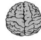

4 - The diagnosis of major depression is made when the patient has either anhedonia (loss of interest or pleasure) or depressed mood and four of the other symptoms of depression (SIG-E-CAPS), lasting ≥ 2 weeks and not explained by other medical or psychiatric conditions.

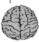

5 - Most patients with depression feel and act sluggish. Typically, this problem is worst in the morning and improves in the evening. Other patients may become agitated. Such behavior changes may be clearer to close family members or friends than to the patients themselves.

1 - Every patient with depression should be assessed for suicidal intent. Asking a patient if he is going to harm himself does not increase the likelihood of completed suicide, and may be life saving. Most patients who attempt suicide have seen their doctor within the past month. The risk of suicide is greater when the patient:

- Has a concrete, doable plan
- Is male
- Has a serious or terminal illness
- Is a substance abuser
- Is out of touch with reality (as might occur with schizophrenia or psychosis)

your day? Do you feel trembly, shaky, have palpitations, or difficulty sleeping?" Such symptoms suggest an anxiety disorder.
- "Do you ever have anxiety attacks?" Evaluate for the presence of panic attacks *(Brain 6)*.
- "Do you fear, avoid, or anxiously anticipate certain situations?" Phobias (avoidance of certain situations or objects) are common and can range from the mildly inconveniencing to devastatingly disabling.
- "Are there certain thoughts, habits or routines that interfere with your day?" Suggests obsessive-compulsive disorder.
- "Do you relive or dream about a highly traumatic event or experience?" Post-traumatic stress disorder frequently happens after a threat to one's life or physical well being (e.g., rape, car accident, trauma).

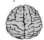

6 - Panic attacks are discrete periods of intense fear or discomfort developing rapidly and peaking within 10 minutes and are associated with symptoms such as sweating, trembling, chest pain, fear of dying, choking, and a pounding heart. Panic attacks can occur in patients with panic disorder, substance abuse, social phobia, depression, and other mental health conditions.

Physical Examination

- General observation. Does the patient appear depressed, weepy, anxious, fidgety? How are they groomed? Do they appear to be in touch with their surroundings?
- Vital signs
- Thyroid (thyroid abnormalities, especially hypothyroidism, can simulate depression)
- Brief physical examination (to evaluate for medical conditions causing depression or anxiety and problems that would influence choice of therapy, such as benign prostatic hypertrophy)
- Mental status examination:
  1. General, including orientation
  2. Attention (e.g., unable to concentrate, recall ability)
  3. Speech (e.g., pressured or fast, sluggish)
  4. Mood and affect (see History)
  5. Thought process (e.g., is thinking logical and coherent, does the patient appear to have racing thoughts?)
  6. Thought content (e.g., preoccupation with death)
  7. Perceptions (e.g., presence of hallucinations)
  8. Insight and judgment (e.g., does the patient grasp the seriousness of the problem?)

Testing

Most patients require no testing other than consideration of an assessment of thyroid function. More elaborate neuropsychologic testing, lab work, or other evaluations are usually predicated on the results of the history and physical examination.

Putting It All Together

The first task in making the diagnosis of depression or anxiety is to uncover underlying medical problems or medications that may account for the patient's symptoms. A thorough history and physical examination and corroboration of information from family and friends are essential. Important life events, such as the loss of a loved one or divorce, substance abuse, and other mental health problems should be assessed.

Further questions can then target the specific mental health condition. The thought content, insight, and judgment of every patient with a significant mental health condition should be ascertained.

Management *(Treatment 1) (Consultation and Referral 1)*

The first priority of management is to treat underlying conditions, including medical problems and substance abuse. In less severe mood disorders, counseling therapies, particularly **cognitive-behavioral therapy** *(Definition 3)* and **interpersonal therapy** *(Definition 4)*, have been shown to be effective in and of themselves. More serious problems are usually treated with a combination of counseling and medications, often agents such as the selective serotonin reuptake inhibitors (SSRIs) that have both anxiolytic and antidepressant properties. Fortunately, a wide variety of medications is available and can be matched to the patient's specific problem and needs. More aggressive treatment, including possible hospitalization, occurs in those individuals who are actively suicidal or have severe impairment of functioning.

Selected Readings

1. American Psychiatric Association: Diagnostic and Statistical Manual of Mental Disorders, Primary Care Version, 4th ed. Washington, DC, American Psychiatric Association, 1995.
2. Ellen FE: Detecting and treating depression. Hippocrates 14(2):30–41, 2000.
3. The Hidden Diagnosis: Uncovering Anxiety and Depressive Disorders. CD-ROM Program. Springfield, NJ, Scientific Therapeutics Information, 1999.
4. Rush AJ, et al: Depression in Primary Care. Washington, DC, Agency for Health Care Policy and Research, U.S. Department of Health and Human Services, 1993, AHCPR publication number 93-0550.
5. Spitzer RL, Kroenke K, Williams JBW, et al: Validation and utility of a self-report version of PRIME-MD: The PHQ Primary Care Study. JAMA 282:1737–1744, 1999.

1 - Treatment of underlying medical conditions, substance abuse, and other primary psychiatric problems will often precede specific therapy for depression and anxiety. Many times brief counseling by the primary care physician will be sufficient to help patients resolve less serious problems. Formal psychotherapy, often done by a counselor, social worker, or therapist, is effective for moderately severe problems and is often an important part of holistic therapy. More serious problems warrant medications, which include a variety of antidepressant and anxiolytics, sometimes in combination.

1 - Consultation or referral should be considered for patients with more serious mood disturbances and in any patient who is deemed a significant suicidal risk. Patients with complicated medical or psychiatric comorbidities or who have failed multiple medications will often warrant consultation. Patients requiring multiple drug therapy or with a diagnosis that is in question will also often be referred. Most primary care physicians will look for help in treating childhood psychiatric disorders. Many patients will see a counselor, psychiatrist, and a primary care physician for their care team.

3 - **Cognitive behavioral therapy:** Counseling that links patients' thoughts and emotional responses, explores their cognitions (ways of thinking) and "self talk," and suggests ways to modify behaviors and practice new ones.

4 - **Interpersonal therapy:** Counseling that focuses on patients' interpersonal relationships and facilitates appropriate changes in communication and relationships.

15. Asthma in Childhood

C. Gerald Judy, MD

Synopsis

Asthma is the most common chronic disease affecting children. The diagnosis of asthma begins with a thorough history and physical examination. It is important to elicit whether symptoms are persistent or intermittent, the frequency of exacerbations, triggers, and the severity of episodes. The physical examination should place special emphasis on all aspects of the respiratory and cardiovascular systems.

The management of asthma is determined by the frequency and severity of exacerbations. A child who has required frequent hospitalizations for severe asthma, pediatric intensive care unit (ICU) admission, mechanical ventilation for respiratory failure, and frequent systemic steroid therapy should be referred for consultation.

Differential Diagnosis

The most common conditions that present with signs and symptoms similar to asthma in infancy and early childhood are:

- **Laryngomalacia *(Definition 1)***
- Airway anomalies
- Gastroesophageal reflux disease (GERD)
- Aspiration
- Bronchiolitis
- Foreign bodies in the airway and cystic fibrosis

1 - Laryngomalacia: The airway is partially obstructed during inspiration by the prolapse of poorly supported aryepiglottic folds, the arytenoids, and the epiglottis. Sometimes called congenital laryngostridor.

In the older child:

- Psychogenic cough
- Tumor
- Recurrent pneumonia

The diseases that may present acutely and with life-threatening consequences are:
- Congestive heart failure
- Bronchiolitis
- Croup syndrome
- Epiglottitis
- Pertussis
- Foreign body aspiration

The disease entities that usually present with more chronic symptoms and that have serious consequences are:
- Cystic fibrosis
- Recurrent aspiration of upper airway secretions or of stomach contents
- Recurrent pneumonia
- Tumors

History

A thorough history is the most important key to the diagnosis of asthma. It is important to elicit when the first symptoms occurred. If the symptoms occurred during early infancy, the possibility of congenital anomalies of the airway, cyanotic congenital heart disease, laryngomalacia, and vascular rings or slings should be considered.

The following questions should be directed at the parent accompanying the infant or child or directly to an older child:

- "Does your baby choke, gag, or cough with feedings or spit up shortly after feedings?" Positive response suggests chronic aspiration (GERD).
- "Does the infant become diaphoretic with feedings or take excessive time to consume 3–4 ounces of formula?" Suggests cyanotic congenital heart disease.
- "Does the 'noisy breathing' or wheeze in an infant disappear with sleep and become more pronounced with agitation?" Consider laryngomalacia.
- "Does the infant have frequent large, bulky, foul-smelling stools and always seem hungry?" Could point to cystic fibrosis.
- "Has the infant or child's growth and development been abnormal?" This could indicate:
      Congenital anomalies
      Neurologic disease to suggest aspiration
      Cystic fibrosis
- "Was the child eating peanuts, popcorn, or soy beans when his symptoms began, specifically cough?" Consider foreign body aspiration.
- "Has the child had recurrent pneumonias?" Rule out:
      Aspiration
      Cystic fibrosis
      Foreign body in the airway
      GERD with aspiration
      Immunologic disorders
- "Is temperature associated with the cough or wheeze?" Infectious etiology is possible.
- "Does the 'noisy breathing' or wheeze occur during inspiration or expiration?" *(Brain 1)*
- "Has the child experienced shortness of breath, difficulty breathing, chest tightness or air hunger or chest pain with viral respiratory illnesses or light, medium, or heavy exercise; during the night; or upon awakening in the morning?" All of these suggest asthma and may be clues as to the severity of the asthma.
- "Does the child cough?" Clarify:
      Day versus night
      Dry versus moist
      Persistent versus episodic
- "What triggers the cough?" These are clues to differential diagnosis and possible therapy.
- "Does the child wheeze?" Wheezing at night with exertion, with laughing, and with viral respiratory illnesses suggests asthma.
- Inquire about the frequency and severity of the wheeze. The severity of the asthma will determine treatment.
- "Is the cough or wheeze responsive to bronchodilator therapy?" Cough and wheeze responsive to bronchodilator therapy suggest asthma.

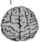
1 - Inspiratory wheeze is more likely to be stridor and suggests an extrathoracic airway obstruction such as croup, epiglottitis, congenital anomaly of the airway, or laryngomalacia.

- "Does the child run and play with inanimate objects in his or her mouth?" This suggests foreign body aspiration.
- "Has the child lost an unusual amount of weight recently?" Suggests systemic disease or tumor.

Physical Examination

General

Although the physical examination may be normal, there may be subtle findings suggesting an underlying disease (e.g., growth failure or cachexia may suggest cystic fibrosis or cancer).

Vitals

- Increased respiratory rate
- Tachycardia
- **Pulsus paradoxus *(Definition 2)***

2 - Pulsus paradoxus: During quiet spontaneous respiration there is a phasic variation of arterial blood pressure. The widening of this normal respiratory variation is known as pulsus paradoxus.

HEENT

- Head (sinus tenderness)
- Ears (otitis media, effusion)
- Eyes (conjunctivitis, allergic shiners [dark rings around orbit])
- Nose (polyps, postnasal drainage, pale boggy mucosa)
- Throat (pharyngeal redness, evidence of infection)

Lungs

- Increased anteroposterior (AP) diameter from air trapping
- Harrison's sulci (anterolateral indentations in the thoracic cage)
- Use of accessory muscles (suggests worsening asthma)
- Auscultation (wheeze) (polyphonic wheeze heard during expiration) *(Brain 2)*
- Stridor heard primarily during inspiration is associated with dynamic collapse from extrathoracic airway obstruction and suggests croup, epiglottitis, vascular ring or sling, or laryngotracheomalacia.
- Coarse crackles may be heard in association with polyphonic wheeze in asthma, whereas fine inspiratory crackles suggest congestive heart failure, pneumonia, or interstitial lung disease.

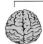

2 - Auscultation of the lungs between asthmatic attacks usually reveals no abnormal breath sounds. The presence of a polyphonic wheeze heard loudest during expiration suggests asthma. A prolonged expiratory phase suggests airway obstruction with air trapping and is compatible with asthma. A monophonic wheeze is heard as a single localized pitch caused by obstruction of one airway as in foreign body aspiration, tracheal or bronchial stenosis, or external compression of the airway by a mass (tumor, enlarged lymph nodes).

Heart

Evaluation of the heart and abdomen are usually normal in an asthmatic. A heart murmur or gallop rhythm suggests heart disease.

Abdomen

Hepatomegaly may be secondary to congestive heart failure or may represent downward displacement of the liver due to hyperinflation seen in asthma.

Skin

- Examination of the skin in an asthmatic may reveal atopic dermatitis or eczema (see Chapter 53).
- Clubbing of the digits is not present in asthma *(Red Flag 1)*.

1 - Clubbing of the digits suggests heart disease or more severe lung disease (CF, bronchiectasis, interstitial lung disease with fibrosis, liver failure, certain tumors, hemoglobinopathies, or other systemic disease processes).

Neurologic

The neurologic examination should reveal any underlying deficit predisposing to chronic aspiration.

Testing

Laboratory tests are rarely helpful in diagnosing asthma and are used only if the diagnosis is unclear or if other diagnoses are suspected.

Chest radiographs are usually normal, but may reveal bronchial wall thickening, hyperinflation, or **atelectasis (Definition 3)** from mucous plugging. With foreign body aspiration, one may see unilateral hyperinflation, a metallic object in the airway, recurrent pneumonia, or atelectasis of the same lobe.

A computed tomography (CT) scan of the sinuses may be obtained to document chronic sinusitis if one suspects the sinusitis is complicating the asthma and has been refractory to medical therapy. CT of the chest is only indicated if parenchymal lung disease, airway anomalies, or external compression of the airways is suspected. Magnetic resonance imaging (MRI) may be used to further delineate vascular rings or slings.

3 - Atelectasis: Collapse of various segments of the lung or of an entire lung due to pressure from an external mass, pleural effusion or blocking of the smaller bronchial tubes with mucus.

Pulmonary function testing is difficulty in young children and usually not necessary. It may be used to support the diagnosis or assess the severity or response to therapy. Baseline spirometry with lung volumes evaluates obstruction to expiratory airflow and air trapping. Asthma causes medium and small airway narrowing. This is reflected by decreased forced expiratory volume in 1 second (FEV_1) and an increased functional residual capacity (FRC), residual volume (RV), and total lung capacity (TLC). Flows may be normal between attacks (see Chapter 70).

Because pulmonary function tests are often normal between attacks, bronchial provocation tests may be used to assess the patient's degree of hyper-responsiveness (methacholine or histamine challenges). A positive test is not diagnostic of asthma but is correlated with an increased likelihood of having disease.

Reversibility of airway obstruction following bronchodilatory therapy (an increase ≥ 15% in two out of three of the following indices: FEV_1, FEV_1 / FVC ratio, and forced expiratory flow [FEF] 25–75%) may support the diagnosis of asthma.

Other tests such as sweat chloride determination, barium swallow, esophageal pH probe study, or appropriate cultures may be indicated depending on clinical suspicion.

Putting It All Together

A diagnosis of asthma is most often made by performing a thorough history. The physical examination may be normal in the physician's office. Pulmonary function tests are difficult to obtain in young children, and laboratory studies are not usually contributory. The physician must elicit a thorough history of the illness and must be aware of the common presentations of asthma, the less common manifestations, and clues to other diagnoses.

The usual chief complaint is recurrent cough or wheeze. Additional symptoms may include chest tightness, air hunger, or shortness of breath. The cough seen in asthma is recurrent, may be dry or productive, and is usually worse at night. The cough and wheeze may be exacerbated by cold air, exercise, or forced expiratory movements such as laughing or crying. The most common trigger of asthma in children is viral respiratory illnesses.

Cystic fibrosis or bronchiectasis should be excluded if purulent sputum is produced on a daily basis. A child need not have failure to thrive or a history suggestive of steatorrhea with cystic fibrosis. Sudden onset of wheezing in a young child may indicate a foreign body, and fever, usually present in pneumonia, is absent with asthma.

A hoarse voice and barking cough are classic symptoms of croup, whereas a spastic staccato cough occurs in pertussis. Psychogenic cough is usually harsh in sound and absent during sleep the majority of the time. Recurrent bronchiolitis with wheezing usually represents early asthma.

Some characteristics found to be associated with asthma mortality in children include:
- Disregard of perceived asthma symptoms
- Poor self care
- Patient–staff conflict
- Patient–parent conflict
- Parent–staff conflict
- Manipulative use of asthma (falsifying asthma symptoms for secondary gain)
- Emotional disturbance
- Depressive symptoms
- History of emotional behavioral reactions to separation or loss
- Family dysfunction

Management

The therapy of asthma is multiphasic and involves environmental control, pharmacologic therapy, and education of the patient and family about the disease, its triggers, and the importance of compliance with therapy. The goal of therapy is to reduce or control symptoms to optimize the patient's lifestyle. In the majority of illnesses, with optimal care, the child should have a reasonably normal and active life.

Environmental control consists of avoidance or limiting the exposure to primary offenders, which in children are cigarette smoke, house dust mites, family pets, seasonal pollens, and emotional disturbances.

Asthmatics classified as **mild-intermittent** have symptoms less than twice weekly, require no daily medications, and can be controlled on intermittent inhaled bronchodilator therapy.

Asthmatics classified as **mild-persistent** have symptoms greater than twice per week, but less than one time per day. These patients may require daily anti-inflammatory therapy in the form of inhaled brochodilator therapy as needed for breakthrough symptoms.

Moderate-persistent asthmatics have daily symptoms and will usually require daily inhaled corticosteroids plus daily long-acting brochodilator therapy (long-acting inhaled brochodilator, sustained-release theophylline, or long-acting beta$_2$-agonist tablets).

Severe-persistent asthmatics have daily, continual symptoms, limited physical activity, and frequent exacerbations. These patients require high-dose inhaled corticosteroids, daily long-acting inhaled brochodilator and sustained-release theophylline, or long-acting beta$_2$-agonist tablets plus systemic (tablets or syrup), long-term corticosteroid therapy.

A child who has required frequent hospitalization for severe asthma, pediatric ICU admission, mechanical ventilation for respiratory failure, and frequent systemic steroid therapy should be referred for consultation.

Selected Readings

1. Chernick D, Boat TF, Kendig EL: Kendig's Disorders of the Respiratory Tract in Children, 6th ed. Philadelphia, W.B. Saunders, 1998.
2. Toussig LM, Landau LI: Pediatric Respiratory Medicine. St. Louis, Mosby, 1999.

16. Back Pain

Jeffrey L. Susman, MD

Synopsis

The vast majority of patients with low back pain (LBP) have a nonspecific strain that will resolve within 4–8 weeks. About 1 of 10 patients will present with leg pain indicative of **radiculopathy** *(Definition 1)*; only about 1 in 100 will have a more severe underlying problem or go on to have more protracted disability. The history and physical examination lay the groundwork for the treatment of the patient with LBP. The history and physical are structured to determine whether the patient has a high likelihood for a serious spinal or nonspinal cause of back pain or radiculopathy. In addition, the evaluation helps to build rapport, emphasize the functional and personal impacts of the problem, and chart a course for education and further therapy. Testing is rarely indicated in the absence of red flags for underlying problems. Immediate referral is indicated in the face of a progressive motor deficit or the **cauda equina syndrome** *(Definition 2)*. Follow-up by phone or in the office should be scheduled to identify early those patients prone to chronic low back pain problems.

1 - Radiculopathy: Disease of the spinal roots indicated by radiating pain (especially below the knee) and motor and sensory deficits.

2 - Cauda equina syndrome: The spinal cord ends at the level of the first lumbar vertebra. From there the cord continues as the filum terminale and, with the dorsal and ventral nerve roots, constitutes the cauda equina. Compression of the cauda equina, as from a central disc herniation, is suggested by severe LBP, saddle anesthesia, progressive neurologic deficits, and loss of bowel or bladder control. This condition is a neurosurgical emergency.

Differential Diagnosis

- "Back strain"
- Radiculopathy
- Nonspinal or serious secondary cause of back pain

History

"Tell me about your back problem. What symptoms are you experiencing?" *(Red Flag 1)* Note any of the following:

- Fever or chills
- Constitutional symptoms (e.g., weight loss, night sweats, anorexia)
- Radiation of pain below knee
- Bowel or bladder complaints
- Duration of pain greater than 4–8 weeks
- No relief with bed rest

"How does your back problem affect your job, school, and household performance? How does your back problem affect your ability to carry out the activities you like to do?" *(Red Flag 2) (Brain 1)*

"Tell me about yourself and your medical history."

- Occupation, job satisfaction, worker's compensation claims
- Family dysfunction

1 - The presence of these symptoms is suggestive of serious underlying conditions (e.g., infection, tumor, fracture, cauda equina syndrome) or of radiculopathy.

2 - These questions further assess the presence of a serious underlying condition that could account for back pain (e.g., metastatic cancer or trauma) or an underlying psychosocial problem that may impair recovery.

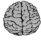

1 - It is important to assess the functional impact of back pain.

- Mood disorder or substance use
- Trauma
- Neoplasm (especially myeloma and adenocarcinomas metastatic from breast, prostate, lung, colorectum, and kidney)
- Systemic rheumatologic condition (e.g., rheumatoid arthritis)
- Metabolic bone disease (e.g., osteoporosis)
- Intravenous drug use
- Use of steroid or other drug that may compromise immune function or increase risk of fracture
- Immunocompromising condition (e.g., AIDS)

"Tell me what you know about back problems."

"Have you known anyone with back problems before? Can you describe their experience?" **(Brain 2)**

"What concerns do you have about this problem? What treatment do you expect?" (e.g., x-rays, bed rest, time off work)

Physical Examination *(Red Flag 3)*

- General observation (e.g., pain behaviors, such as grimacing or moaning, abnormal gait, atrophy)
- Vital signs, including temperature
- Screening examination of abdomen, flanks
- Palpation of the spine and back
- Range of motion of spine
- **Straight leg-raising** and **crossed-straight leg-raising test** *(Definition 3) (Table 1) (Figure 1)*
- Lower extremity reflexes
- Lower extremity motor function
- Lower extremity sensation
- Babinski sign
- Gait
- Rectal and genital examination if cauda equina syndrome suspected

Testing

No testing is necessary, unless secondary cause of back pain, cauda equina syndrome, or rapidly progressive neurologic syndrome is suspected.

Putting It All Together

The vast majority of patients presenting with low back pain have a nonspecific "back strain." However, the physician should be alert to:

- Underlying occupational and psychosocial issues that may predispose the patient to chronic problems
- Masqueraders (nonspinal causes of pain) of LBP such as an abdominal aortic aneurysm and serious causes of back pain such as an underlying malignancy, fracture, or infection
- Nerve root entrapment or radiculopathy, particularly in patients with the cauda equina syndrome or a rapidly progressive neurologic deficit

2 - These questions help manage expectations and address patient concerns to provide patient education.

3 - The physical examination is targeted to uncover signs of other conditions causing LBP (e.g., infection, tumor, fracture, cauda equina syndrome) or signs of radiculopathy.

3 - Straight leg-raising test: This test determines impingement on the sciatic nerve, usually by a herniated disk. With the patient either seated or lying supine, the examiner raises the patient's leg on the affected side. Pain in a sciatic distribution, particularly below the knee, constitutes a positive test. This test is relatively sensitive for sciatic nerve root impingement. Pain elicited in the opposite leg denotes a positive **crossed straight leg-raising test** and is less sensitive, but even more specific.

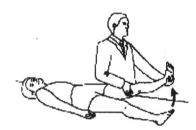

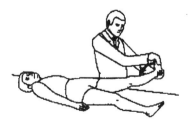

Figure 1: Straight leg-raising test.
(From Bigos SJ, Bowyer O, Braen GE, et al: Acute Low Back Problems in Adults. Clinical Practice Guideline 14. Rockville, MD, US Department of Health and Human Services, Public Service, Agency for Health Care Policy and Research, AHCPR publication 95–642, 1994, with permission.)

Table I. Changes Associated with Nerve Root Impingement

Involved Nerve Root	Sensory Changes	Deficits in Strength	Reflex Changes	Atrophy
L4	Anteromedial thigh and medial foot	Quadriceps weakness	Patella	Quadriceps
L5	Lateral leg, dorsum of foot	Dorsiflexion of great toe, difficulty walking on heel	None	None
S1	Posterior calf and lateral foot	Plantar flexion of foot, difficulty walking on toes	Ankle	Gastrocnemius and soleus
Cauda equina (massive midline)	Variable: buttocks, thighs, feet, perineum	Variable paralysis and paresis; urinary retention	Diminished sphincter tone; variable reflex loss	May be present

Management *(Treatment 1) (Consultation and Referral 1)*

The history and physical exam are geared to uncovering serious causes of LBP rather than making a specific diagnosis. The physician should focus on understanding the patient's concept of illness, addressing occupational and psychosocial issues, providing education, and activating the patient. Diagnoses such as "degenerative changes" or "subluxations" are nonspecific, cannot be reliably diagnosed on the history and physical exam, and do not have prognostic value. Individuals may be reassured that most back pain resolves within 4–8 weeks and that additional evaluation (with laboratory, imaging studies, or other tests) is unwarranted. The patient should be encouraged to remain active; however, no specific set of exercises has been shown to hasten recovery.

Follow-up with the patient should be scheduled either by phone or in the office. The reevaluation should focus on ongoing discomfort, functional status, the presence of red flags, and factors suggesting a risk for chronic problems.

1 - Acetaminophen, aspirin, and nonsteroidal anti-inflammatory drugs (NSAIDs) are usually effective. Other medications, such as muscle relaxants, are best avoided. Manipulation is another proven option. Prolonged bed rest, traction, and braces are ineffective.

1 - Referral should be considered in patients with persistent, functionally disabling radiculopathy or a more serious cause of LBP.

Selected Readings

1. Bigos SJ, Bowyer O, Braen GE, et al: Acute Low Back Problems in Adults. Clinical Practice Guideline 14. Rockville, MD, US Department of Health and Human Services, Public Health Service, Agency for Health Care Policy and Research, 1994, AHCPR publication 95-642.
2. Carey TS, Garrett J, Jackman A, et al: The outcomes and costs of care for acute low back pain among patients seen by primary care practitioners, chiropractors, and orthopedic surgeons. N Engl J Med 333:913, 1995.
3. Deyo RA, Rainville J, Kent DL: What can the history and physical examination tell us about low back pain? JAMA 268:760–765, 1992.
4. Malmivaara A, Hakkinen U, Aro T, et al: The treatment of acute low back pain with bed rest, exercises or ordinary activity? N Engl J Med 332:351, 1995.
5. Weber H: The natural course of disc herniation. Acta Orthop Scand Suppl 251(64):19–20, 1993.

17. The Birth Control Visit

Keith B. Holten, MD

Synopsis

Many patients who would not otherwise be seen by a health care provider schedule a visit for birth control advice. Most commonly, women seek this care, so this chapter will give priority to the risk factors affecting women's health *(Brain 1)*.

The birth control visit is an opportunity to provide appropriate educational and preventive services, including contraceptive care. This encounter usually occurs after sexual activity has begun, many times without the use of contraception. Fear of an unintended pregnancy may have prompted the visit.

Establishing rapport during this visit can lead to a lifetime of good health care. During the history, sexual behaviors and screening for partner violence can be considered. A physical examination can be performed and cancer and sexually transmitted disease (STD) screening provided. Contraceptive prescriptions can be made available. Education can be offered regarding reproductive health, general healthy behaviors, and follow-up care.

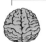

1 - Risk factors affecting women's health
- Unintended pregnancy
- Exposure to sexually transmitted diseases
- Cigarette smoking
- Substance use
- Violence
- Accidents
- Poor nutrition and exercise behaviors
- Poverty

Differential Diagnosis

- Pregnancy "scare"
- Preconception care
- Family planning
- Prevention visit

History

Medical History

- "Do you have a history of any medical problems?" Focus on a history of migraine headaches, blood clots, stroke, high blood pressure, blood sugar problems, or liver disease *(Red Flag 1)*.
- "Do you take any medications?"

1 - These medical problems signal additional risk associated with hormonal contraception containing estrogen.

Reproductive and Sexual History

- "Tell me about your periods." Determine onset, flow, frequency, last period, and use of tampons and pads *(Red Flag 2)*.
- "Are you sexually active now? How many sexual partners have you had?" Determine age of first activity, practices, number of partners.
- "When was your last Pap smear?" Some patients may be here for their first Pap smear and require special education before proceeding.

2 - Women presenting for birth control may be pregnant. A careful menstrual history should be obtained and a urine pregnancy test performed.

- "Have you ever been pregnant?" Determine number of pregnancies, pregnancy problems, and type of deliveries.
- If applicable, "Are you nursing a child?" *(Red Flag 3)*
- "Do you use birth control? What type are you interested in?" Explore her knowledge of contraceptives and ways to reduce the risk of acquiring a sexually transmitted disease.
- "Have you ever been treated for a sexually transmitted disease?" Is there a history of chlamydia, gonorrhea, warts, abnormal Pap smear, syphilis, or pelvic infections? (see Chapters 40 and 56)

3 - Lactating women should not take estrogen-containing oral contraceptives.

Family and Social History

- "Are there diseases that run in your family?" Is there a history of stroke, high blood pressure, blood clots, or migraines?
- "Do you use drugs or alcohol?"
- "Do you smoke?" *(Red Flag 4)*
- "Who is in your household?" *(Brain 2)*

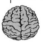

4 - Smokers should be advised to quit, and those 35 and older should not be prescribed estrogen-containing oral contraceptives.

2 - Pursuing this history can make it easier to screen for risk of partner violence.

Physical Examination

The physical examination provides baseline health status information and allows for cancer and STD screening. Thyroid enlargement may be detected with a careful neck examination.

- Vital signs—check blood pressure and pulse
- HEENT (head, ears, eyes, nose, throat)—check dental health
- Neck—check for thyromegaly
- Cardiac—check for murmurs
- Lungs—check for abnormal sounds
- Abdomen—check for hepatomegaly, obesity
- Pelvic exam
    - Vulva—check for lesions
    - Vagina—note any discharge. If present, do wet prep.
    - Cervix—with Pap test. Do cultures if at risk for STDs (see Chapter 56).
    - Uterus—check position and size
    - Adnexa—check for ovarian enlargement
- Extremities—note any varicose veins or palpable cords

Testing

These must be decided on an individual basis. Women with heavy menses should be encouraged to have a hematocrit to screen for anemia. Lipids levels are controversial but are indicated for a family history of premature coronary artery disease.

- Pap smear
- Hematocrit
- Cervical cultures for chlamydia and gonorrhea
- Urine pregnancy test
- HIV testing (see Chapter 40)
- Syphilis screening—rapid plasmin reagin (RPR) test or Venereal Disease Research Laboratory (VDRL) test
- Lipid screening

Putting It All Together

Patients presenting for birth control are usually healthy. This is an opportunity to build rapport with the patient and do appropriate history taking, physical screening, and appropriate education. An optimal approach can lead to a lifetime of good health.

Management

The focused history and physical examination is useful to prioritize the time available for the visit. After risk factors for various methods of birth control are eliminated, the provider can give the most appropriate contraception prescription *(Treatment 1)*, discuss appropriate screening laboratories, spend time educating the patient, and recommend a reasonable follow-up plan *(Treatment 2)*.

Combination oral contraceptives are commonly prescribed, but appropriate education must be provided to users to maximize efficacy *(Treatment 3)*.

Selected Readings

1. Hatcher RA, Trussell J, Stewart F, et al: Contraceptive Technology, 17th revised ed. New York, Ardent Media, 1998.
2. Hatcher RE, Zieman M, Walt A, et al: Managing Contraception. Tiger, GA, Bridging the Gap Foundation, 1999.
3. Rieder J, Coupey SM: Contraceptive Compliance in the Adolescent Patient. Female Patient 24:19–31, 1999.

1 - Methods of birth control:
- Abstinence
- Barrier methods
  - Male condom
  - Female condom
  - Spermicides
  - Diaphragm
  - Intrauterine device (IUD)
- Hormonal
  - Medroxyprogesterone acetate (Depo-Provera)
  - Oral contraceptives (combination estrogen and progesterone or progestin only)
  - Emergency contraception
- Sterilization
- Abortion

2 - Educational topics:
- Sexual and reproductive health
- Partner violence
- Smoking and drugs avoidance
- Exercise
- Healthy diet and weight control
- Accident prevention (seat belts, bicycle helmets)
- Age-appropriate guidelines for preventive care (visits, vaccines, cancer screening)

3 - Patient information: birth control pills
- How should I take the pills?
- What if I forget to take it?
- When should I use a back-up method?
- What minor side effects should I expect?
- What things should I report to my doctor?

18. Breast Masses

Julie A. Hobart, MD

Synopsis

Patients who present with a breast mass will have a benign process approximately 90% of the time. The differential diagnosis of a breast mass includes a **fibroadenoma *(Definition 1)*, fibrocystic changes *(Definition 2)*,** and malignant tumors. Breast cancer is the most common cancer diagnosed in women, with 1 out of every 8 women developing breast cancer in their lifetime if they live to age 85. Both the history and physical examination will be helpful in distinguishing between benign and malignant conditions.

A targeted personal and family history along with the breast exam will determine whether further evaluation of the breast mass is needed. Some of the most common risk factors include a personal history of cancer, family history in a first-degree relative, and increasing age *(Table 1)*. If a cyst is suspected, fine-needle aspiration can confirm the diagnosis quickly and inexpensively. If a solid mass is more likely, ultrasound, mammogram, or referral for biopsy may be more appropriate interventions.

1 - Fibroadenoma: A benign neoplasm arising from glandular epithelium that is commonly found in breast tissue.

2 - Fibrocystic breast disease: Cystic lesions contained within an area of fibrous tissue. Symptoms of painful, tender breasts that increase around the time of menses are typical of this disease.

Table 1. Incidence of Breast Cancer within 1 Year for Women at a Given Age

Age (Years)	Breast Cancer Incidence
30	1 in 4000
40	1 in 800
50	1 in 400
60	1 in 300
70	1 in 200
80	1 in 200

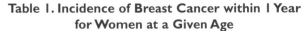

Adapted from Barton MB, Harris R, Fletcher SW: Does this patient have breast cancer? The screening clinical breast examination: Should it be done? How? JAMA 282:1270–1280, 1999.

Table 2. Representative Findings of Women with Breast Lumps

Finding	Likelihood
Fibrocystic changes	40%
No disease	30%
Miscellaneous benign changes	13%
Cancer	10%
Fibroadenoma	7%

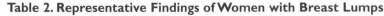

Adapted from Contran RS, Kumar V, Robbins SL, Schoen FJ: Robbins' Pathologic Basis of Disease, 5th ed. Philadelphia, W.B. Saunders, 1994.

1 - These symptoms may indicate malignancy. If these symptoms are present, more urgent evaluation with fine-needle aspiration, mammography, or surgical referral for open biopsy should be considered.

Differential Diagnosis *(Table 2)*

- Cyst
- Fibroadenoma
- Cancer
- Plugged milk duct
- Intraductal papilloma

History

"Tell me about the lump in your breast. What other symptoms are you having?" Keep alert for the following red flags *(Red Flag 1)*:

- Nipple discharge (especially if it is blood-tinged or unilateral) *(Brain 1)*
- Skin changes: retraction or thickening, **p'eau d'orange** *(Definition 3)*
- Lump increasing in size
- Associated constitutional symptoms: weight loss, malaise, and anorexia
- Other important symptoms to review include location, duration, tenderness, and changes with the menstrual cycle. Breast tenderness and masses that occur only with a menstrual cycle are more likely to be related to fibrocystic breast disease and are most likely benign *(Brain 2)*.

"Let's review your past medical history" *(Red Flag 2)*

- Family history of breast cancer. A first-degree relative, mother or sister, with a history of breast cancer can double the patient's risk of a malignant mass.
- Previous history of breast masses and final outcome of evaluation. Some atypical cells on a previous biopsy may increase the patient's risk 4–6 times above normal.
- Recent pregnancy
- Recent or current breast-feeding
- Other medical problems. Any personal history of cancer puts the patient in a higher risk category.
- Caffeine use. Patients who drink larger amounts of caffeine may experience more tenderness of their breasts.

"What are you most concerned about?" (e.g., cancer, surgery, changed physical appearance, ability to breast-feed or have children)

Physical Examination *(Brain 3)*

- General appearance (cachectic, pale, presence of pain)
- Vital signs
- Inspection: sitting with arms at side (note: inspection is not shown to increase diagnostic sensitivity)
- Examination of the skin of the breast for thickening or retractions
- Examination of the nipple for discharge, retraction
- Palpation of the breast: lying with arms at shoulder height *(Brain 4)*, *(Figures 1 and 2)*
- Examination of the axillary and supraclavicular region for lymph nodes

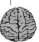

1 - If nipple discharge is present, it is important to ask the patient about color, duration, unilateral or bilateral, spontaneous or with stimulation, and whether or not the patient is currently breast-feeding. Pathologic nipple discharge is defined as bloody, unilateral, or associated with a breast mass. Physiologic discharge is discharge that is only present with compression and is often bilateral.

3 - P'eau d'orange: Skin changes resembling the surface of an orange peel. This is the result of cancerous cells infiltrating and shortening Cooper's ligaments and causing puckering of the skin.

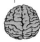

2 - If breast pain is present, cancer is the etiology in < 5%. One study noted that 10–15% of women with benign breast disease had mastalgia and only 2.5–3% of women with breast cancer did.

2 - These questions further assess concern about a malignant lesion. A positive family history in a first-degree relative or a previous history of breast cancer increases the risk of malignancy.

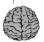

3 - In one study, the HIP trial, the clinical breast exam (CBE) alone was responsible for 45% of all the breast cancer diagnoses.

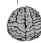

4 - Clinical breast exam key points:
- Recognize breast borders and do a complete exam:
    - Superior: clavicle
    - Medial: midsternum
    - Inferior: Inferior bra line
    - Lateral: Midaxillary line
- Be systematic with pattern of exam: circular vs. lawn mower vs. quadrants.
- The circular or lawn mower techniques are more complete.
- Use finger pads of middle three fingers.
- Vary amounts of pressure: superficial, intermediate and deep.
- A chaperone may be appropriate for this exam.
- Appropriate draping during the exam will keep the patient at ease throughout the exam
- Use an adequate amount of time. Studies have shown an increase in sensitivity with increased duration of the exam suggest 3 minutes per side.

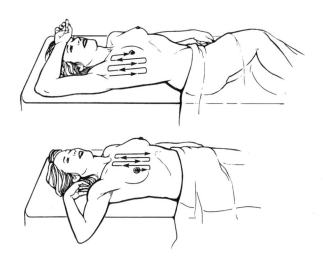

5 - For example, a well-circumscribed 1.5–cm mass is located 2 cm from the nipple at 3 o'clock. It is freely movable and nontender.

Figure 1: Position of patient and direction of palpation for the clinical breast exam. The top figure shows the lateral portion of the breast; the bottom shows the medial portion. Arrows indicate vertical strip pattern of examination.
(From Barton MB, Harris R, Fletcher SW: Does this patient have breast cancer? The screening clinical breast examination: Should it be done? How? JAMA 282:1270–1280, 1999, with permission.)

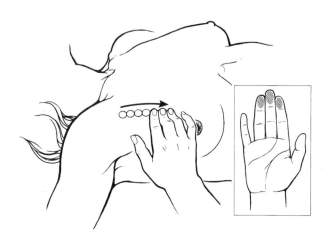

Figure 2: Palpation technique. Pads of the index, third, and fourth fingers (inset) make small circular motions, as if tracing the outer edge of a dime.
(From Barton MB, Harris R, Fletcher SW: Does this patient have breast cancer? The screening clinical breast examination: Should it be done? How? JAMA 282:1270–1280, 1999, with permission.)

Documentation of a breast mass is usually best using the size of the mass, distance from the nipple, and location by times on a clock. Also, notation of the presence of tenderness, firmness, mobility, and shape of the mass should be included *(Brain 5)*. Drawings can also be helpful.

4 - Fine-needle aspiration: A procedure in which a small needle is passed several times through a breast mass in order to obtain a sample of cells or fluid to evaluate.

Testing *(Figure 3)*

Fine-needle aspiration (FNA) *(Definition 4)* of the breast should be considered if the mass is easily palpable and potentially cystic in origin.

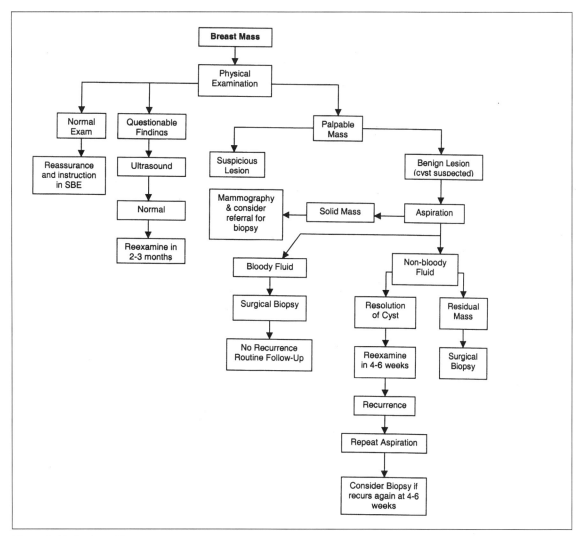

Figure 3: Evaluation of breast masses.

Some recommend sending aspirated fluid for evaluation only when it is bloody. Nonbloody fluid is rarely associated with malignancy, and sending all fluid is not cost-effective. Clinical follow-up in 4–6 weeks should be scheduled for any cyst that has been successfully aspirated.

The triple diagnostic technique of clinical breast exam (CBE), mammography, and FNA can be used to rule out malignancy. If all three modalities favor a benign process, the patient has a 99% chance of having a benign lesion.

Mammography should be considered if the mass is fixed, hard, associated with skin changes or lymphadenopathy, the family history for breast cancer is significant, or the patient is 40 years or older. In some cases, surgical referral may also be appropriate for prompt biopsy and diagnosis *(Brain 6)*.

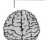

6 - Recently, genetic testing for breast cancer has become available. Only 10–15% of all breast cancer is familial, and only one third of those are associated with the *BRCA 1* or **2** *(Definition 5)* mutations. The cost of this testing is approximately $2600 and could potentially affect the patient's ability to get future insurance policies, so all factors should be considered before ordering such testing.

5 - *BRCA 1* and 2: *BRCA 1* is a gene on chromosome 17 involved in tumor suppression and has a lifetime risk of 55–85% for breast cancer. *BRCA 2* is found on chromosome 13 and also is associated with an increased risk of breast cancer.

Putting It All Together and Management

The majority of patients presenting with a breast mass will have a benign process, but the physician must be alert for those patients at risk

Table 3. Risk Factors for Breast Cancer

- Female gender
- Older age
- Previous history of breast cancer
- Family history for breast cancer in a first-degree relative
- History of a breast lesion with atypical hyperplasia on breast biopsy
- Age > 30 for first pregnancy
- Menarche at younger than age 12
- Menopause after age 50
- Nulliparity
- History of exposure to high-dose radiation
- Obesity
- History of ovarian or endometrial cancer
- Hormone replacement therapy (data are inconclusive but suggest a relative risk of 1.14, which is not significant under greater than 5 years of treatment)
- Ductal or lobular carcinoma in situ (cancer that has not spread beyond that one area)

for malignancy *(Table 3)*. Physical exam can heighten your suspicion if any of the following are present: a fixed hard mass, skin changes, bloody nipple discharge, or lymphadenopathy.

Remember, normal breast tissue sometimes will feel lumpy. Your job as the clinician is to distinguish normal from abnormal lumps. Time and practice will increase your comfort with this examination.

In those masses where the suspicion for malignancy is high, further evaluation with mammography or referral for biopsy would be indicated. If suspicion is lower, ultrasound or needle aspiration would be more appropriate.

In any patient with a breast mass, fear of cancer is likely to be an underlying concern. Acknowledgment of this fear and letting the patient know that you will be investigating this together will reassure the patient and help to establish a trusting relationship.

Selected Readings

1. Barton MB, Harris R, Fletcher SW: Does this patient have breast cancer? The screening clinical breast examination: Should it be done? How? JAMA 282:1270–1280, 1999.
2. Cotran RS, Kumar V, Robbins SL, Schoen FJ: Robbins' Pathologic Basis of Disease, 5th ed. Philadelphia, W.B. Saunders, 1994.
3. Lieu D: Fine needle aspiration: Technique and smear preparation. Am Family Physician 55:839–846, 1997.
4. Morrow M: The evaluation of common breast problems. Am Family Physician 61:2371–2378, 2000.

19. Chest Pain

David V. O'Dell, MD

Synopsis

Chest pain is a common problem. It is important to determine quickly whether the pain is due to a potentially catastrophic process (i.e., myocardial infarction, dissecting aneurysm, or pulmonary embolism) or if the pain is a symptom of a less serious but more common problem. The vast majority of patients presenting to a primary care office with chest pain do not end up having a serious cause. Even patients presenting to the emergency room with chest pain are not likely to have a serious problem. The most important initial step is to determine if the chest pain is immediately life-threatening. A good history is the key to sorting out the etiology of the chest pain, and a targeted physical examination completes the initial evaluation. In some patients, an electrocardiogram (EKG), a chest x-ray, and laboratory tests may provide essential diagnostic information. For patients with classic crushing substernal chest pain who also have an EKG diagnostic for an acute infarction or who are hemodynamically unstable, expeditious management is essential. Establishing the etiology of a patient's chest pain is one the most important challenges faced by health care workers, and when a serious cause cannot be reliably excluded, it is best to err on the side of caution by admitting a patient for further observation and testing.

Differential Diagnosis *(Table 1)*

Conditions that are potentially immediately life-threatening are indicated with an asterisk (*).

Cardiovascular
- Myocardial ischemia (angina, unstable angina, myocardial infarction)*
- Aortic stenosis*
- Hypertrophic cardiomyopathy*
- Severe hypertension*
- Aortic dissection*
- Pericarditis*

Pulmonary
- Pneumothorax*
- Pulmonary emboli*
- Cancer (primary or metastasis)
- Pneumonia
- Bronchitis
- Pleuritis

Gastrointestinal
- Esophageal rupture*
- Esophageal reflux or spasm
- Peptic ulcer disease
- Cholecystitis
- Diaphragmatic inflammation

99

Musculoskeletal/Neuromuscular

• Muscle strain
• Rib fracture
• Costochondritis
• Herpes zoster
• Osteoarthritis of spine

Psychological

• Anxiety
• Depression
• Secondary gain

History *(Red Flag 1)*

"Describe your chest pain." Remember to let the patient tell his or her story but be sure to touch on the following areas:

• Severity of the pain. "On a scale of 1 to 10, with 1 being hardly noticeable and 10 being severe, how severe is your pain?"
• Location. "Where is it? Does it radiate (or go anywhere)?" Ask the patient to point to the site. Consider **pleuritic chest pain (Definition 1)**.
• Characteristic or quality of the pain. "Is it a burning, squeezing, pressure or crushing, vice-like, knife-like, or dull or sharp pain?" *(Brain 1)*
• Duration
   "How long does the pain last?" Try to ascertain seconds, minutes, hours, or days.)
   "When did you first notice the pain?"
   "Have you ever had this type of pain before? (Any previous episodes of chest pain? If so, is it worse?"
• Exacerbating factors. "What brings on the pain? Exertion, emotional stress, lifting, twisting, or deep breathing?" Note **atypical chest pain (Defintion 2)**.
• Alleviating factors. "What makes the pain better?" (e.g., rest, relaxing, antacids, nitroglycerin).
• Associated symptoms. "Do you have fevers, chills, sputum production, cough, sweating, shortness of breath, belching, or sour taste in the throat? Do you have **palpitations (Definition 3)**? If so, when? How fast? Is the heart beat regular or irregular?"

"Tell me about your medical history." Pay particular attention to history of coronary artery disease, chronic obstructive pulmonary disease (COPD), pneumonia, ulcer disease, gastroesophageal reflux disease (GERD), anxiety, recent stressors, and history of trauma.

Other helpful questions:

• "What is the most physically active thing you do, and does it predictably bring on the pain?" If physical activity prompts the pain, **angina (Definition 4)** becomes more likely.
• "What do you think is wrong?" A family member who just had a heart attack last week might prompt a visit.

1 - If the patient is in obvious physical distress or is hemodynamically unstable, *immediate* help should be sought from a more seasoned professional.

1 - Pleuritic chest pain: Pain that is predictably brought on by deep breathing and can often be localized to a specific area (pleurisy, rib fracture, pneumonic process).

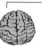

1 - Patients often describe angina as a pressure or discomfort, but deny they have pain.

2 - Atypical chest pain: Chest pain that is not predictably brought on by exertion or does not fit the classic definition of angina.

3 - Palpitations: Abnormal awareness of the heart beating.

4 - Angina: Transient chest pain caused by myocardial ischemia. It is typically substernal in location and may radiate to the left shoulder, jaw, or back. It is exacerbated by physical exertion, cold, and emotional stress. Patients often describe it as a pressure, heaviness, or band-like discomfort, and some patients hesitate to call it a pain. Angina typically lasts from 1 to 20 minutes and is relieved by rest or nitroglycerin.

Unstable angina (USA): Chest pain characteristic of angina occurring at rest (thus, all chest pain occurring at rest is not USA).

Physical Examination *(Table 1)*

Although the physical exam in patients presenting with chest pain is often unremarkable, it may help diagnose or exclude other causes. For example, herpes zoster may be diagnosed by its characteristic rash; a patient with costochondritis will be diagnosed with focal chest wall pain. Particular attention should be paid to the following:

General Status of Patient
- Alert or somnolent?
- Writhing in pain or comfortable?
- Anxious or unconcerned?

Vital Signs
- Temperature
- Pulse
- Blood pressure
- Respiratory rate

Chest *(Red Flag 2)*
- Observe movement. Look for symmetrical movement with respirations, tracheal deviation, labored breathing, signs of trauma, skin lesions, and chest pain change with positions.
- Percuss. Is it dull / hyperresonant?
- Palpate the chest wall. Remember to focus on the area where the patient reports the pain *(Brain 2)*

Cardiovascular
- Heart. Check rate and rhythm (is it regular?). Check for murmurs (particularly new), gallops, and jugular venous distention *(Brain 3).*
- Peripheral pulses? If present, check for equality and upstrokes.
- Peripheral edema? If so, is it unilateral or bilateral?

Lungs
- Check respiratory rate, breath sounds throughout, air movement, and inspiratory-to-expiratory ratio.
- Are there wheezes, rales or crackles, rhonchi, or pleural rubs? If so, where and when (inspiratory or expiratory)?

Abdomen
- Check for distention, tenderness, bowel sounds, organomegaly, signs of trauma, and hematomas.

Testing

If the history or physical exam is diagnostic, additional evaluation may not be necessary. For example, if the patient has classic costochondritis, pleurisy, herpes zoster, or a rib fracture, no specific testing is needed. However, if there is suspicion that the chest pain is of cardiac origin, an EKG should be obtained immediately *(Consultation and Referral 1)*. A chest x-ray, cardiac enzymes (creatine phosphokinase [CPK] with

2 - If the patient has no breath sounds over one side of the chest, has tracheal deviation, or is having significant difficulty breathing, *immediate* help should be sought (pneumothorax).

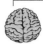
2 - If you are able to reproduce a patient's exact pain with palpation, this finding suggests a chest wall cause (costochondritis, muscle strain, or rib fracture).

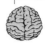
3 - The presence of a fourth heart sound (S_4) during chest pain suggests angina.

1 - Emergent echocardiography or coronary angiography is sometimes necessary to make or exclude a diagnosis of cardiac chest pain.

Table 1. Differential Diagnoses of Chest Pain

Disorders (Not Mutually Exclusive)	Clinical Setting	Location	Characteristic/ Quality	Severity	Timing/ Duration	Exacerbating Factors	Relieving Factors	Associated Symptoms and PE Findings	Diagnostics
Myocardial ischemia: Angina Infarct	Rare in younger patients (<30–35) Hx of CAD or cardiac risk factors*	Substantial, may radiate to the neck, shoulder, arms, back	Pressure, heavy, band-like, weight, ache	Angina: Discomfort (not a pain) Infarct: Severe	Angina: 2–20 min Infarct: Min to hrs	Exertion, cold emotional stress	Angina: Rest, NTG Infarct: NTG, morphine	Dyspnea, nausea, sweating, Anxious PE: S4–sometimes but often normal	EKG Cardiac enzymes: CPK LDH Troponins
Atypical chest pain	Any age	Variable	Often sharp	Mild–severe	Fleeting to hrs	Moving arms twisting	Not correlated with exertion	Palpitations PE: Often unremarkable	Negative EKG and cardiac enzymes
GERD Esophageal spasm	Follows large meals/ alcohol use	Retrosternal Epigastrium Sternal notch	Burning, squeezing	Mild–severe	Variable	Swallowing	Antacids, Sometimes belching	Dysphagia Belching PE: Normal	Negative cardiac studies
Bronchitis Pneumonia	Coryza, cough, fevers, sputum	Middle of chest	Burning irritation	Mild	Persistent	Coughing cold air	Sometimes humidified air	Respiratory illness PE: Rhonchi or crackles	Infiltrates on CXR
Chest wall pain	Hx of trauma, viral infection	Variable	Knife-like	Variable	Variable	Twisting, bending	Stationary posture	PE: Reproduction of pain with palpation	
Anxiety	Variable (anxious patient)	Middle of chest/ variable	Stabbing, aching, dull	Variable	Fleeting to continuous	Emotional stress	Decrease stress exercise	Palpitations at rest, anxiety PE: Unremarkable but anxious	Negative evaluation
Pericarditis	Often follows viral illness	Precordial, may radiate to back	Sharp, knife-like	Mild–severe	Variable	Position changes coughing	Sitting up	PE: Pericardial friction rub	Characteristic EKG ESR
Dissecting aortic aneurysum	Older patients often with hx of CAD or cardiac risk factors*	Precordial radiation to back or abdomen	Tearing, ripping	Severe	Persistent			PE: hemi/paraplegia, syncope, loss of femoral pulses or unequal arm/leg pulses, murmur of aortic regurgitation	Widened mediastinum on CXR Diagnostic chest/abdomen CT

PE = physical examination, Hx = history, CAD = coronary artery disease, NTG = nitroglycerin, EKG = electrocardiogram, CPK = creatine phosphokinase, LDH = lactate dehydrogenase, GERD = gastroesophageal reflux disease, ESR = erythrocyte sedimentation rate, CXR = chest x-ray, CT = computed tomography

*Cardiac risk factors include smoking, hypertension, diabetes, hypercholesterolemia, positive family history.

Adapted from Bates B: A Guide to Physical Examination and History Taking. Philadelphia, JB Lippincott, 1991.

isoenzymes, troponin T or I, lactate dehydrogenase [LDH]) **(Brain 4)**, complete blood count (CBC), and oxygen (O_2) saturation measure can be very helpful. The chest x-ray (infiltrates, effusions, cardiomegaly, widened mediastinum, pneumothorax), CBC (e.g., leukemoid reaction, left shift, anemia), and O_2 saturation (hypoxia) are more likely to be helpful in noncardiac cases. If there is still significant concern that the chest pain is cardiac related, the standard course of action is to admit the patient to a telemetry unit and obtain serial cardiac enzymes and EKGs. At least 8–12 hours of observation and serial enzymes are necessary to rule out myocardial damage. If there is no damage, patients often will undergo a functional cardiac test (treadmills, echocardiograms, or nuclear studies) to exclude ischemic myocardium as the cause of the pain. Use Table 1 to correlate the patient's history, physical findings, and laboratory results, and point to a likely diagnosis.

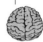

4 - Cardiac enzymes are markers for ischemic injury. The enzymes leak out when a cell is damaged or dies and are therefore unlikely to be elevated (positive) when drawn immediately after the onset of chest pain. Repeating the enzymes 6–12 hours after the initial measurement is critical to determine if damage has occurred.

Putting It All Together

The majority of patients presenting with chest pain to a primary care clinic will not have a serious condition. The history is key and often suggests an underlying problem. The physical may be diagnostic but, on the other hand, may be entirely normal in the patient with significant cardiac ischemia. Older patients and patients with a history of heart disease need to be evaluated much more cautiously.

Management

The initial evaluation is geared to exclude serious causes, and once this task is accomplished, management should be directed at the presumed cause **(Brain 5)**. If there is a high degree of suspicion for cardiac disease, patients should be started on aspirin (barring a contraindication) and a beta-blocker and then admitted for observation. If the initial evaluation excludes a cardiac etiology and the patient is thought to have GERD, a therapeutic trial of acid suppression with either a histamine$_2$ blocker (e.g., cimetidine, ranitidine) or a proton pump inhibitor (omerprazole, lansoprazole) is reasonable. If the patient has chest wall pain, nonsteroidal anti-inflammatory drugs (e.g., ibuprofen, naproxen) can be helpful. If the patient has pneumonia or bronchitis, a beta-agonist inhaler (albuterol) and appropriate antibiotics are indicated. If the etiology of the pain remains elusive, consider referring the patient for further evaluation **(Treatment 1)**.

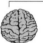

5 - A therapeutic trial of nitroglycerin that relieves the discomfort is strongly suggestive of angina but can also relieve pain caused by esophageal spasm. A therapeutic trial of antacids that relieves the pain suggests GERD.

1 - For patients with angina, nitroglycerin often relieves the discomfort, and, if the pain persists, aspirin, beta-blockers, and heparin can be useful. Unstable angina requires hospitalization and similar medications. Thrombolytic therapy is reserved for patients with an EKG diagnostic of a myocardial infarction.

Selected Readings

1. Barker LR, Burton JR, Zieve PD: Ambulatory Medicine. Baltimore, Williams & Wilkins, 1995.
2. Bates B: A Guide to Physical Examination and History Taking. Philadelphia, JB Lippincott, 1991.
3. Kuntz KR, Fleischmann KE, Hunink MG: Cost-effectiveness of diagnostic strategies for patients with chest pain. Ann Intern Med 130:709–718, 1999.
4. Noble J: Primary Care Medicine. St. Louis, Mosby, 1996.

20. Child Abuse and Neglect

Michael J. Moran, MD

Synopsis

Child abuse is one of the more frequent diagnoses one will encounter in primary care medicine *(Red Flag 1)*. Child maltreatment is divided into four categories: **physical abuse, sexual abuse, emotional** or **psychological abuse,** and **neglect** *(Definition 1)*. Emotional or psychological abuse is most often seen as coincident with other types of abuse. The differential diagnosis is quite extensive and depends on the type of abuse incurred. This is one area where a thorough history and physical examination must be done. If child abuse is suspected, some limited diagnostic testing may be necessary. Management of child abuse involves treatment of the injury or condition and reporting the abuse to proper law enforcement authorities for investigation. Physicians must be on the lookout for signs and symptoms of child abuse and be willing to make this diagnosis. When the diagnosis is missed, children are at significant risk of returning with more serious injury or death.

1 - In 1998, there were 2 million reports of child abuse in the United States involving 3 million children. Nine hundred thousand were substantiated; 1087 deaths were reported in forty-nine states. The majority of deaths were under age 3.

1 - Physical abuse: The infliction of physical injury as a result of punching, beating, kicking, biting, burning, shaking, or otherwise harming a child.

Sexual abuse: Includes fondling a child's genitals, intercourse, incest, rape, sodomy, exhibitionism, and commercial exploitation through prostitution or the production of pornographic materials.

Emotional or psychological abuse: Acts or omissions by the parents or other caregivers that have caused, or could cause, serious behavioral, cognitive, emotional, or mental disorders in a child. Examples include confinement to a closet, habitual scapegoating, belittling, and rejecting treatment.

Child neglect: Failure to provide for the child's basic needs. Neglect can be physical, educational, or emotional.

Differential Diagnosis

Physical Abuse

Skin Conditions
- Accidental injury
- Bleeding disorders
- Birthmarks
- Connective tissue disorders

Fractures
- Accidental
- Congenital disorders
- Infectious

Sexual Abuse

- Congenital conditions
- Accidental trauma
- Infectious diseases
- Behavioral problems

Child Neglect

- Failure to thrive (see Chapter 32)
- Delay in care

History

An abused child may present with any constellation of symptoms, including severe life-threatening injuries and death. Initial management is to provide emergency care, but as soon as possible, a thorough history needs to be taken *(Brain 1)*. One of the frequent indicators of child abuse is an account of the incident that does not match the injury to the child. If there is more than one parent or caretaker, they should be interviewed separately for a detailed history of the injury to see if there are consistencies or discrepancies in their stories *(Brain 2)*.

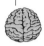

1 - Interview of the child should be without parents present if he or she is able to answer questions.

"Tell me about the injury."

- "How, when, and where did the injury occur?" These questions give the basis for the injury and which physical findings can be seen as compatible or not compatible with the injury.
- "Who witnessed the injury?" If witnessed by more than one person this adds credibility. If not, the sole witness may be the perpetrator.
- "When did symptoms occur? Immediately or delayed?" Often there is a delay in seeking medical care when abuse occurs. Also, injuries are sometimes attributed to a remote minor injury.
- "Is there a history of previous injuries?"

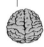

2 - Risk Factors
- National rate of child victimization: 13.9/1000 children
- Child in poverty 22 times more likely to suffer abuse
- Boys are more likely to be seriously hurt
- Girls are three times more likely to suffer sexual abuse
- 75% of perpetrators are parents and 10% are relatives
- Child risk factors—prematurity, twins, chronic illness, slow development, retardation, hyperactivity, perceived as different, previous injuries.
- Abuser risk factors—unwanted or unplanned pregnancy, single parent, youth, closely spaced children, abused as a child, stress, substance abuse, domestic violence, isolation, poor parenting skills, illness, and emotional disturbance.

"Tell me about your child."

- "How was the pregnancy? Was the pregnancy planned?"
- "Has he been sick recently? Does he have a chronic illness?" Added stress on the family may lead to abuse, but the illness needs to be ruled out as the cause of problem.
- "Is the child on any medicines?" Side effects can cause bruising or symptoms.
- "Is he a fussy baby? What do you do to comfort him?" (Often, abused children are described as fussy and hard to comfort.)
- "Has the child been growing normally?" Failure to thrive is a symptom of neglect.
- "What are the child's developmental capabilities?" Could the child be capable of being injured this way?
- "Does the child have all his immunizations?" (possible neglect issue)
- "Is the child toilet trained?" A high percentage of physical abuse occurs around toilet training and diaper changing.
- "Does the child have any behavior problems? Is he a discipline problem?" Determine if the parents feel they need to discipline this child more or if he is viewed as being "different".

"Tell me about your family."

- "Any history of members of parents' families having trouble with bleeding or bruising?" Rule out coagulation problems.
- "Is there anyone in the extended family who has a history of a large number of bone breaks or easily breaks bones?" Consider **osteogenesis imperfecta** *(Definition 2)*.
- "Any history of infants born with abnormalities in the extended family?"
- "Any sibling had a previous serious injury?"
- "Who lives in the home?"
- "Do parents work?" Try to get a sense of economic ability of the family and the level of stress.
- "Do parents generally agree on parenting issues and discipline?"
- "How is baby-sitting handled? Do parents share or is there an outside source?" This can be a measure of stress on the family.
- "Has anyone in the home been hit, kicked, or punched?" Reveal any domestic violence.

2 - **Osteogenesis imperfecta:** A disorder of bone growth that causes fragile bones and easy breakage.

Questions specific to child sexual abuse

- What are the allegations?
- If the child is verbal, a history should be obtained in a separate interview with the child. Try to determine:

    Does child know difference between truth and lie? (age related)

    When did it occur?

    What occurred and who did it?

    How often did this occur?

    Was pain or bleeding associated with the incident? (significant for trauma)

    Was someone told about the incident? Was the child told to keep a secret?

Physical Examination

The physical exam must be done in a thorough and stepwise fashion. The exam must be comprehensive to document areas of injury or abuse and also to rule out any other cause of the child's illness or injury. All parts of the exam must be documented carefully and described in the narrative. Adjuncts to the written record are photographs and drawings or diagrams. These should be used whenever possible. The physical examination gives documentation of the injuries that have occurred and possible description of the mechanism of action of the injury.

- **General appearance:** Is the child obtunded? Is she able to answer questions? Does she appear afraid, in pain, happy, sad? How is the interaction between parent and child? Are the child's actions and demeanor appropriate for age? Does the child appear emaciated?
- **Vital signs:** Are they stable or do they need immediate attention? Height, weight, and head circumference should be plotted on growth curves because they are important to rule out nutritional deprivation.
- **Head, eyes, ears, nose, mouth, and throat (HEENT):** Are there bruises, swollen areas, bruises or tears on the inner lips, loose teeth? A funduscopic exam with pupil dilatation should always be done to rule out retinal hemorrhages.
- **Chest:** Is there pain on palpation or with movement? Is there difficulty with breathing? Consider fractured ribs.
- **Heart:** Are there signs of shock, poor perfusion, increased pulse, or thready pulse? Look for shock secondary to blood loss or brain injury.
- **Abdomen:** Is the exam painful? Is there guarding? Is there distention? Are bowel sounds present? Check for inter-abdominal injury and bleeding)
- **Genitalia:** Is there bruising or bite marks? (This area is often abused when sexual abuse occurs or when there is anger related to toilet training) *(Brain 3)*.
- **Extremities:** Is there painful motion? Is there swelling or bruising? Is patient using all extremities? Is she favoring an arm? Does she have a limp? (These are all signs of injury to extremities.)
- **Neurologic:** Is the child alert, arousable, unresponsive? (brain injury). Does the child have seizures as presenting symptom? (brain injury or not taking seizure medications)
- **Skin:** Are there bruises? What size are they? What color? What shape are they? Where are the bruises? Are there any burns? *(Brain 4)*. Is there a rash? (possible sign of neglect)

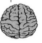

3 - Girls should always have a colposcopic exam with video capability done when there is concern about sexual abuse.

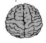

4 - Children commonly get bruised but usually only in very specific areas, such as forehead, bony prominences of arms, lower legs, or back.

Testing

The use of laboratory testing and x-ray needs to be individualized based on the presentation of the child and the differential diagnosis considered. A thorough history and physical exam will reduce the amount of testing needed.

If bleeding or bruising is present, consider:

- Complete blood count (CBC) with platelets
- Partial thromboplastin time (PTT) and prothrombin time (PT)
- Bleeding time

If serious injuries or fractures, consider:

- Skeletal survey *(Brain 5)*
- Thorough exam for possible osteogenesis imperfecta and lab testing if needed

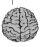

5 - A skeletal survey is done to identify any old fractures or other recent fractures. Fractures of various ages are a significant sign of possible child abuse. Skeletal surveys are done only for children less than three years old.

If concerned about internal injury (i.e., brain or abdomen), consider:

- Computed tomography (CT) scan
- Magnetic resonance imaging (MRI)

If concerned about sexual abuse, consider:

- Vaginal cultures
- Rape kit *(Brain 6)*

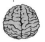

6 - A rape kit contains all that is necessary to send to law enforcement and/or the lab for evaluation of an acute sexual assault.

Putting It All Together

Child abuse is more common than previously believed, and one must be aware of its signs and symptoms. To make the diagnosis of child abuse, the physician must always have an index of suspicion. The physician must also be aware that serious injury is not caused by a trivial action. Child abuse is a broad category, and often more than one type of abuse is seen.

The history and physical are extremely important in the evaluation. The history gives us a clear picture of what happened in the usual accidental injury. In child abuse, the history is often inconsistent with the physical exam. The physical exam tells us the extent of the injury, but also, in case of bruising, may provide some information about the timing of the injury. Laboratory testing and x-rays finish the picture and allow us to put it all together in a diagnosis. If child abuse is the diagnosis, appropriate evaluation to rule out other possible diagnoses must be done. This is to ensure that the diagnosis is as certain as possible because of the long-term implications of this diagnosis. Documentation of findings is an absolute must when dealing with child abuse. The history and physical exam records must be thorough and legible. Photographic documentation should be used whenever possible to back up the narrative description. The physician may be involved in court proceedings and will find it easier when observations have been recorded in an objective manner.

Management

Management of the child who has suffered inflicted injuries is twofold. Initial care focuses on the child's medical condition. The actual treatment of the injury due to child abuse is the same as if it had been accidental. If the child had a fracture or burns or bruises, these are all treated per protocols presented elsewhere in this book.

To ensure long-term success of the care, one must ensure that the child will be safe from injury in the future. To do this, law enforcement and social services need to be involved in the patient's care *(Brain 7)*. Law enforcement officials look for evidence of a crime, and the department of social services evaluates the home for the safety of the child or of other children present in the home. The physician provides valuable information to law enforcement in the form of the history and physical exam and whether the injury is consistent with the history given.

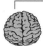

7 - It is mandatory in all 50 states that anyone who cares for children must report anything that is suspicious of child abuse. The physician does not need to prove abuse, only to be suspicious of it.

The primary care physician must provide for the immediate medical management of the child and the child's long-term care. The long-term care would involve advocacy for the child and treatment of any sequelae of the initial injury. This would also involve coordinating care with social service personnel for proper evaluation and treatment of future needs of the child. It is likely that the child will need some type of counseling in the future. Many children who have been abused show evidence of post-traumatic stress disorder, attachment disorder, and a variety of behavioral disorders. The child and caretakers will benefit from long-term therapy for these problems.

Prognosis in child abuse is guarded. If it is properly diagnosed, and appropriate intervention by the courts and social services occurs, the child's future can be improved. If the diagnosis is missed, the risk of greater injury is high.

Selected Readings

1. Behrman RE, Kliegman R (eds): Nelson Textbook of Pediatrics, 15th ed. Philadelphia, W.B. Saunders, 1996.
2. Briere J, Berliner L, Bulkly J, et al: The APSAC Handbook on Child Maltreatment. Thousand Oaks, CA, Sage Publications, 2001.
3. Reece R: Child Abuse: Medical Diagnosis and Management. Philadelphia, Lea & Febiger, 2000.

Informational Web Sites

American Professional Society on Abuse of Children (APSAC): http://www.apsac.org.

National Clearinghouse on Child Abuse and Neglect Information: http://www.calib.com/nccanch/.

21. Chronic Obstructive Pulmonary Disease

Debra J. Romberger, MD

Synopsis

Chronic obstructive pulmonary disease (COPD) is characterized by the presence of **emphysema** or **chronic bronchitis** *(Definition 1)*. It is defined by the presence of **airflow obstruction** *(Definition 2)*. The airflow obstruction of COPD can be accompanied by **airway hyperreactivity** (such as seen in asthma) and may be partially reversible. Emphysema and chronic bronchitis have unique descriptions, but any one patient may have components of both processes. Patients with COPD experience slowly progressive loss of lung function, which is measured by pulmonary function tests (PFTs) *(Brain 1)* (see Chapter 70). Patients typically complain of shortness of breath with exertion, cough, and sputum production. Physical examination may demonstrate decreased air movement in the lungs or coarse rhonchi, with or without wheezing. Cigarette smoking is a major cause of COPD, and smoking cessation is key to reducing the rate of the lung function decline. Medications are available to ease symptoms, but they do not completely reverse COPD once it occurs. Prevention of pulmonary infections through the use of influenza and pneumococcal vaccines is important in limiting further damage to the lungs. Oxygen therapy improves survival in patients with documented hypoxemia.

1 - Emphysema: Destruction of alveolar air spaces in the lung.

Chronic bronchitis: A clinical condition characterized by chronic cough and sputum production occurring on most days for at least 3 months in a year for at least 2 successive years.

2 - Airflow obstruction: A reduction or limitation in the ability to exhale gas from the lungs. This may occur because bronchial tubes have increased mucus blocking bronchioles or bronchi. Edema of bronchial walls, which occurs in inflammation, may also cause airflow obstruction. Destruction of the lung tissue tethering open small airways can also lead to airflow obstruction.

Airway hyperreactivity: Spasm of bronchial smooth muscle that causes constriction of bronchial tubes and, thus, airflow obstruction.

Differential Diagnosis

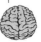

1 - Airflow obstruction is measured by PFT using a spirometer. It is performed by taking a deep breath in and exhaling as much air as possible quickly. Airflow obstruction is present if the FEV_1 (forced expiratory volume of air in first 1 second of exhalation) is reduced in comparison to the FVC (forced vital capacity or total volume of air exhaled in the manuever). In other words, the amount of air that is exhaled in the first second of the forced exhalation manuever is reduced because of the presence of obstruction to airflow. If the FEV_1/FVC ratio is less than 75%, airflow obstruction is likely present. The percent (%) of predicted value for FEV_1 is used in staging COPD:
Stage I: $FEV_1 > 50\%$ (of predicted value)
Stage II: $FEV_1 > 35–49\%$ (of predicted value)
Stage III: $FEV_1 < 35\%$ (of predicted value)

- **Asthma.** Asthma is characterized by inflammation and airflow obstruction that has a significant reversible component, reversing either spontaneously or with treatment.
- **Congestive heart failure (CHF).** Patients with CHF may experience dyspnea on exertion but do not usually have significant airflow obstruction on PFTs. Patients occasionally may experience wheezing.
- **Cystic fibrosis (CF).** Although most patients with CF are diagnosed as children, some patients are not diagnosed until young adulthood.
- **Primary pulmonary hypertension (PPH).** Patients present with dyspnea on exertion. However, patients with PPH are more likely to be women in their 30s or 40s who do not have airflow obstruction on pulmonary function testing.
- **Recurrent pulmonary emboli.** Patients experience shortness of breath but should not have significant airflow obstruction on PFTs.
- **Idiopathic pulmonary fibrosis.** This condition tends to occur in patients as they age and is characterized by dyspnea. The PFTs show restriction and not obstruction.
- **Physical deconditioning.** People who are very sedentary may experience shortness of breath with exertion due to respiratory muscle weakness.

History

"Tell me about your breathing problems. What type of symptoms are you experiencing?" Determine the following:

- Sudden onset of shortness of breath versus slowly developing **(Red Flag 1)**
- Examples of activities that cause shortness of breath (helps assess severity of condition and gives insight into physical routine of patient)
- Cough with or without sputum production (defines chronic bronchitis)
- Associated symptoms such as chest pain or hemoptysis **(Red Flag 2)**

"Are you a smoker or have you smoked in the past?" (Review smoking status on follow-up visits with COPD patients.)

- Approximate the amount of smoking (how many packs per day for how many years)
- Has the patient ever been able to stop smoking and for how long?
- What tools, if any, has the patient used to help stop smoking in the past (e.g., nicotine gum or patch, other medications, or behavior techniques such as hypnosis)?

"Have you had problems with your lungs before, in childhood or as an adult?"

- Patients with repeated chest infections as children, especially if untreated, may have damage to airways, which leads to chronic bronchitis.
- Frequent episodes of acute bronchitis as an adult also leads to chronic airway injury.
- " Do other persons in your family have lung disease?" **(Brain 2)**

"What type of work have you done? How do you like to spend your free time? "

- Persons who have worked (or played) in certain environments may be at risk for a variety of lung diseases, including occupational asthma, hypersensitivity lung disease, and chronic bronchitis.
- Examples of exposures associated with lung diseases include dusts (grain dust, livestock confinement facilities), silica, birds (feathers and droppings), asbestos, and some chemicals.

" Are you taking any medicines now? Any drug allergies?" (Review type and frequency of use of all medications) **(Red Flag 3)**.

Physical Examination

Look (Inspection)

Does the patient look as though he or she is short of breath?

- Rapid breathing
- Use of accessory muscles (retraction of lower intercostal interspaces and supraclavicular fossae during inspiration)
- Pursed lip breathing
- Difficulty completing sentences when talking

1 - Sudden onset of shortness of breath is more likely associated with an acute condition such as pulmonary embolus or acute infection, which may be life-threatening. COPD tends to be a slowly progressive condition.

2 - Chest pain can be a sign of either cardiac or pulmonary disease, including angina, pulmonary embolus, pleurisy, and pneumonia. The most common cause of hemoptysis (coughing up blood) in the United States is bronchitis. However, tuberculosis is the most common cause worldwide. Hemoptysis can be seen with other conditions, including lung cancer.

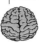

2 - There are genetic forms of emphysema. The most important one is alpha1-antitrypsin deficiency. This should be considered especially in persons with early onset of COPD (in their 30s–40s), even if they are smokers. It should also be considered in all patients with COPD who have been non-smokers and in patients with a strong family history of emphysema.

3 - Angiotensin-converting enzyme (ACE) inhibitors are a category of drugs associated with cough and commonly used for hypertension. Beta-adrenergic blockers are recommended for some patients with heart disease and can cause increased wheezing and shortness of breath in some patients with COPD or asthma.

What is the patient's general physical condition? *(Brain 3)*

- Frail and deconditioned or obese?
- Any difficulty moving from chair to exam table?
- Is there cyanosis of mucous membranes or nail beds?
- Is peripheral edema present? (This may occur with complications of COPD such as right-sided heart failure.)
- What is shape of patient's chest? (Patients with emphysema trap air in their lungs, and the chest may appear barrel-shaped on exam.)

Listen (Auscultation)

- Patients with significant airflow obstruction may have reduced movement of air. Breath sounds may be reduced throughout all lung fields and seem to be nearly absent.
- Other lung sounds that may be heard include:
  Rhonchi, a snoring sound
  Wheezing, a hissing or musical sound, commonly heard on expiration
  Crackles (sometimes called *rales*) and broadly classified as coarse (more suggestive of COPD and congestive heart failure) vs. fine (Velcro sound, suggesting interstitial lung disease)
  Cardiac sounds may be muted in COPD because of air trapping within the lungs

Testing

COPD is defined by the presence of airflow obstruction, which is measured by PFT using a spirometer. Thus, a diagnosis of COPD should not be given unless spirometry has been performed *(see Brain 1)*. If the presence of significant airflow obstruction is unclear with spirometry alone, measurement of **lung volumes** and **diffusion capacity** may be of benefit *(Definition 3)*. Lung volumes better assess whether any restriction of the lungs that is present occurs in other pulmonary diseases, such as interstitial lung diseases. In COPD, lung volumes may show air trapping with an increase in the residual volume (RV) of air present in the lungs. Diffusion capacity assesses the ability of gases to cross the air-capillary barrier in the lung and may be reduced in a variety of diseases, including interstitial lung diseases, recurrent pulmonary emboli, and emphysema.

Reduced oxygen level in the blood (hypoxemia) occurs as COPD progresses. In patients with an FEV_1 of 35–49% of predicted, an arterial blood gas is recommended to look for reduced oxygen level (pO_2) and elevation in carbon dioxide (pCO_2). Oximeters measure oxygen saturation (SaO_2) as opposed to pO_2 and can also be used to follow oxygen status. Patients with chronic hypoxemia are at risk to develop secondary polycythemia; a hematocrit is used to evaluate this condition.

A chest radiograph may show evidence of COPD, although it is not a sensitive test for this disease process. Hyperinflation of the lungs with flattened diaphragms and an increased retrosternal airspace may be seen on a chest x-ray in a patient with emphysema. Patients with chronic bronchitis tend to have increased markings on chest x-ray, which correlates to airways that are thickened from chronic irritation. Chest x-rays are helpful in looking for the presence of other disease processes such as CHF, pulmonary fibrosis, or tumors.

3 - Patients with emphysema are classically described as "pink puffers," whereas patients with chronic bronchitis are known as "blue bloaters." The mechanisms that account for these changes are not completely understood. "Pink puffers" are often very thin and do not appear cyanotic. "Blue bloaters" are often overweight and appear cyanotic in their nailbeds and mucous membranes.

3 - Lung volumes: The actual volumes of different compartments within the lungs (lung volumes) can be measured using specialized equipment. These compartments include total lung capacity (TLC), which is the total volume of air in the lungs at full inspiration, and residual volume (RV), the volume of air left in the lungs after emptying the lungs as much as possible with forced expiration. Both of these values may be increased in emphysema.

Diffusion capacity: A measurement of how well oxygen can diffuse across the alveolar epithelium into pulmonary capillaries within the alveolar space. It is actually measured by using small quantities of carbon monoxide. Because of the destruction of alveolar tissue in emphysema, the diffusion capacity may be significantly reduced.

Putting It All Together

Patients with COPD often present after 50 years of age, with progressive shortness of breath with activity and, possibly, chronic cough. They often attribute their symptoms to aging and may not seek medical attention until the dyspnea is severe enough to interfere with their activities of daily living. In addition, patients with COPD typically become much more symptomatic when they develop an acute respiratory tract infection (viral or bacterial) and often seek medical attention at that point. Spirometry is essential in making the diagnosis of COPD and can be done by a hand-held device in the office. Patients with asthma will also show airflow obstruction with spirometry during an asthma attack. However, their airflow obstruction usually improves significantly with asthma treatment. Some patients with COPD also have a component of asthma and will demonstrate partial, but not complete, improvement in airflow obstruction with the same medications.

Patients with cardiac disease, especially CHF, may also present with dyspnea on exertion. Physical examination findings of CHF, such as bibasilar rales on lung exam or an S_3 on cardiac exam, and chest x-ray changes of interstitial edema may help distinguish these patients from those with COPD.

Smoking is clearly the most important risk factor for COPD. However, only about 15% of smokers will develop significant COPD. There is currently no good marker to identify which smokers will progress to COPD. Yearly spirometry is useful to assess how much lung function patients who continue to smoke are losing and can identify patients who are most susceptible to the damaging effects of smoke. Loss of lung function is slowed by smoking cessation, and ex-smokers lose function at nearly the same rate as persons who never smoked.

Management

Smoking cessation is critical for patients diagnosed with COPD because this is the only therapy that will reduce their continued loss of lung function. Inhaled bronchodilators (both selective beta$_2$-adrenergic agonists and ipratropium bromide) typically provide improvement in symptoms, but education of proper technique for inhaler use is important to maximize usefulness of these medications. Oral bronchodilators such as theophylline may be helpful for some patients, but do have a higher incidence of side effects (nausea, nervousness). The role of drugs, such as inhaled glucocorticoids (steroids), to reduce airway inflammation of COPD continues to be defined. There is a clear role for systemic steroids in acute exacerbations of COPD. The benefit of chronic use of oral steroids is unclear for most patients and must be weighed against the side effects of the medication. Prevention of recurrent respiratory tract infections is important to reduce further lung damage; yearly influenza vaccination and pneumococcal vaccination every 5–6 years are recommended.

COPD in patients who develop hypoxemia (currently defined as pO$_2$ ≤ 55 or SaO$_2$ ≤ 88% while breathing room air) is associated with substantial morbidity and mortality that can be improved with the use of oxygen therapy at home. Patient survival is better if they wear the oxygen mask

24 hours per day. In addition, many patients with COPD lose skeletal muscle mass and strength, including respiratory muscles, because of the inactivity caused by dyspnea. In pulmonary rehabilitation programs, with proper instruction and the use of oxygen as needed, many patients with COPD experience improved exercise capacity and quality of life, despite no significant change in lung function. The education about lung disease and the social interactions that occur in rehabilitation may contribute to enhanced quality of life as well. Furthermore, a small number of patients with COPD may be candidates for single lung transplantation *(Consultation and Referral 1)*.

1 - Patients with significant COPD (stage II and stage III) who are not responding to therapy may benefit from consultation with a pulmonary specialist.

Selected Readings

1. American Thoracic Society: Standards for the diagnosis and care of patients with chronic obstructive pulmonary disease. Am J Respir Crit Care Med 152:S77–S120, 1995.
2. Ball P: Epidemiology and treatment of chronic bronchitis and its exacerbations. Chest 108:43S–52S, 1995.
3. Clinical reprint series: Chronic obstructive pulmonary disease. J Respir Dis 1:R1–R40, 1996.
4. Nocturnal Oxygen Therapy Trial Group: Continuous or nocturnal oxygen therapy in hypoxemic chronic obstructive lung disease. Ann Intern Med 93:391–398, 1980.

22. Congestive Heart Failure

David V. O'Dell, MD

Synopsis

Congestive heart failure (CHF) is the clinical diagnosis given to patients who present with evidence that the heart is unable to meet the metabolic needs of the body. Most often this deficiency is due to poor left ventricular function, but there are many causes. The clinical presentation can vary from minimal symptoms (mild dyspnea on exertion, ankle edema, orthopnea) to life-threatening pulmonary edema. Initial management is geared at stabilizing the patient and relieving symptoms. Once this is accomplished, a diligent search should be undertaken to determine both the underlying cause and the precipitating cause of the CHF. An echocardiogram is the key component of this evaluation. For patients with stable heart failure, therapy is geared toward maintaining cardiac function and being ever vigilant for signs of worsening heart failure.

Background Terminology (Table 1)

Clinicians divide heart failure into various categories. Although these categories are not specific diagnoses, they are clinically useful, particularly early in the patient's course, and can help point to the underlying etiology of the CHF. *Left-sided* and *right-sided HF* are used to describe a patient's symptoms, and *systolic* and *diastolic HF* are used to refer to the underlying function of the heart. As patients with CHF progress, these forms often blur together and the terms become less helpful; hence, the common clinical adage: the most common cause of right-sided HF is left-sided HF.

- *Left-sided HF* refers to patients who primarily have signs of pulmonary congestion (dyspnea, orthopnea, PND) and is commonly associated with compromised left ventricular function (after an infarct or with an underlying **cardiomyopathy *[Definition 1]*** or an overloaded left ventricle (severe aortic stenosis or systemic hypertension).
- *Right-sided HF* refers to patients primarily with venous distention (peripheral edema, jugular venous distention [JVD], distended liver) and is commonly caused by pulmonary hypertension or a right ventricular infarct.
- The term *systolic HF* is used when the heart is unable to pump (decreased ejection fraction) an adequate amount of blood forward (dilated cardiomyopathies).
- The term *diastolic HF* is used when the primary problem is that the left ventricle is unable to relax and thus impairs filling of the ventricle (restricted ventricular filling) *(Brain 1).*

1 - Cardiomyopathy: A disease of the myocardium. Most often this term is used to refer to a disorder that impairs the ability of the heart muscle to contract normally.

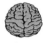

1 - Patients with diastolic HF typically have preserved left ventricular ejection fractions and are usually asymptomatic at rest but become symptomatic with exertion.

When the CHF is due to left ventricular dysfunction, the ventricle begins to dilate, setting in motion a complex cascade of events that lead to increased vascular resistance and salt and fluid retention. Initially, the

Table 1. Common Terms Used in CHF Patients

Term	Definition
Dyspnea	Difficulty breathing including an abnormal awareness of breathing or unexpected shortness of breath
Orthopnea	Dyspnea or shortness of breath on reclining (2, and 3-pillow orthopnea refers to the elevation necessary to relieve the dyspnea)
Paroxysmal nocturnal dyspnea (PND)	Awakening suddenly (often 2–3 hours after retiring) from severe orthopnea that is characteristically improved with sitting upright
Dyspnea on exertion (DOE)	Difficulty breathing after minimal exertion
Nocturia	Necessity to get up at night to urinate
Edema	Excessive accumulation of fluid in tissues, commonly seen about the ankles
Dependent edema	Edema in the lowest portion of the body (ankles if upright, back and buttocks if supine) as influenced by gravity
Pitting edema	Edema that retains a dent after pushing on it with a finger

heart is able to compensate as predicted by Frank-Starling curve, and the amount of blood ejected remains relatively constant *(Figure 1)*. Ultimately, however, without intervention the myocardium stretches until it decompensates, resulting in pulmonary edema *(Brain 2)*.

The degree of disability a patient suffers is commonly quantified by the New York Heart Association Scale. This classification has important prognostic implications *(Table 2)*.

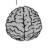

2 - The Frank-Starling curve is the result of plotting the cardiac output as a function of left ventricular end diastolic pressure. Normal ventricular muscle responds differently than that of patients with chronic CHF (see Figure 1).

Table 2. New York Heart Association Classification for Cardiac Patients

Grade	Description
I	No functional limitation of physical activity
II	Dyspnea or chest pain with moderate activity
III	Dyspnea or chest pain with minimal activity
IV	Dyspnea or chest pain at rest

Differential Diagnosis

Volume-overloaded Conditions
(e.g., peripheral swelling or edema, ascites)

- Renal failure
- Liver failure with cirrhosis
- Nephrotic syndrome (proteinuria, hypoalbuminemia, and hyperlipidemia)
- Venous insufficiency

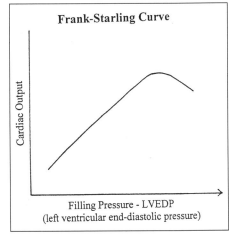

Figure 1: Frank-Starling curve.

Other Common Causes of Dyspnea

- Pneumonia
- Chronic obstructive pulmonary disease (COPD)
- Reversible ischemic heart disease
- Pulmonary embolism
- Restrictive pulmonary conditions
  (scarring that decreases lung volumes, e.g., sarcoidosis)
- Severe anemia
- Poor physical conditioning
- Anxiety

Underlying Causes of CHF

- Dilated cardiomyopathies (poor pump function)
    - Ischemic heart disease (resulting from heart attacks)
    - Viral
    - Alcoholic
    - Drugs (e.g., anthracyclines [chemotherapeutic agents], cocaine)
    - Pregnancy
- Increased workload
    - Hypertension
    - Anemia
    - Valvular lesions (aortic stenosis, mitral regurgitation)
    - Hyperthyroidism
    - Hypertrophic heart disease
    - Arteriovenous fistulas
- Restricted ventricular filling
    - Stiff ventricle (concentric hypertrophy, hypertrophic heart disease)
    - Pericardial constriction (cardiac tamponade, chronic constriction)
    - Mitral or tricuspid stenosis
    - Infiltrations (e.g., hemochromatosis, amyloidosis)
    - Atrial myxoma

Precipitating Causes of Exacerbations of CHF

- Dietary or medication nonadherence
- Onset of new arrhythmia (e.g., atrial fibrillation, atrioventricular block)
- Myocardial infarction or ischemia
- Uncontrolled hypertension
- Anemia
- Infections
- Pulmonary embolism
- Renal disorder

History

For patients who present with shortness of breath or a volume-overloaded condition, the initial history is geared to help establish the diagnosis of CHF and then to identify the underlying cause. For patients with an established diagnosis of CHF, the history is aimed at identifying what precipitated the exacerbation.

"What symptoms are you experiencing?" Inquire about:

- Ankle swelling/edema
- Shortness of breath and dyspnea
- Orthopnea

- Paroxysmal nocturnal dyspnea
- Change in exercise tolerance and dyspnea on exertion (DOE)
- Nocturia
- Cough (particularly nocturnal)
- Chest pain
- Palpitations
- Sputum production, fevers, chills
- Abdominal pain or distention
- Fatigue
- Change in weight

"Do you have a history of . . ."

- Coronary artery disease (CAD) or chest pain?
- Hypertension?
- History of lung disorders (COPD, sarcoidosis, restrictive lung diseases)?
- Diabetes?
- Renal disease?
- Liver disease?
- Anemia?
- Hypercholesterolemia?
- Drug or alcohol use?

For patients with known heart failure:

- "Do you know why you have CHF?" (Looking for the underlying etiology)
- "Are your symptoms [dyspnea, ankle edema, orthopnea, weight gain] worsening?"
- "How have your symptoms changed?" *(Brain 3)*
- Assess the functional impact of the CHF. Patient comments such as the following are significant: "Last week I could walk up the hill to get my mail without stopping, but now I have to stop and rest." or "I used to sleep with one pillow but now I feel better with two pillows."

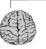

3 - It is important that patients with established CHF be alert to changes in their symptoms so they can seek medical care.

For patients with an exacerbation of CHF:

- "Have you had chest pain or palpitations? Have you run out of medications or changed your diet [e.g., increased intake of salty foods]?"
- "What have you done differently?"

Physical Examination

- Vital signs. Pay particular attention to respiratory rate, heart rate, and any change in weight.
- Observe the patient's breathing. Is it labored? The vitals and respiratory effort may give important clues to the etiology or might suggest another cause *(Red Flag 1)*
- Does the respiratory rate change with reclining? Does the patient have more dyspnea on reclining? Orthopnea is very suggestive of a diagnosis of CHF.
- Ankle swelling or edema. Is it pitting? How high does it go (e.g., ankle, calf, knee) *(Brain 4) (Figure 2)*
- Lung exam. Note rales/crackles (particularly in the bases), wheezes, or dullness on percussion. Fever, sputum production, and crackles and wheezes suggest a pulmonary cause of the dyspnea, not CHF.

1 - Tachypnea (> 24 breaths/min), tachycardia (> 100 bpm), and use of accessory muscles to breathe require immediate definitive intervention.

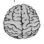

4 - Generalized edema or anasarca suggests a primary renal etiology, not CHF. Peripheral edema alone without dyspnea is common and often due to venous insufficiency or a side effect of medication. Nifedipine and nonsteriodals are common causes.

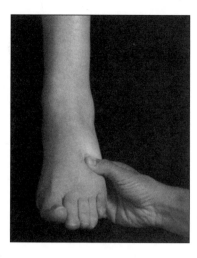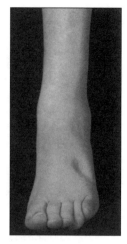

Figure 2: Pitting edema.
(From Bates B: A Guide to Physical Examination and History Taking. Philadelphia, JB Lippincott, 1991, with permission.)

- Heart exam. Note regularity, murmurs, S_3 and S_4.
- Jugular venous distention *(Figure 3)*
- Abdominal exam
    - Hepatojugular reflux
    - Hepatomegaly. Is the liver edge tender? This is consistent with a swollen liver secondary to CHF.
    - Ascites

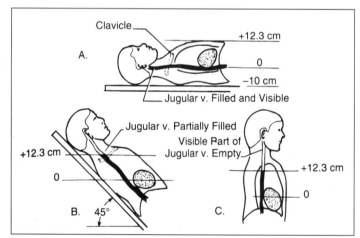

Figure 3: Jugular venous distention. The sagittal section is drawn to scale from a lateral x-ray film of a normal adult male thorax. The anteroposterior diameter of the thorax at the level of the fourth interspace is 20 cm; from this point, the vertical distance to the superior border of the clavicle is 15 cm in the erect position. The right atrium is located at the midpoint of an anteroposterior line from the fourth interspace to the back. In any posture, a horizontal plane through this point is the "phlebostatic" or "zero level." In this figure, a slightly elevated venous pressure of 12.3 cm is assumed. *A*, With the patient supine, the horizontal plane (12.3 cm is above the zero level) is above the neck, so the jugular vein is filled; normal venous pressure also should fill the vein in this position. *B*, With the thorax at 45°, the blood column extends midway up the jugular, so the head of the column is visible. *C*, In the erect position, the head of the column is concealed within the thorax, 2.7 cm below the upper border of the clavicle, although the venous pressure exceeds the normal.
(From DeGowin RL, Brown RD: Degowin's Diagnostic Examination. New York, McGraw-Hill, 2000, with permission.)

Testing

In patients with established stable heart failure with an identified underlying cause, no further diagnostic studies may be indicated. Patients who present with dyspnea and peripheral edema and in whom the diagnosis of CHF is being considered need a thorough evaluation including a complete blood count (CBC), electrolytes, creatinine, blood urea nitrogen (BUN), blood glucose, thyroid-stimulating hormone (TSH), liver function tests, albumin, urinalysis, electrocardiogram (EKG), chest x-ray, pulse oximeter or arterial blood gas (ABG), and ultimately an echocardiogram *(Brain 5)*. For patients with established heart failure who suffer an exacerbation, repeating part or all of this work-up may be appropriate, but checking the renal function and the electrolytes is often all that is needed. Patients with a new diagnosis of CHF or with CHF without an identified cause should also have serum iron and ferritin levels checked and consideration given to cardiac stress testing, coronary arteriography, and very rarely an endomyocardial biopsy *(Consultation and Referral 1)*.

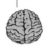

5 - The echocardiogram often points to the underlying cause, such as the diagnosis of aortic stenosis, ischemic heart disease, or cardiomyopathy.

1 - Sorting out a patient with dyspnea can be challenging. Consultation, admission, and additional testing (e.g., pulmonary function testing, pulmonary angiogram, immediate echocardiogram) should be considered if the etiology cannot be determined.

Putting It All Together

Patients with an established diagnosis of CHF should be asked if they are experiencing any of the classic symptoms of heart failure (shortness of breath, leg swelling, orthopnea, nocturia, or a nocturnal cough) and should have a focused physical examination, including weight, vital signs, lung and heart exam, and a check of neck veins and for peripheral edema. Follow-up appointments are opportunities to reinforce the importance of adhering to the treatment plan and to note any changes in the patient's symptoms, making early intervention possible. Patients who are doing well may only need to have their prescriptions refilled or adjusted and ongoing follow-up arranged. Patients with worsening symptoms should be evaluated more thoroughly, and a careful search should be undertaken to identify precipitating causes. In patients for whom a diagnosis of CHF is being seriously considered, an echocardiogram is essential and to help confirm the diagnosis and can often suggest the underlying cause.

Management

Patients presenting with acute heart failure or pulmonary edema should be given IV diuretics, placed on oxygen, and hospitalized. Once the patient has been stabilized and the underlying etiology has been established, treatment should be directed at the primary cause. The goal of chronic therapy for left ventricular dysfunction is to improve the ability of the heart to pump effectively. This can be accomplished by afterload reduction (with angiotension-converting enzyme [ACE] inhibitors), removal of excess fluid (with diuretics), and increasing cardiac contractility (with digoxin) *(Treatment 1)*. Excellent long-term studies have shown consistent benefit from the use of ACE inhibitors, beta blockers, and, most recently, spironolactone. Early initiation of ACE inhibitors is particularly important and may be related to the drug's ability to decrease the ventricle from stretching out or remodeling. Digoxin therapy has been shown to decrease the frequency of hospitalization. For patients with diastolic dysfunction, therapy is aimed at relaxing the

1 - An empiric trial of furosemide is often helpful both therapeutically and diagnostically and can quickly relieve a significant amount of distress.

ventricle to improve ventricular filling, and beta blockers and calcium channel blockers are recommended *(Brain 6)*.

6 - A comprehensive management plan should include dietary consultation (avoiding sodium), daily weighing, and, if necessary, periodic home nursing visits.

Selected Readings

1. Barker LR, Burton JR, Zieve PD: Ambulatory Medicine. Baltimore, Williams & Wilkins, 1995.
2. Bates B: A Guide to Physical Examination and History Taking. Philadelphia, J.B. Lippincott, 1991.
3. DeGowin RL, Brown RD: Degowin's Diagnostic Examination. New York, McGraw-Hill, 2000.
4. Isselbacher KJ, et al (eds): Harrison's Principles of Internal Medicine, 15th ed. New York, McGraw-Hill, 2001.
5. Williams JF, et al: American College of Cardiology/American Heart Association Task Force report: Guidelines for the evaluation and management of heart failure. Circulation 92:2764–2784,1995. Also viewable online at http://www.americanheart.org/Scientific/statements/.

23. Constipation

Dale R. Agner, MD

Synopsis

Constipation is described as difficult, painful, or incomplete defecation or decreased stool frequency *(Definition 1)*. Patients are often embarrassed to ask about constipation, so the examiner should ask about difficulties with stools and what is normal for the patient. Water is reabsorbed from stool in the colon. If the voluntary anal sphincter resists the colonic urge to defecate, or if stool remains in the rectal vault, then the stool continues to lose water, hardens, and gains in size. If this cycle continues, the colon dilates and rectal tone is lost. Low fiber, dehydration, immobility, medications, and cancer can delay intestinal transit time. Poor bowel habits, psychosocial issues, and pain from anal fissures, hemorrhoids, or previous hard bowel movements can lead to retention in pediatric or adult patients. Muscle dysfunction from sphincter trauma, chronic stimulant-laxative use, or chronic rectal vault distention by large stools can lead to rectal outlet delay *(Definition 2)*. Exercise, fiber, hydration, good bowel habits, and avoidance of constipation medication are the backbones of treatment.

1 - Functional constipation:
- Straining at least 25% of the time
- Lumpy or hard stools at least 25% of the time
- Feeling of incomplete evacuation at least 25% of the time
- Fewer than 2 bowel movements a week greater than 25% of the time

2 - Rectal outlet delay: (1) Anal blockage > 25% of the time and prolonged defecation or (2) manual disimpaction (when necessary)

Differential Diagnosis

Personal and Psychosocial Habits

- Low fiber intake
- Decreased fluid intake
- Sedentary lifestyle
- Laxative abuse
- Retention-conscious or unconscious (e.g., professional drivers, history of sexual abuse)

Over-the-Counter Medications

- Iron supplements
- Calcium supplements
- Antidiarrheals
- Antihistamines
- Nonsteroidal anti-inflammatory drugs (e.g., ibuprofen)

Prescription Medication

- High blood pressure agents (e.g., diuretics or calcium channel blockers)
- Anticholinergic side effects from medications (e.g., antihistamines, antipsychotics, antiparkinsonian medications, tricyclic

antidepressants)
- Opioid pain medications, especially codeine (which is more constipating than other opioids and frequently prescribed)

Chronic Diseases
- Parkinson's disease
- Dementia
- Physical immobility
- Spinal cord injuries
- Hypothyroidism

Anorectal Pathology

- Hemorrhoids
- Rectal fissure
- **Rectocele *(Definition 3)***

Colon Cancer

3 - Rectocele: A thinned rectovaginal septum with an enlarged rectal vault, often due to multiple vaginal deliveries or birth trauma. A rectocele often decreases the ability to defecate except with extra straining or maneuvers (e.g., digital disimpaction or providing digital support to the rectovaginal septum while defecating).

History

"Do you have any difficulties with bowel movements?"

- "Is the constipation new? Did it begin recently?" (to rule out new medications)
- "Is it a marked change from previous bowel habits?" (to determine fissure, neoplasm) *(Red Flag 1) (Consultation and Referral 1)*
- "Do you have any hemorrhoids or protrusions at the rectum?" (anorectal pathology)

"What symptoms do you have? What is normal for you?" (functional constipation or rectal outlet delay)

- "Any straining to defecate?"
- "How often do you have a bowel movement?"
- "Do you feel like you have 'emptied'?"
- "Are the stools hard, lumpy, or like pellets?"
- "Do you feel 'blocked'?"
- "Is there any blood?" (Blood indicates hemorrhoid, fissure, or neoplasm.)
- "Do you have any pain with defecation?" (Pain indicates hemorrhoid or fissure.)

"What medications are you taking, including over-the-counter or home remedies?"

- Iron supplements, cold medications, and antihistamines are often overlooked.
- Prescription medications may have constipating side-effects.

"Do you have to do anything to help have your bowel movements?"

- If so, how often do you have to use a laxative, enema, or suppository? (loss of tone, decreased motility, or enlarged rectal vault)

1 - New-onset constipation should prompt an investigation. A change in bowel habits for a person at risk for colon cancer needs endoscopic evaluation. Constipation can be the result of emotional factors, a rectal fissure, the addition of a new medication, or a neoplasm.

1 - Colonoscopy should be obtained for patients with risk factors for colon cancer, including blood in stools, anemia, or patients with unexplained weight loss.

If constipation is severe or longstanding, or the patient is at a unique risk (e.g., opioid analgesics medications for cancer or spinal cord injuries):

"Do you ever have to loosen up the stool or use extra maneuvers to remove the stool?" (possible fecal impaction)
"Is there any history of colorectal cancer in your family?" Ask the patient to include brothers, sisters, parents, aunts, or uncles *(Red Flag 2)*.

- Any red blood or dark tarry stools
- Weight loss or anemia (neoplasm)
- Any history of colon polyps or colon evaluation (colonoscopy evaluation)

"Is there any history of rectal problems?"

- Hemorrhoids or hemorrhoidectomy
- Anal fissures or perirectal abscesses (anorectal pathology)
- Birth trauma, tears during vaginal delivery, or forceps or vacuum delivery (rectocele)

2 - Risk factors for colon cancer include age over 50, family history of colorectal cancer, weight loss, blood in stool, or iron-deficiency anemia. Screening for colorectal cancer should begin at age 50 or 10 years younger than the age a relative was diagnosed with colon cancer, whichever is sooner.

Physical Examination

- General. Note conditions that can predispose, such as paraplegia or Parkinson's disease.
- Vital signs and weight. Note any weight loss secondary to cancer in the elderly or an eating disorder.
- Abdominal examination. Look for masses that might represent a large stool amount or cancer.
- Anorectal inspection for hemorrhoids, fissures, and skin tags. A skin tag is usually from a resolved hemorrhoid; a fissure may be from a few hard stools. Hemorrhoids are thought to be "cushions" developed from frequent hard or painful stools.
- Digital rectal examination for pain, sphincter tone, rectocele, stool character (e.g., stool present or not, hard or soft), and possible impaction

Testing

- Order stool guaiac for occult gastrointestinal bleeding in the adult population.
- Office anoscopy should be performed for fissures, hemorrhoids, or bleeding (for children, gentle inspection and digital examination with the little finger is usually sufficient).
- Order colonoscopy for those at risk for cancer or unexplained bleeding. Use of flexible sigmoidoscopy with an air-contrast barium enema is decreasing; it costs less, but it is less sensitive.
- A complete blood cell count (CBC) and a thyroid-stimulating hormone (TSH) may be considered.
- If laxative abuse is suspected or multiple medications are being used, a serum electrolyte evaluation is prudent.
- An abdominal x-ray can help show the amount of stool if impaction or severe constipation is suspected.

Putting It All Together

Most constipation is due to functional causes that may be easily remedied with changes in exercise, hydration, increased fiber intake, and avoidance of constipating medications. However, one should remain alert for occult physical causes and more complex psychosocial issues, such as laxative abuse in the patient with an eating disorder (body-image) or sexual abuse *(Consultation and Referral 2)*.

Chronic constipation often leads to habitual over-the-counter stimulant-laxative use. Chronic stimulant-laxative use actually impairs colonic motility. Stimulants often have the quickest "results," and patients may be reluctant to discontinue their use. Therefore, education regarding prevention, treatment, and laxative misuse is paramount.

Those who have experienced impaction or long-term obstipation have special concerns and warrant different approaches regarding management. This group can include the physically impaired patient or patients requiring long-term opioid pain medications. Impaction or chronic obstipation causes the colon and rectal vault to become dilated, and return to normal tone and motility can take several months *(Brain 1)*.

Patients with physical causes not amenable to outpatient treatment *(Consultation and Referral 3)*, complex psychosocial issues, reimpaction, concern for cancer, or chronic constipation not responding to treatment should be referred for further evaluation. *(Figure 1)*.

Management

Treatment is focused on identifying causes and trying to remove them, if possible. If the rectal and colonic tone are normal, bulk-fiber fluids, exercise, stool softeners, lubricants, eliminating or modifying precipitant causes, and education are usually sufficient.

If complicating factors are present or the rectal-colonic tone is diminished, as in obstipation or impaction, then osmotic agents (e.g., lactulose), lubricants, and lifestyle modifications are used as appropriate. Developing good bowel habits is important— for example, using the toilet after a meal, when the colon's natural motility helps assist the defecation process. Once the process is regular, transition to softeners, lubricants, and fiber may occur. Stimulants may be used intermittently and judiciously. This approach works for children and adults.

If impaction is encountered, enemas are used first until the "results" are clear *(Brain 2)*. Then osmotics are used to flush the system. Careful attention must then be given to regulate the stools to about one soft stool per day. Opioid-induced constipation can quickly lead to obstipation or impaction *(Definition 4)*. Once tone is restored, usually after 30–90 days, bulk fiber may be resumed *(Brain 3)*.

2 - Laxative abuse often has many underlying complex social-emotional issues. An eating disorder with laxative abuse or a history of sexual abuse can lead to constipation. Referral to a mental health specialist should be considered.

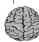

1 - Dietary fiber is indicated only after normal bowel tone has been restored. This process can take several months after longstanding constipation or fecal impaction. Dietary fiber or bulking agents given after disimpaction can lead to reimpaction and an unhappy patient.

3 - Patients with constipation secondary to possible muscle dysfunction or rectocele should be evaluated by a gastroenterologist or a colorectal surgeon.

2 - When obstipated or impacted, patients should be given enemas until clear "from below," *before* anything is given by mouth "from above." Giving a stimulant or osmotic agent when blocked or impacted can lead to bowel perforation.

4 - **Obstipation:** Intestinal obstruction, impaction, or severe constipation.

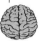

3 - Returning to normal bowel function after longstanding constipation requires patient education about the etiology, prevention of constipation, and good bowel habits.

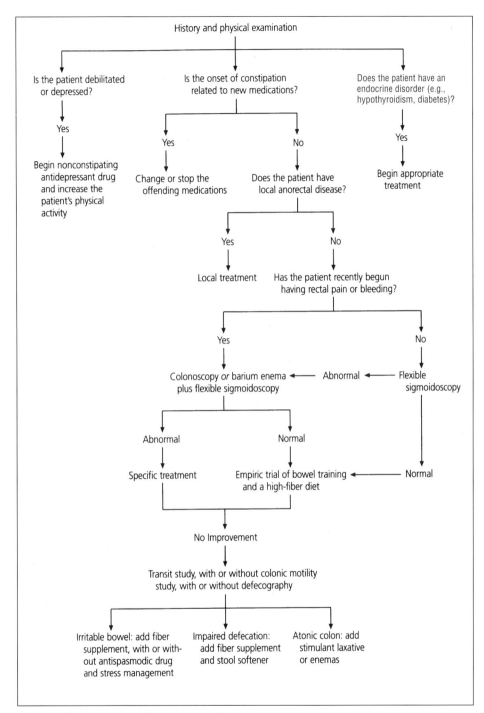

Figure 1: Evaluation of constipation in the elderly.
(From Schaefer DC, Cheskin LJ: Constipation in the elderly. Am Fam Physician 588:907–919, 1998, with permission.)

Selected Readings

1. Abi-Hanna A, Lake AM: Constipation and encopresis in childhood. Pediatr Rev 19:23–31, 1998.
2. Schaefer DC, Cheskin LJ: Constipation in the elderly. Am Fam Physician 58:907–919, 1998.
3. Whitehead WE, Chaussade S, Corazziari E, et al: Report of an international workshop on management of constipation. Gastroenterol Int 4:99–113, 1991.

24. Coronary Artery Disease

David V. O'Dell, MD

Synopsis

Coronary artery disease (CAD), *coronary heart disease* (CHD), and *ischemic heart disease* (IHD) are all terms that refer to the disease state resulting from inadequate blood flow through the arteries that supply the heart. Most often these coronary arteries become narrowed by **athero-sclerotic plaque** *(Definition 1)*. CAD is the leading cause of death for both men and women in America. The most feared complication of CAD is a **myocardial infarction** (MI) *(Definition 2)*, commonly referred to as a heart attack. The classic symptoms of a heart attack are crushing subster-nal chest pain radiating to the neck and jaw. However, most patients will present with much subtler complaints, ranging from a slight pressure or heaviness in their chest, upper arm or shoulder, indigestion, to no pain at all. The physical examination in patients with CAD is often unimpressive. An electrocardiogram (EKG) can be diagnostic in the setting of an acute MI, but most often more sophisticated testing is required to define the CAD *(Red Flag 1)*. Beta-blockers, aspirin, cholesterol-lowering medica-tions, and angiotensin-converting enzyme (ACE) inhibitors have all been shown to improve prognosis. Finally, all of a patient's risk factors, including hypertension, diabetes, smoking, hyperlipidemia, and sedentary lifestyle, should be aggressively addressed.

1 - Atherosclerosis: A complex process involving the deposition of cholesterol, lipids, calcium, and other cellular products on the inside surface of arteries forming focal plaques.

2 - Myocardial infarction (MI): Actual death of myocardial cells due to ischemia. An MI is most commonly caused by the rupture of an atherosclerotic plaque on the wall of a coro-nary artery and the subsequent formation of an occluding thrombus at that site. Cells do not die immediately, and timely intervention (reperfusion) saves heart muscle. MIs are diagnosed by having two of the following three criteria: classic story of substernal chest pain, characteristic EKG changes, and positive cardiac enzymes.

1 - A patient with a suspected myocardial infarction should immediately be referred to a center for definitive treatment.

Differential Diagnosis

Not all "heart problems" are caused by blockage of the coronary arteries. Patients will often describe any chest disorder as a problem with their heart or even refer to it as a heart attack. Other possibilities include:

- Valvular heart disease (e.g., aortic stenosis, mitral regurgitation). Typically a significant murmur will be present on physical exam.
- Pulmonary insufficiency or emboli. Primary presenting concern is usually shortness of breath.
- Cardiac electrical conduction disorders. Typically presenting concerns are palpitations; irregular, slow, or rapid rhythms; premature beats; syncope (fainting) episodes; or even sudden death *(Brain 1)*.
- Congenital heart disease. Typically diagnosed in childhood, and the patient may have a healed chest incision.
- Severe anemia. Patients often will appear quite pale, and their symp-toms resolve with replenishment of their blood mass.

1 - Although electrical conduction disorders are more common in patients with CAD, dsyrhythmias can occur in anyone.

Not all MIs are caused by atherosclerosis. Other pathophysiologic caus-es of coronary artery blockage include:

- Cocaine-induced spasm
- Inflammation of the artery (vasculitis)
- Coronary aneurysms
- Congenital abnormalities

History

Remember, many patients with heart disease will have atypical symptoms!

"Tell me about your symptoms. Do you have any chest discomfort, heaviness, pressure, or pain? Is this your heart pain?" Note signs of angina *(Red Flag 2).*

- "Does the chest discomfort occur with exercise, cold, or emotional stress?"
- "Does it occur at a certain time of the day?" (mornings versus evenings)
- "Has the pattern of your angina changed?" (accelerated angina)
- "Is there pain at rest? (unstable angina)

"Tell me about your heart problems."

- "Have you had a myocardial infarction or heart attack? Was it proven?" (need evidence from EKGs or cardiac enzymes, such as creatine phosphokinase (CPK) with isoenzymes, troponin T or I)
- Ask about previous cardiac procedures or operations, including echocardiograms, stress tests, holters, event recorders, catheterizations, angioplasty, stents, coronary artery bypass grafting, and cardiac arrests *(Tables 1–3).*
- "What heart medications are you taking? What have you taken in the past?"
- "Have you ever had **congestive heart failure** (CHF)? *(Definition 3)* (see Chapter 22).
- "Do you know how well your heart pumps blood?" (**ejection fraction**) *(Definition 4)*
- "Have you ever had problems with your heart rhythm? Have you had **palpitations** *(Definition 5)*?"

Define the patient's cardiac risk factors.

- "Do you have diabetes (see Chapter 27) or hypertension (see Chapter 42)? For how long?"
- "How are these managed?" (e.g., medications, diet)
- "Do you smoke? Have you ever smoked? How much [packs per day for how long]? Have you tried to quit? What methods have you tried?"
- "What is your cholesterol?"
   "Do you watch your diet?"
   "Are you on cholesterol-lowering medication?"
- "How much exercise do you get?"
- "Is there a history of premature CAD in your family?" (onset prior to age 55)
- "What medications are you taking?" Be sure to ask about aspirin.

Review the patient's past medical history with particular attention to other illnesses that are linked with atherosclerosis or hypertension, thus CAD. For example, inquire about a history of strokes, peripheral vascular disease or claudication symptoms, kidney disease, and peripheral edema. Also, include medication allergies or intolerance (i.e., aspirin or beta blockers).

2 - A significant change in a patient's angina pattern should prompt a thorough evaluation.

3 - Congestive heart failue (CHF): The clinical diagnosis given to patients who present with evidence that the heart is unable to meet the metabolic needs of the body.

4 - Ejection fraction: The percentage of blood in the left ventricle ejected by the contraction of the heart.

5 - Palpitation: An abnormal awareness of the heart beating.

Table 1. Common Definitions and Terms in Coronary Artery Disease

Term	Definition
Angina	Transient chest pain caused by myocardial ischemia, most often because of inadequate blood flow past a stable atherosclerotic lesion. It is typically substernal in location and may radiate to the left shoulder, jaw, or back. Angina is exacerbated by physical exertion, cold, and emotional stress. Patients often describe it as a pressure or heaviness, or band-like discomfort, and some patients hesitate to call it a pain. Angina typically lasts 1–20 minutes and is relieved by rest or nitroglycerin.
Unstable angina (USA)	Chest pain characteristic of angina occurring at rest (thus, all chest pain occurring at rest is not USA).
Accelerated angina	Commonly used to describe a patient who has known stable angina and now has a change in the pattern, frequency, or severity of the angina. For example, a patient who usually experiences angina only when climbing a significant hill is now getting angina with much less exertion.
Prinzmetal's (variant) angina	Transient chest pain caused by a focal coronary artery spasm in a vessel without a hemodynamically significant atherosclerotic lesion. The spasm results in myocardial ischemia of the tissue distal to the spasm. This form of angina can occur at any time (exertional or nonexertional) and is rare.
Transmural MI	This type of infarction is caused by the occlusion of an epicardial (larger) vessel. It results in the death of the entire thickness of the myocardium, and thus formation of Q waves in the appropriate EKG leads (i.e., inferior, anterior, or posterior MI).
Subendocardial or non–Q wave MI	This type of infarction is usually the result of blockage of distal (smaller) vessels or nonocclusive thrombus causing myocardial cell necrosis limited to a relatively small area. This diagnosis can only be made with enzymes and clinical history because EKG findings are nonspecific.
Acute coronary syndrome	Chest pain and evidence of a very small climb in the cardiac enzymes (e.g., troponins or CPK isoenzymes).

MI = myocardial infarction; CPK = creatine phosphokinase.

Table 2. Diagnostic Cardiac Procedures

Procedure	Definition
Cardiac catheterization—left	Insertion of a catheter into an artery (usually the femoral) and then advancing it to both the right and left coronary arteries. Contrast (dye) is then infused and fluoroscopic (x-ray) images are taken. This is the gold standard test for confirming and defining CAD.
Cardiac catheterization—right (Swan Ganz)	Insertion of a catheter into a vein (usually either the subclavian or internal jugular) to measure the pressure in the various chambers of the heart.
Echocardiography (echo)	An ultrasound probe is placed against the chest and used to take pictures of the heart. When the probe is placed in the esophagus, the procedure is called a transesophageal echocardiography (TEE).
Exercise tolerance test (ETT) Dobutamine stress test Nuclear stress test	A patient is asked to exercise (on the treadmill most commonly) while their vitals, EKG tracings, and sometimes echocardiogram are monitored. These tests can suggest CAD. If a patient is unable to exercise, IV dobutamine can be infused to mimic exercise. Other variations include using a nuclear medicine tracer to determine blood flow to specific areas of the heart during and after exercise.
Holter monitoring and cardiac event recorder	Outpatient recording devices attached to electrodes on the patient's chest that record the heart's rhythm.

Table 3. Therapeutic Cardiac Procedures

Procedure	Description
Angioplasty (balloon)/ percutaneous transluminal coronary angioplasty (PTCA)	Insertion of a catheter into a coronary artery to the precise area of blockage and then blowing up a balloon to open up the area of stenosis.
Angioplasty with stent	As above, but once the stenosis is relieved, a wire stent is inserted in this area to prevent restenosis.
Atherectomy	Removal of a blockage in a coronary atery by using a catheter with a device that shaves away atherosclerotic plaque.
Coronary artery bypass graft (CABG)	Venous grafts that are sown between the aorta and coronary arteries and bypass the area of atherosclerotic blockage and supply blood to ischemic areas. Arteries, specifically the left internal mammary artery (LIMA), can also be used.
Cardioversion	Electric shock applied to the chest in an attempt to restore sinus rhythm.
Reperfusion therapy	Refers to efforts to reopen a stenotic coronary artery using either drugs (thrombolysis) or angioplasty to break up a clot.

Physical Examination

- How does the patient look? Comfortable versus writhing in pain, anxious or unconcerned, diaphoretic?
- Review the patients vitals: temperature, pulse, blood pressure, and respiratory rate.
- Examine the chest and lungs:
  1. Symmetrical movement with respirations? Is the breathing labored?
  2. Dull or hyperresonant on percussion? Is the chest wall tender?
  3. Are there wheezes, rales/crackles, rhonchi, or pleural rubs?
- Examine the heart and vessels:
  1. Is the heart rhythm regular? If not, are all the contractions conducted to the radial artery?
  2. Check for murmurs, gallops, and jugular venous distention (JVD) (see Chapter 22).
  3. Check carotids and femoral arteries for bruits and good upstrokes.
  4. Peripheral pulses: present, diminished, or absent?
  5. Is there peripheral edema? Unilateral/bilateral?
- Examine abdomen. Check for distention, tenderness, bowel sounds, organomegaly, and bruits.

Testing

For patients with established CAD without any significant change in their symptoms, no further diagnostic studies may be indicated. All patients with CAD need to have **lipid profiles** *(Definition 6)* and occasionally have a liver profile checked if they are on lipid-lowering medications that can be hepatotoxic. For patients with hypertension, periodic monitoring of electrolytes and kidney function is prudent. Patients with diabetes should also have blood sugars closely monitored, routine hemoglobin A_{1c} (HgA$_{1c}$), and

6 - Lipid profile: Reports a patient's total cholesterol, high-density lipoprotein (HDL) (so-called good cholesterol), low-density lipoprotein (LDL) (so-called bad cholesterol), and triglycerides.

urinalysis. For patients with stable CAD, routine EKGs, chest x-rays, exercise tolerance tests (ETT), and echocardiograms are not indicated.

Patients with a change in their chest pain pattern need additional work-up. An EKG is the initial step *(Brain 2)*. Patients with atypical chest pain (see Chapter 19) are usually best evaluated with some type of exercise stress testing. If the patient has unstable or accelerated angina, the best course is to obtain routine lab tests (cardiac enzymes, electrolytes, blood urea nitrogen [BUN], serum creatinine, and complete blood cell count [CBC]), appropriate consultation, and then to proceed directly to heart catheterization or an appropriate imaging study. For patients with suspected CAD, a complete evaluation should include lab, x-ray, and an imaging study. All common cardiac risk factors should be assessed. Common useful tests include a lipid profile, CBC, blood sugar, electrolytes, thyroid-stimulating hormone (TSH), electrolytes, BUN, and a serum creatinine.

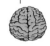

2 - Localized ST segment elevation with or without hyperacute T waves are classic EKG findings indicating an acute infarct **(Figure 1)**.

Putting It All Together

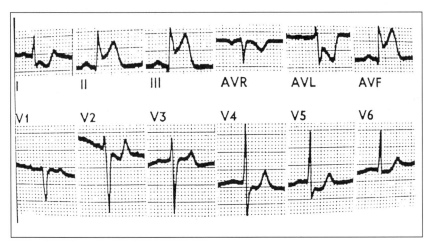

Figure 1: Twelve-lead EKG showing an acute inferior myocardial infarction with ST segment elevation (II, III, and AVF) and reciprocal ST segment depression (I and AVL).

Most patients presenting to clinic with known CAD are stable and will have had no significant change in their symptoms. These patients need to have their medications reviewed or refilled and previous education reinforced. Diligently addressing each of a patient's risk factors on routine clinic visits is important and ultimately pays off in better patient outcomes. Stress the benefits of consistent exercise and encourage your patients to adhere to a low-fat, low-cholesterol diet. For patients who smoke, urge them to quit or at least cut down. Patients with a change in their angina pattern or with new or different chest pain warrant further evaluation.

Management

In the past, most of the effort for patients with CAD was geared toward decreasing symptoms. Although controlling or relieving the patient's symptoms is obviously important, there is compelling evidence that aggresively addressing risk factors improves the patient's prognosis. Beta-blockers, aspirin, and the cholesterol-lowering statins have all been shown to decrease recurrent CAD events and improve prognosis. All patients with known CAD should be on both beta-blockers and aspirin unless there is a contraindication to these agents. Cholesterol should be lowered to the levels suggested by the National Cholesterol Education Program (NCEP). Patients who smoke should be encouraged to quit. Hypertension and diabetes should be aggressively treated, and, at least for individuals with diabetes, the goal should be a blood pressure of < 130/85. ACE inhibitors have also been shown to decrease CAD events and are a particularly good choice in hypertensive diabetics. In addition to beta-blockers, for patients with chronic stable angina, long-acting nitrates and calcium channel blockers are useful in decreasing the frequency and severity of angina. All patients with angina should have a prescription for nitroglycerin, either sublingual or spray, and know how to use it in case of chest pain *(Brain 3)*. Finally, all patients with CAD should be encouraged to engage in some form of exercise. Physically active patients likely will do better, in part because exercise promotes the development of collateral arteries to areas of the ischemia.

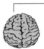

3 - Nitroglycerin (NTG) instructions for patients: Place a tablet under your tongue when you have chest pain. If chest pain is still present after 5 minutes, take another NTG tablet. If after an additional 5 minutes chest pain is still present, take a third tablet. If the chest pain is still not relieved, proceed directly to the nearest emergency room.

Patients with unstable angina should be hospitalized in a monitored bed (telemetry) and started on beta-blockers, aspirin, and heparin. Strong consideration should be given to starting a 2b/3a antiplatelet agent (eptifibatide). For patients with acute MIs, reperfusion should be aggressively pursued with either a thrombolytic agent *(Treatment 1)* or angioplasty. Timely consultation and appropriate use of interventions are key in assuring good outcomes.

1 - Tissue plasminogen activator (TPA) and streptokinase are the most widely used thrombolytic agents (clot busters).

Common additional issues encountered in managing patients with CAD include rhythm disturbances and congestive heart failure (CHF). The most common rhythm disturbances seen are premature ventricular contractions (PVCs) and atrial fibrillation. PVCs are very common and are usually benign unless the patient has a significantly damaged left ventricle. Atrial fibrillation is also very common and most often occurs in patients with dilated left atria. For the management of CHF please refer to Chapter 22.

Selected Readings

1. American College of Cardiology/American Heart Association: 1999 update: ACC/AHA guidelines for the management of patients with acute myocardial infarction. J Am Coll Cardiol 34:890–911, 1999.
2. National Cholesterol Education Program Expert Panel: Summary of the second report of the National Cholesterol Education Program (NCEP) Expert Panel on Detection, Evaluation, and Treatment of High Blood Cholesterol in Adults (Adult Treatment Panel II). JAMA 269:3015–3023, 1993.
3. Noble J: Primary Care Medicine. St Louis, Mosby, 1996.
4. The Sixth Report of the Joint National Committee on Prevention, Detection, Evaluation, and Treatment of High Blood Pressure. Arch Intern Med 157:2413–2446, 1997.
5. UK Prospective Diabetes Study Group: Tight blood pressure control and risk of macrovascular and microvascular complications in type 2 diabetes: UKPDS 38. BMJ 317(7160):703 713, 1998.

25. Cough in Adults

J. Scott Neumeister, MD

Synopsis

Respiratory complaints are the most common reason patients visit a physician's office. Cough is the most common symptom.[1] Most coughs are acute (< 3 weeks' duration) and require little evaluation. They are typically due to a respiratory infection such as the common cold or bronchitis. When a cough becomes chronic (> 3 weeks), other diagnoses need to be considered. Keep in mind that cough after upper respiratory infection can persist for many weeks (postviral bronchitis). Although by definition this is a chronic cough, evaluation is usually not done until an 8-week period has passed. The history and physical examination are designed to elicit the possible diagnoses, which will then determine appropriate testing and management. The impact a cough has on a patient's personal life and occupation also should be considered. This will help build rapport with the patient and help understand expectations of the patient in seeking help for the cough. The history and physical should not only gather information regarding the common diagnoses (postnasal drip, gastroesophageal reflux disease [GERD], asthma), but also screen the patient for serious underlying disorders (congestive heart failure [CHF], pneumonia, cancer). Cough can also cause serious complications *(Brain 1)*. Screening for complications such as pneumothorax, rib fracture, or urinary incontinence is important because management of these issues, in addition to the cough, can make a tremendous impact on the patient's quality of life.

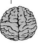 **1** - Serious complications such as a pneumothorax, arrhythmia, and laryngeal trauma are unusual. Patients can suffer a rib fracture or urinary incontinence. Headaches and syncope are also reported.

Differential Diagnosis

Acute Cough

Upper Respiratory Tract Infection
- Otitis
- Rhinitis
- Pharyngitis
- Sinusitis

Lower Respiratory Tract Infection
- Bronchitis
- Laryngitis
- Pneumonia

Aspiration
- Foreign body
- Secretions
- Noxious fumes

Chronic Cough (> 3 weeks)

- Postnasal drip
- GERD *(Brain 2)*
- Asthma
- Smoking
- **Chronic bronchitis** *(Definition 1)*
- Postviral bronchitis
- Medication (angiotensin-converting enzyme [ACE] inhibitors)
- Congestive heart failure
- Malignancy (primary lung or metastatic disease)
- Psychogenic
- **Brochiectasis** *(Definition 2)*
- *Bordetella pertussis*
- Pulmonary fibrosis
- Sarcoid
- Vasculitis

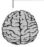 **2** - Cough can occur because of chemical irritation from aspirated gastric contents.

 1 - Chronic bronchitis: Chronic obstructive pulmonary disease characterized by a productive cough 3 months out of the year in 2 consecutive years.

 2 - Bronchiectasis: Permanently dilated bronchi usually secondary to chronic or recurrent infections. Secretions pool in the dilated bronchi.

History

"Tell me about your cough and what symptoms you are having."

- Time of day *(Brain 3)*
- Association with meals or acid reflux (GERD)
- Recent colds or flu (postviral bronchitis)
- Fever or chills (infections)
- Hemoptysis *(Red Flag 1)* (cancer, infections)
- Sputum production (infections)
- Nasal congestion or pressure (postnasal drip)
- Weight loss (cancer)
- Medications
- Duration (acute vs. chronic cough)
- Shortness of breath (cancer, chronic obstructive pulmonary disease [COPD], CHF)
- Leg swelling (CHF)
- Wheezing (asthma, COPD, foreign body)
- Chest pain
- Past medical history

 3 - When a cough occurs predominantly at night, consider GERD, asthma, or CHF.

 1 - Hemoptysis, weight loss, and shortness of breath may signify a more serious underlying problem. Malignancy or serious infections such as pneumonia or tuberculosis need to be considered.

"What makes it better?"

"What makes it worse?"

"How is your cough affecting your lifestyle, job, school, or household performance?" Ask about:

- Occupation and satisfaction with work
- Work environment and triggers (dust, chemicals)
- Interference with social activities
- Concern for serious underlying disease

Physical Examination

- General appearance of the patient
- Observation of respiratory effort, accessory muscle usage
- Vitals and temperature (infections)

- Cardiac auscultation (CHF)
- Pulmonary auscultation and percussion (asthma, COPD, CHF)
- Extremities: note edema (CHF)
- Abdominal palpation: note mid-epigastric pain (GERD)
- HEENT
    Nares, pharynx, and ears *(Brain 4)*
    Lymph nodes (cancer, sarcoid, infections)

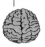

4 - Irritation of the tympanic membrane (from a hair or foreign body) can cause a cough.

Testing

The majority of patients do not require extensive testing. A medication trial based on the suggested diagnosis from the history and physical is all that is needed (e.g., decongestants or first-generation antihistamines *[Brain 5]* for postnasal drip). If this is not helpful, tests should follow in accordance with the abnormal historical or physical findings. If no specific disorder is suggested, postnasal drip, asthma, GERD, and chronic bronchitis should be of concern. They can all present without other symptoms except for the presence of cough. Sinusitis can cause occult postnasal drip. Sinus x-rays or a CT of the sinuses can diagnose this disorder. Other tests to consider are an esophageal pH probe for GERD, a **methacholine challenge test** *(Definition 3)* for asthma, or pulmonary function tests for chronic bronchitis. A chest x-ray can also be obtained for chronic cough. Although this does not diagnose the common disorders that cause the chronic cough (postnasal drip, GERD, asthma), it does help to rule out serious causes of cough. These include malignancies, CHF, pulmonary fibrosis, bronchiectasis, or occult infection. If any red flags are present (see Red Flag 1), a chest x-ray should definitely be ordered.

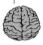

5 - The newer nonsedating antihistamines help postnasal drip only when dealing with histamine-mediated conditions such as allergic rhinitis. The first-generation antihistamines work via their anticholinergic actions.

3 - Methacholine challenge test: Inhalant stimulating bronchoconstriction in patients with occult asthma.

Putting It All Together

Patients who present with a cough generally require no intervention other than symptomatic care. With a history of a current or recent infection, reassurance is all that is necessary. Cough secondary to a respiratory infection usually is self-limited. If the cough lasts more than 8 weeks, further evaluation is required. Appropriate testing is guided by the history and physical exam. In the absence of abnormal findings, the first step is to stop any offending medications. ACE inhibitors are the most common medications to cause a cough. A cough due to a medication generally subsides within a few days. Smoking cessation should also be encouraged. Cough secondary to smoking will usually be better in a few weeks. If cough does not improve, a chest x-ray should be ordered to rule out serious underlying disease. The next step is to search for the common causes of cough. Postnasal drip, GERD, asthma, and chronic bronchitis account for 90% of chronic coughs. Cough can be a source of lost productivity and cause concern that a serious medical problem exists. The tests mentioned in the previous section will allow you to quickly evaluate the patient and perhaps minimize their psychosocial issues.

Management

Therapy for cough will be effective only if treating the underlying cause. Antitussive therapy for a cough that serves no useful function (clearing foreign matter), such as a postviral bronchitis, can be achieved with dextromethorphan *(Brain 6)*. Other options include the use of narcotics. Codeine is the most common and can be used in combination with dextromethorphan.

Postnasal drip is best treated with decongestants. However, antihistamines can also be used. The newer, nonsedating antihistamines are effective only in histamine-mediated conditions such as allergic rhinitis. Many patients request antibiotics to treat their cough. This may be appropriate if the underlying condition is sinusitis or otitis. Other upper respiratory tract infections, laryngitis, and bronchitis are usually viral. Thus, they require only symptomatic care.

Asthma is initially treated with inhaled beta$_2$ agonists. If cough persists, inhaled corticosteroids can be added. GERD initially should be managed with lifestyle changes *(Brain 7)* with consideration of medications to block acid production or a prokinetic agent. Chronic bronchitis is approached by removing the stimuli (cigarettes or other chemical irritants) or treating with an ipratropium bromide inhaler. Failure of a specific treatment suggests that the diagnosis of the underlying cause is incorrect or that a second process exists. Common pitfalls include forgetting that the above disorders often present with minimal historical or physical exam findings and can coexist. Other pitfalls include failure to stop smoking, not recognizing a medication side effect, or using inappropriate antitussive therapy. Expectorants and mucolytics will not suppress a cough. Do not forget to consider other underlying diseases. Although they tend to present with historical and physical exam findings, the other diagnoses listed in the differential diagnosis section can be silent, too! Patients can be reassured that a diagnosis can be made 90% of the time. Patience is required because it can take months for a cough to subside even with appropriate therapy. For coughs that elude diagnosis, consider referral to a specialist or that the cough is psychogenic.

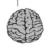

6 - Ipratropium bromide has also been shown to be effective for a cough that follows a respiratory infection (postviral bronchitis).

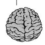

7 - Lifestyle changes include weight loss, elevating the head of the bed, and avoiding products that promote reflux. Common triggers include caffeine, mint, alcohol, chocolate, and cigarettes.

Selected Readings

1. Dowell SF, Schwartz B, Phillips WR: Appropriate use of antibiotics for uris in children: Part II: Cough, pharyngitis, and the common cold. Am Fam Physician 58:1335–1343, 1998.
2. French CL, Irwin RS, Curley FJ, Krikorian CJ: Impact of chronic cough on quality of life. Arch Intern Med 158:1657–1661, 1998.
3. Irwin RS: Silencing chronic cough. Hosp Practice 34:53–60, 1999.
4. Irwin RS, Madison JM: The diagnosis and treatment of cough. N Engl J Med 343:1715–1721, 2001.
5. Meyer AA, Aitken PV: Evaluation of persistent cough in children. Primary Care 23:883–891,1996.
6. Schappert SM: National ambulatory medical care survey: Summary. Vital Health Stat 230:1–20, 1993.
7. Smyrnois NA, Irwin RS: Approach to the patient with cough. In Kelly WN (ed): Kelly's Textbook of Internal Medicine, 3rd ed. Philadelphia, Lippincott-Raven, 1997.

26. Cough in Infants and Children

C. Gerald Judy, MD

Synopsis

Cough is a symptom of respiratory disease and is not an illness in itself. It is one of the most frequent symptoms in pediatric illnesses *(Definition 1)*. A cough that persists beyond the duration that one would expect from a viral respiratory illness (7 days to 3 weeks) warrants a thorough diagnostic investigation. Common causes of chronic or recurrent cough include respiratory tract infections at any level, asthma, foreign body inhalation, cystic fibrosis (CF), bronchopulmonary dysplasia (chronic lung disease of infancy), chronic sinusitis, smoking (active and passive), gastroesophageal reflux disease (GERD), and psychogenic cough.

If the cough persists for more than 6 weeks, rare causes of chronic cough should be considered. These include congenital anomalies of the airways and lung parenchyma, trauma, uncommon infections, immunologic abnormalities, tumor, and chronic interstitial lung disease.

The differential diagnosis of chronic cough is extensive. A thorough history and physical examination should guide the diagnostic approach. Treatment is based on the etiology and not the symptom (cough). Referral or consultation should be considered if the diagnosis remains unclear after the initial work-up or if the patient presents with respiratory distress without an obvious cause or failure to thrive, steatorrhea *(Definition 2)*, or digital clubbing *(Definition 3) (Red Flag 1)*.

 1 - Chronic cough: A sudden, explosive forcing of air through the glottis, excited by an effort to expel mucus or other matter from the bronchial tubes or larynx, persisting longer than 3 weeks.

 2 - Steatorrhea: Fatty stools; the passage of large amounts of fat in the feces.

 3 - Digital clubbing: Broadening and thickening of the ends of the fingers, seen in, but not limited to, chronic pulmonary diseases.

 1 - The infant or child that presents with cyanosis, severe respiratory distress, or stridor may require hospitalization.

Differential Diagnosis

Because the differential diagnosis of chronic cough is so extensive, the history and physical examination should guide the work-up in order to limit the number of diagnostic tests.

The most common etiologies of chronic cough are viral respiratory tract infections of the airways and lung parenchyma, asthma, GERD, and CF. Persistent or recurrent pneumonia, congestive heart failure (CHF), foreign body aspiration, CF, asthma, and immune deficiency disorders are the most likely disorders to cause potentially serious problems either acutely or long-term.

Common Causes of Cough in Childhood

- Trauma: foreign body in tracheobronchial tree
- Infection: pneumonia, pharyngitis, laryngotracheobronchitis, sinusitis, pertussis, and influenza
- Toxin: hydrocarbon ingestion, tobacco, wood-burning stove
- Inflammatory: asthma, allergy

- Metabolic-genetic: CF
- Circulatory: CHF
- Multiple etiologic causes: GERD, bronchopulmonary dysplasia (BPD), and psychogenic cough

Uncommon Causes of Cough in Childhood

- Trauma: foreign body in the ear or esophagus
- Infection: tuberculosis, *Pneumocystis carinii,* cytomegalovirus (CMV), visceral larva migrans, schistosomiasis, psittacosis, mycosis, humidifier fever (protozoa), rickettsiae, and hydatid cyst
- Immunologic: AIDS, congenital and other immune deficiency disorders, vasculitis, sarcoidosis, and hypersensitivity pneumonitis
- Tumors: T-cell leukemia, lymphoma, and teratoma
- Congenital: tracheoesophageal (TE) fistula vascular rings and slings, laryngomalacia, tracheomalacia, tracheobronchomalacia, bronchogenic cysts, pulmonary sequestrations, and cystic adenomatoid malformations
- Multiple etiologic causes: bronchiectasis, chronic interstitial lung disease

History

The medical history usually begins with the history of present illness. If the chief complaint is chronic cough in an infant, it may be more appropriate to begin with the antenatal, birth, and neonatal history.

- "What was the duration of pregnancy?"
    Full-term (suggests no prenatal or perinatal risk factors)
    Prematurity and degree of prematurity are risks for hyaline membrane disease (HMD) or respiratory distress syndrome (RDS)
- "What medicines did you take during pregnancy?" (Medicines may contribute to congenital anomalies.)
- "Did you smoke during your pregnancy, or does anyone in the house smoke now?" (Passive and second-hand cigarette smoke is an irritant to the airway.)
- "Was meconium suctioned from the airway at birth?" (possible meconium aspiration pneumonitis and its complications, i.e., BPD)
- "Did the baby require intubation and mechanical ventilation?" (Length of ventilation > 7 days has risk for BPD.)
- "What was the duration of oxygen requirement?" (> 30 days has increased risk for BPD.)
- "Does the baby have 'noisy breathing' while awake that disappears with sleep?" (laryngomalacia)
- "What age did the cough begin?" (Differentiate congenital from acquired etiologies.)
- "Describe the cough [dry, hacking, brassy, wet sounding]?" (infectious vs. noninfectious etiology)
- "When does the cough occur?" (Psychogenic cough typically occurs only during the day and in the presence of others.)
- "Is cough present at night or associated with wheezing, dyspnea, exercise, laughing, and exposure to cold air?" (asthma)
- "Is cough seasonal?" (allergy, asthma)
- "Does cough occur with feedings or shortly after feedings?" (aspiration, TE fistula, GERD)

Findings Associated with Cough That May Give Clue to Etiology

- Cough occurs in paroxysms followed by redness of face, cyanosis, ending with a "whoop" (pertussis or parapertussis)
- Cough produces green-brown, foul-smelling sputum with malodorous breath **(bronchiectasis)** *(Definition 4)*
- Temperature (infectious etiology)
- Hemoptysis (trauma, infection, congenital anomalies, hemosiderosis)
- Hemoptysis with anemia and recurrent pneumonia **(hemosiderosis)** *(Definition 5)*
- Diarrhea, steatorrhea, failure to thrive (CF)

- Recurrent pneumonia (immune deficiency, CF, anatomic abnormalities, dysfunctional swallowing, aspiration, bronchiectasis, GERD, **primary ciliary dyskinesia** *[Definition 6])*
- Neurodevelopmental delay and muscular dystrophies (aspiration syndromes)
- History of atopy, eczema, atopic dermatitis, hay fever (asthma)
- History of frequent infections, poor growth or failure to thrive, one or both parents having numerous sexual partners, parental substance abuse (HIV or AIDS)
- Exposure to gaseous toxins or hydrocarbon ingestion (chronic interstitial lung disease)
- Exposure to sick birds **(psittacosis)** *(Definition 7)*
- Exposure to tuberculosis (TB)
- Currently living or ever lived in an area endemic to TB
- History of TE fistula repair (tracheomalacia and GERD)

4 - Bronchiectasis: Dilation of a bronchus or the bronchial tubes commonly described as being cylindrical or saccular and resulting from chronic infection.

5 - Hemosiderosis: The accumulation of hemosiderin (an iron-containing substance) in any tissue.

6 - Primary ciliary dyskinisia: An inherited disorder characterized by specific ultra-structural defects of the cilia causing associated impairment of ciliary motion and mucociliary clearance.

Dietary History

- In children younger than 5–6 years: "Does the child consume nuts or soybeans?" (foreign body aspiration)
- "Does the child place toys or inanimate objects in mouth frequently while playing?" (foreign body aspiration)

7 - Psittacosis: A form of pneumonitis caused by the bacteria *Chlamydia psittaci*, usually transmitted to humans by inhalation of the bacteria from bird droppings, feathers, and dust.

Family History

- "Has any relative had chronic bronchitis, wheezy bronchitis, asthmatic bronchitis, asthma, eczema, tuberculosis, or other chronic lung disease?"
- "Are the child's immunizations current?" (pertussis)

Social History

- Parent's employment (possible exposure to toxins causing chronic interstitial lung disease or hypersensitivity pneumonitis)
- "Does the child attend day care? (increased exposure to viral respiratory illnesses)
- In older children, it is important to elicit hobbies (exposure to dusts, paint, glue, and other fumes)
- Age of dwelling, presence of basement, recent renovations, number and type of animals in the home, the presence of composite furniture, waterbeds, carpets, ceiling tile (all of which contain volatile aldehydes that may complicate asthma)

Physical Examination

General Appearance

- Cachexia (malnutrition, muscle wasting, and pallor all suggest a serious, chronic illness)
- Respiratory distress, difficulty breathing **(Red Flag 2)**

2 - Tachypnea; nasal flaring; suprasternal, supraclavicular or suprasternal notch; sternal, intercostal, or subcostal retractions and paradoxic respirations all suggest respiratory distress and warrant immediate evaluation.

HEENT

- Foreign body in the external canal (cough receptors located in external canal)

- Transverse nasal crease (inhalant allergies)
- Dark circles under the eyes ("allergic shiners")
- Widening of nasal bridge and "grape-like clusters" observed in nasi (nasal polyps suggesting chronic allergic disease or CF)
- Nasal mucosa edematous, boggy, and pale in appearance with clear secretions (allergic rhinitis)
- Inflamed nasal mucosa with edema, mucopurulent, foul-smelling blood-tinged discharge (infectious process such as chronic sinusitis or foreign body)
- Retrognathia, micrognathia, macroglossia (all contribute to upper airway obstruction, which may contribute to chronic aspiration of upper airway secretions and chronic aspiration pneumonitis)
- State of oral and dental hygiene (dental caries causing increased volume of bacteria with chronic microaspiration may cause chronic pneumonitis)
- Oral thrush and leukoplasia (immune deficiency disorders)
- Size of uvula (long uvula may cause chronic cough)
- Abnormal or poor motion of uvula (suggests cranial nerve palsy, which may be associated with dysfunctional swallowing and aspiration)
- Foul breath (bronchiectasis)
- Tracheal deviation (neck mass, foreign body aspiration with atelectasis or hyperinflation due to air trapping, lymphoma, or other tumor-causing external tracheal compression, and chronic cough)
- Character of voice (hoarseness or weak cry suggests vocal cord dysfunction and recurrent aspiration)

Chest

- Barrel-chest deformity (chronic obstructive lung disease such as CF or poorly controlled asthma)
- Asymmetry of chest (cardiomegaly and congestive heart failure)
- Harrison's groove or sulcus (horizontal depression in lower thoracic cage at the site of diaphragmatic attachment suggesting chronic increased work of breathing (pulmonary fibrosis, CF, poorly controlled asthma)
- Shallow, rapid respirations (parenchymal lung disease)
- Prolonged expiration (obstructive lung disease)
- Decreased fremitus (airway obstruction, pleural fluid, and pleural thickening)
- Increased fremitus (parenchymal consolidation)
- Dullness to percussion (pleural fluid or parenchymal consolidation)

Lungs

- Bronchial breath sounds in periphery of lung (parenchymal consolidation)
- Bronchovesicular breath sounds (lung consolidation)
- Wheezing (polyphonic suggests obstructive lung disease such as asthma)
- Stridor (extrathoracic airway obstruction)
- Fine inspiratory crackles (bronchitis, pneumonia, pulmonary infarction, atelectasis, and chronic interstitial lung disease)
- Coarse crackles (bronchiectasis such as one would find in advanced CF)

Heart

- Murmurs (CHF)

Abdomen

- Masses (lymphoma and other tumors)

Lymph Nodes

- Peripheral adenopathy (lymphoma, HIV)

Extremities

• Digital clubbing (chronic lung disease such as CF)

Neurologic

• Muscle weakness, localized or generalized neurologic signs (aspiration pneumonitis)

Diagnostic Tests

The diagnostic tests should be guided by the findings of a thorough history and physical examination. Diagnostic tests should begin with the least invasive. A minimal exam would be a chest x-ray. Other diagnostic studies may include:

• Barium esophagram (TE fistula, vascular rings and slings, GERD)
• Feeding and swallowing study (aspiration, laryngeal webs, and clefts)
• Computed tomography (CT) scan of the sinuses (chronic sinusitis)
• CT scan of the neck and chest (suspected masses, adenopathy, interstitial lung disease, congenital anomalies)
• Magnetic resonance imaging (MRI) (vascular anomalies, including vascular ring)
• Pulmonary function tests, including bronchoprovocation, basic spirometry, pre- and postbronchodilator spirometry, lung volumes and diffusion capacity (asthma, CF, restrictive lung disease, chronic interstitial pneumonitis and fibrosis)
• Esophageal pH monitoring (GERD)
• Allergy testing (asthma)
• Complete blood count (CB) (anemia, leukocytosis, leukopenia, eosinophilia)
• Quantitative/immunoglobulins (IgA, IgG and subclasses, IgM, IgE)
• Sputum culture and sensitivity (infections)
• Sweat chloride test (CF)
• TB skin test (tuberculosis)
• Lymph node biopsy (lymphoma, sarcoidosis, histoplasmosis)
• Sedimentation rate (chronic inflammatory diseases)
• Serum angiotensin-converting enzyme (ACE) (sarcoidosis)
• HIV testing
• Nasal epithelial scrapings or airway biopsy (ciliary evaluation)
• Bronchoscopy and bronchoalveolar lavage (BAL) (infections, airway anatomy, foreign body)
• Open lung biopsy (interstitial lung disease, uncommon infections or opportunistic infections
• More complete immune work-up

Putting It All Together

Cough is one of the most common chief complaints in pediatrics and has a long list of causes. Without some guidance the evaluation of this complaint could consume a lot of valuable time and resources.

The majority of time, the etiology of cough can be determined by the history and physical examination with few diagnostic tests required. Important clues to etiology can be obtained by noting the age at the onset of cough, the character of the cough, whether or not the cough occurs only during the day, and whether or not there is any associated temperature *(Red Flag 3)*. A cough that is continuous day and night but worse at night suggests asthma, CF, or other processes causing bronchiectasis. Cough absent during sleep is highly suggestive of psychogenic cough. The presence of family or school conflicts may support the suspicion of psychogenic cough. A history of choking or gagging episodes with the occurrence of the cough suggests possible foreign body aspiration. Signs or symptoms of chronic illness such as poor growth, recurrent fevers, and purulent sputum should prompt a search for more severe pulmonary or systemic disease. A careful feeding and neurologic history may point to chronic aspiration or GERD as a cause of the cough.

The physical examination should be complete, with emphasis on the head and neck, chest, and cardiovascular examination.

3 - In infants, persistent cough (> 3 weeks) should always be considered abnormal. For children older than 1 year of age, a cough that persists for more than 6 weeks is uncommon and should be taken seriously.

The laboratory evaluation should be directed by findings elicited in the history and physical examination. The more common tests will include a chest radiograph, pulmonary function testing, CT, MRI, barium esophagram, esophageal pH monitoring, and bronchoscopy. Laboratory studies that may be helpful include a CBC with differential, quantitative immunoglobulins, sweat test, TB skin test and other skin tests, ciliary epithelial scrapings, or biopsies and allergy testing. It may also be reasonable to include an empiric trial of bronchodilator therapy or a short course of systemic steroids to prove or disprove asthma as an etiology for the chronic cough.

Management

Therapy of chronic cough is targeted at the cause. A trial of therapy (e.g., a beta-agonist for presumptive asthma) is often helpful.

Consultation may be necessary if the diagnosis remains unclear after the initial work-up or if the patient presents with respiratory distress without an obvious cause, failure to thrive, steatorrhea, finger clubbing, or poor general health.

The infant or child who presents with cyanosis, severe respiratory distress, or stridor may require hospitalization.

Selected Readings

1. Behrman RE (ed.): Nelson Textbook of Pediatrics, 14th ed. Philadelphia, W.B. Saunders, 1992.
2. Chernick D, Boat TF, Kindig EL (eds): Kindig's Disorders of the Respiratory Tract in Children, 6th ed. Philadelphia, W.B. Saunders, 1998.
3. Taussig LM, Landau LI (eds): Pediatric Respiratory Medicine. St. Louis, Mosby, 1999.

27. Diabetes

Douglas H. Wheatley, MD

Synopsis

Diabetes is a disease of abnormal glucose metabolism resulting in high blood sugars and is diagnosed on the basis of standardized criteria. The history and physical examination are the cornerstones for treating the diabetic patient. The goals of the visit with the diabetic patient are to gather information, set treatment goals, and motivate adherence. Treatment goals and strategies vary depending on whether the patient has type 1 or 2 diabetes mellitus, age, economic resources, educational background, presence of diabetic complications, and personal motivation to achieve glycemic control. Important issues to explore during the visit include blood sugar records, diet, foot care, blood pressure, and other diabetic standards. Optimal diabetic care is often best achieved with a coordinated team approach. The diabetic care team consists of a physician, nutrition specialist, pharmacist, nurse, mental health professional, and diabetic educator. When treatment goals are not met, consultation with an endocrinologist may be helpful.

Differential Diagnosis

Diabetes mellitus is a group of diseases characterized by hyperglycemia. This differential includes:

- **Type 1 diabetes.** Commonly diagnosed in children or young adults. Is thought to be immune mediated with total destruction of the insulin-producing cells in the pancreas. Exogenous insulin therapy is essential for treatment.
- **Type 2 diabetes.** This is usually diagnosed in persons older than 40, but can occur at younger ages. This is the largest group of patients with hyperglycemia. Obesity and insulin resistance are often seen in these individuals.
- **Gestational diabetes.** This is defined as hyperglycemia during pregnancy; it usually resolves after delivery. Many patients will go on to develop gestational diabetes with subsequent pregnancies and often type 2 diabetes later in life.
- **Secondary causes of diabetes.** Hyperglycemia may develop with other disease states such as cirrhosis of the liver, pancreatitis, hemochromatosis, Cushing's syndrome, acromegaly, pheochromocytoma, glucagonoma, and other endocrine abnormalities.

History

The medical history can uncover the presence of symptoms suspicious for diabetes in patients not yet diagnosed. For those with an established diagnosis of diabetes, the history helps assess the patient's compliance and understanding of their individual care plan. Routine questions may include:

- "Are you experiencing any unusual symptoms?" (symptoms suggestive of high blood sugar) *(Red Flag 1)*
- "Have you experienced any symptoms suggestive of low blood sugars?" *(Red Flag 2)*
    "What is the frequency and timing of low blood sugars?"
    "Is there any relationship with the timing of food intake?"
    "Do your low blood sugars occur after exercise?"

"Has there been a change in the dose of medication used to lower your blood sugar?"

"How do you manage your low blood sugar?"

- "Have you had other recent medication changes?"
- "How often and how do you test your blood sugar?"
- "Have you experienced a **coma** associated with diabetes?" *(Definition 1)* Ask about frequency, severity, and probable cause.
- "What medication do you take to control your blood sugar?
    - *Insulin.* Inquire about the type and dose of insulin taken, the time of daily administration, and the method of delivery (e.g., intermittent subcutaneous injections, continuous delivery wit an insulin pump).
    - *Oral glucose-lowering agents.* Inquire about the name(s), dosage strength, time and frequency of administration.
- "Tell me about other medications you take regularly" (both prescription and nonprescription)
- "Do you have any medication allergies?"
- "Tell me about other health problems, particularly risk factors for heart attacks and hardening of the arteries?" *(Red Flag 3)*
- "Do you have any medical complications secondary to your diabetes?" *(Red Flag 4)*
- Inquire about habits of healthy living.
    - "Tell me about your diet?" (total calories per day and timing of consumption)
    - "When do you exercise?" (type, frequency, and time commitment)
    - "Do you smoke?" (type and frequency of use) *(Brain 1)*
    - "How much alcohol do you drink?" (type and frequency) (see Brain 1)
    - "How do you manage stress?"
    - "How often do you have a **glycated hemoglobin** obtained?" *(Definition 2).* Ask for results
    - "Are your immunizations current?" *(Red Flag 5)*
    - "Do you wear a diabetic identification bracelet or necklace?"
- Ask about factors that may influence the patient's ability to manage his or her diabetes (e.g., cultural, educational, economic, health insurance availability, psychosocial).
    - "Do you have support from family, friends, and coworkers with your diabetes?"
    - "Overall, are you pleased with the way you are managing your diabetes?"

Physical Examination

The physical examination should pay close attention to organ systems in which patients with diabetes may experience complications. Generally, one should evaluate the following:

- General observation (does the patient appear in any distress?)
- Complete set of vital signs with temperature *(Red Flag 6)*
- Eye examination (with ophthalmoscope) looking for **retinopathy** *(Definition 3) (Figures 1 and 2)*
- Oral exam: check dentition
- Neck: palpate thyroid

1 - Symptoms of hyperglycemia include excessive thirst, excessive urination, blurred vision, fatigue, and unexplained weight loss.

2 - Symptoms suggestive of hypoglycemia include fatigue, shaking, sweating, irritability, impaired cognition, and loss of consciousness. These symptoms are neither sensitive nor specific.

1 - Ketoacidosis: A complex metabolic disturbance developing as a consequence of insulin deficiency and an excess of insulin counterregulatory hormones, usually occurring in individuals with type 1 diabetes.

Hyperosmolar coma: A problem of hyperglycemia and hyperosmolarity, occurring in individuals with poorly controlled type 2 diabetes. Like ketoacidosis, this can be fatal if not aggressively managed. It often is precipitated by an underlying problem such as infection.

3 - Atherosclerosis, commonly described as "hardening of the arteries," is one of the many complications patients with diabetes may develop after several years of uncontrolled blood sugars. Other risk factors for atherosclerosis include obesity, smoking, hypertension, hyperlipidemia, and a family history of atherosclerotic cardiovascular disease.

4 - Medical complications secondary to years of uncontrolled blood sugars include blindness, renal failure, nerve damage, heart disease, and skin changes. It is important to evaluate these symptoms during the history, physical examination, and laboratory assessments.

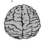
1 - Diabetics, at risk for morbidity and premature death from atherosclerosis, should avoid addictive behaviors that may accelerate this process.

2 - Glycated hemoglobin (sometimes called HbA$_{1c}$): A blood test that estimates a patient's average glucose for the prior 3 months.

5 - Patients with diabetes should receive all routine immunizations, including a pneumococcal vaccine, and a yearly influenza vaccine.

6 - The target blood pressure for an adult diabetic is 130/80 or less.

- Heart exam: auscultate for rhythm and murmurs
- Abdomen: auscultate for bowel sounds and bruits, palpate for masses or organomegaly
- Pulses: palpate for peripheral pulses, auscultate for presence of bruits)
- Skin: check for presence of rash, examine injection sites if the patient is receiving insulin
- Hands and feet: evaluate for infection or dermal ulcers, check for sensation
- Neurologic: screen for possible neuropathy by checking sensation in the upper and lower extremities—a special monofilament is available to test for **neuropathy (Definition 4)**

 3 - Retinopathy: Damage to the retina of the eye in diabetics who have experienced several years of poorly controlled blood sugars. This results in damaged blood vessels to the eye and can lead to blindness.

 4 - Neuropathy: Degenerative changes in the peripheral nerves involving both sensory and motor function. The most typical pattern is sensory loss involving the hands and feet.

Testing

The diagnosis of diabetes rests with the demonstration of abnormal blood glucose *(Table 1)*. The clinic should be capable of performing immediate blood sugar and urine ketone results. Other tests used to assess the diabetic include:

- Glycated hemoglobin (quarterly, if treatment goals not met; twice yearly, if goals met)
- Fasting lipid panel (yearly; less frequently if normal)
- Urinalysis (check for presence of glucose, ketones, and protein)
- Serum creatinine and blood urea nitrogen (to evaluate renal function)
- Urine test for microscopic albumin (yearly, if urinalysis negative for protein)
- Electrocardiogram (baseline, for adults)
- 24-hour urine collection to determine creatinine clearance and total protein excretion

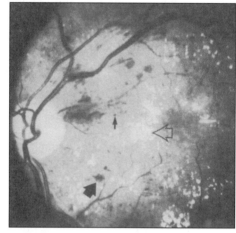

Figure 1: Nonproliferative diabetic retinopathy with abundant mascular exudate *(open arrow)*, microaneurysms *(small arrows)*, and intraretinal hemorrhage *(large arrow)*.
(From Vaughan D, Asbury T, Riordan-Eva P: General Ophthalmology, 14th ed. Stamford, CT, Appleton & Lange, 1995, with permission.)

Table 1. Criteria for the Diagnosis of Diabetes

Normoglycemia	Impaired Glucose Metabolism	Diabetes Mellitus*
FPG < 110 mg/dl	FPG ≥ 110 and < 126 mg/dl	FPG ≥ 126 mg/dl
2-hr PG < 140 mg/dl	2-hr PG ≥ 140 and < 200 mg/dl	2-hr PG ≥ 200 mg/dl** or Symptoms of diabetes and a random PG of ≥ 20 mg/dl

FPG = fasting plasma glucose; PG = plasma glucose.

*A diagnosis of diabetes must be confirmed, on a subsequent day, by measurement of fasting glucose, 2-hour plasma glucose, or random plasma glucose (if symptoms present). Fasting is defined as no caloric intake for at least 8 hours.
**This test requires the use of a glucose load containing the equivalent of 75-g anhydrous glucose dissolved in water.

Adapted from American Diabetes Association: Clinical practice recommendations 1998: Screening for type 2 diabetes. Diabetes Care 21(S1):S21, 1998.

Putting It All Together

An organized medical record, with an individualized therapeutic plan, is essential to ensure that goals to achieve glycemic control are being reached. Impress upon the patient that individuals who meet guidelines

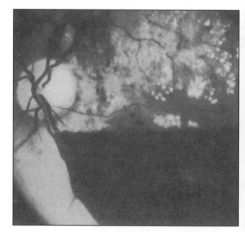

Figure 2: Proliferative diabetic retinopathy with preretinal hemorrhage obscuring the inferior macula. Macular exudate, microaneurysms, and intraretinal hemorrhages are also present.
(From Vaughan D, Asbury T, Riordan-Eva P: General Ophthalmology, 14th ed. Stamford, CT, Appleton & Lange, 1995, with permission.)

for controlling their blood sugars may delay or postpone the onset of diabetic microvascular complications. Also, empower the diabetic patient to be an active participant in management decisions.

Management

The history and physical examination are geared to assess diabetic patients' knowledge of their disease, determine how well they are controlling their blood sugar, and identify diabetic complications. The goals for glycemic control are outlined in *Table 2*. Additionally, goals for blood pressure, lipids *(Table 3)*, and smoking cessation (as appropriate) are important. Remember to address psychosocial or occupational issues that may hinder the patients' ability to manage their diabetes well. Standardized guidelines for the care of adults with diabetes, available from the American Diabetes Association, are helpful to ensure that therapeutic recommendations are being addressed *(Table 4)*. Encourage diabetic patients to be actively involved in the management of their disease. Don't forget to utilize the team approach to care, with input from other health care professionals, to assist the diabetic with disease management.

Follow-up with the diabetic should be scheduled periodically in the office and may be supplemented by phone or electronic mail. How well the disease is managed, the type of diabetes the patient has, and the presence of diabetic complications are all factors that help determine the frequency of office visits. When treatment goals are not achieved, consultation with an endocrinologist is appropriate.

Table 2. Glycemic Control for People with Diabetes (Plasma Values)

Biochemical Index	Normal	Goal	Action Suggested
Preprandial glucose	< 110 mg/dl	80–120 mg/dl	< 80 or > 140 mg/dl
Bedtime glucose	< 120 mg/dl	100–140 mg/dl	< 100 or > 160 mg/dl
Glycated hemoglobin	< 6%	< 7%	> 8%

Adapted from American Diabetes Association: Clinical practice recommendations 1998: Standards of medical care for patients with diabetes mellitus. Diabetes Care 21(S1):S24, 1998.

Table 3. Lipid Levels for Adult Diabetics

Risk	HDL Cholesterol* (mg/dl)	LDL Cholesterol (mg/dl)	Triglycerides (mg/dl)
High	< 35	> 130	≥ 400
Borderline	35–45	100–129	200–399
Low	> 45	< 100	< 200

*For women, HDL cholesterol values should be increased by 10 mg/dl.

From American Diabetes Association: Standards of medical care for patients with diabetes mellitus. Diabetes Care 22(suppl 1):S57, 1999.

Table 4. Diabetes Continuing Care Standards

Parameter	ADA Recommended Frequency
Glucose Control*	
HbA$_{1c}$	2–4 times a year
Self-monitoring of blood glucose	As directed
Cardiovascular Assessment*	
Blood pressure	Every visit
Lipids	Annually
EKG	As needed
Other Exams*	
Eyes dilated	Annually
Feet	At least annually
Urinalysis for protein	Annually
Weight**	Every visit
Microalbumin	At least annually if urinalysis negative for protein
Other Goals*	
Exercise	
Smoking cessation	
Improve nutrition	
Education*	
Knowledge of diabetes	Annually
Knowledge of self-management skills	Annually

*Special attention, specialist referral, or counseling may be necessary.
**Nondiabetic range of HbA$_{1c}$ is 4–6%.

Adapted from American Diabetes Association: Clinical practice recommendations 1998: Standards of medical care for patients with diabetes mellitus. Diabetes Care 21:S1, 1998.

Selected Readings

1. American Diabetes Association: Standards of medical care for patients with diabetes mellitus. Diabetes Care 22(suppl 1):S32–S41,1999.
2. American Diabetes Association: Implications of the diabetes control and complications trial. Diabetes Care 22(suppl1):S26,1999.
3. American Diabetes Association: Diabetic nephropathy. Diabetes Care 22(suppl1):S66–S69,1999.
4. American Diabetes Association: Tests of glycemia in diabetes. Diabetes Care 22(suppl1):S77–S79,1999.
5. Haffner M: Management of dyslipidemia in adults with diabetes. Diabetes Care 21:160–178,1998.
6. Vaughan D, Asbury T, Riordan-Eva P: General Ophthalmology, 14th ed. Stamford, CT, Appleton & Lange, 1995.

Web Sites

American Diabetes Association: www.diabetes.org

National Kidney Foundation: www.kidney.org

28. Difficulty Breathing and Shortness of Breath

Debra J. Romberger, MD

Synopsis

Many clinical conditions cause patients to complain of shortness of breath. The most common causes are related to either pulmonary or cardiac conditions, but disorders involving skeletal muscles and **respiratory drive** *(Definition 1)* may also cause this symptom. The history and physical exam are very important in determining if the underlying cause is acute and potentially life threatening in contrast to either a less severe acute problem or a progressive chronic condition. Common causes of shortness of breath in adults include infections such as bronchitis and pneumonia, asthma, chronic obstructive pulmonary disease, coronary artery disease, congestive heart failure, and pulmonary embolus. Although a variety of tests may be appropriate, testing useful in most patients includes a chest x-ray, spirometry, and an assessment of oxygenation with either oximetry or an arterial blood gas. Management often includes medications, but is focused on the most likely diagnosis based on both history and physical examination. Smoking cessation should be addressed with all patients who are still smoking. Other lifestyle issues, such as exposures at work or in the home environment, may also be important.

1 - Respiratory drive: Respiratory drive refers to the central nervous system control of breathing. Several types of receptors respond to changes in chemical composition of blood and mechanical changes of lung tissue, for example, and provide feedback to the regions of the brain that control breathing.

Differential Diagnosis

The differential diagnosis for patients with **dyspnea** *(Definition 2)* is broad and includes diseases affecting the lungs, heart, respiratory muscles, central nervous system, and hematologic (blood) system.

Lung Diseases

2 - Dyspnea: A sensation of breathlessness.

- Airflow obstruction. Examples include aspiration of a foreign body, asthma, chronic obstructive pulmonary disease (COPD), and cystic fibrosis.
- Restrictive lung conditions. Restriction of the lungs can be caused by changes in the pleural space from fluid (pleural effusions) or air (pneumothorax). Restriction within the lung interstitium may be related to infections (pneumonia), occupation (e.g., asbestos) or organic dust exposures (hypersensitivity pneumonitis), systemic diseases (e.g., sarcoidosis, systemic lupus erythematosus), cancer (primary lung cancer or metastases from other sources), or idiopathic pulmonary fibrosis (IPF) (scarring of the lung of unknown etiology).
- Vascular diseases. Examples include pulmonary embolus and pulmonary hypertension.

Cardiac Diseases

- Congestive heart failure with pulmonary edema (fluid in lung tissue)

- Coronary artery disease
- Valvular heart disease
- Pericardial effusion (fluid around the heart)
- Pericarditis (inflammation of the lining of the heart)

Respiratory Muscle Diseases

- Neuromuscular diseases, such as myasthenia gravis, Guillain-Barré syndrome, and amyotrophic lateral sclerosis (ALS)
- Muscular dystrophies and muscle disorders (or myopathies) such as those induced by medications including glucocorticoids
- Physical deconditioning

Central Nervous System Diseases

- Metabolic conditions such as diabetic ketoacidosis and fever increase respiratory drive, which causes patients to feel short of breath.
- Panic attacks are associated with shortness of breath.

Hematologic System

Anemia can cause dyspnea related to reduction in the oxygen carrying capacity of blood *(Brain 1)*.

History

- "When did you first notice feeling short of breath? Did it begin suddenly or slowly become noticeable?" This helps distinguish between an acute or chronic process *(Red Flag 1)*.
- "When does the shortness of breath occur? Does it occur with exertion, at rest, or both? Does it awaken you from sleep?" *(Brain 2)*
- "Does anything seem to bring on the shortness of breath?" Possible triggers especially for asthma include walking outside in the cold, strong smells such as perfumes, smoky rooms, exercise, certain foods, work environments, stressful situations.
- "Are you experiencing other symptoms?"
  1. Fever, chills, night sweats (signs of infection or other systemic illnesses)
  2. Cough with or without sputum (Discolored sputum may sugge bacterial infection.)
  3. Hemoptysis *(Red Flag 2)*
  4. Weight loss, change in appetite, skin rashes, joint pains, muscle weakness (Such constitutional symptoms may indicate a systemic disease process.)
  5. Chest pain or chest tightness (Substernal chest pain or pain that radiates into the arm or jaw may suggest angina.)
  6. Heartburn, nausea, or vomiting (Gastroesophageal reflux disease can exacerbate asthma.)
  7. Swelling of legs (This may be a sign of heart failure if it is bilateral or a sign of deep venous thrombosis if unilateral.)
- "Have you ever had trouble with your breathing before?"
  1. Asthma as a child (Some asthmatics have symptoms in childhood that remit in young adulthood and then later recur.)
  2. Previous hospitalizations for lung or cardiac problems

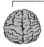

1 - Pulmonary and cardiac causes of dyspnea are most common and should be considered first. Conditions affecting respiratory muscles or the central nervous system should be considered when the history, exam, and testing do not suggest primary lung or heart disease.

1 - Sudden onset of significant shortness of breath is often associated with potentially life-threatening acute conditions such as pulmonary embolus, myocardial infarction, pulmonary edema, pneumothorax, an asthma attack, and severe allergic reactions with swelling of vocal cords. All of these conditions require prompt evaluation and treatment.

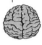

2 - Awakening at night short of breath may be a symptom of poorly controlled asthma. Paroxysmal nocturnal dyspnea (PND), episodes of awakening short of breath that improves by sitting up on the edge of the bed, is also seen in congestive heart failure.

2 - The most common cause of coughing up blood (hemoptysis) in the United States is bronchitis. However, tuberculosis is the most common cause of hemoptysis worldwide. Hemoptysis can be seen with a variety of other conditions, including lung cancer.

- "Have you had other medical problems?"
  1. Past history of other major medical problems such as blood cl cancer, diabetes, kidney or liver disease
  2. Current medications
  3. Drug, food, or other types of allergies
- "Have you tried any medications for your breathing, either over the counter or prescription? (If the patient suspects asthma, he or she may have tried over-the-counter bronchodilators such as Primatene.)
- "Do any of your family members have lung or heart problems? Do allergies and hayfever run in your family? Has anyone had trouble with blood clots?" (Asthma and allergies may be, in part, inherited. Similarly, some disorders of blood clotting are also inherited.)
- "Are you a smoker or have you smoked in the past? " *(Brain 3)*
- "What kind of work do you do? Have you done similar work in the past or different types of jobs? What about your hobbies?" (Look for exposures that are associated with lung diseases such as asbestos, certain types of dusts, or animal or bird exposures.)

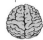
3 - Smoking is the major risk factor for COPD and lung cancer. Smoking history is typically recorded in pack years. *Example:* 1 pack per day for 20 years = 20 pack years.

Physical Examination

Look (Inspection)

Does the patient look short of breath? Note:
- Rapid breathing
- Use of accessory muscles (retraction of lower intercostal interspaces and supraclavicular fossae during inspiration)
- Pursed lip breathing (lips puckered with prolonged exhalation)
- Difficulty completing sentences when talking

What is the patient's general physical condition?
- Well-developed, frail and deconditioned, obese, etc.
- Any difficulty moving from chair to exam table?
- Is there **cyanosis** of mucous membranes or nail beds? *(Definition 3)*
- Is there **clubbing**? *(Definition 4)*
- Is the thoracic cage abnormal such as in kyphoscoliosis (backward and lateral curvature of the spine) or a barrel chest in COPD?
- Is there leg swelling?

3 - Cyanosis: Bluish discoloration of skin and mucous membranes due to excessive concentration of reduced hemoglobin in the blood. This can occur with deficient oxygenation of the blood.

4 - Clubbing: An enlargement of subcutaneous tissue in the ends of the fingers and toes.

Listen (Percussion and Auscultation)

Percussion
Solid organs (the heart) or consolidated lung tissue (firm dense material within the lung such as occurs in pneumonia) will sound dull on percussion compared to typical air-filled lungs. Percussion can be described as normal, impaired, or absent.

Breath Sounds
Determine type and location (diffusely present or localized to one area, heard during inspiration, expiration, or both). Note any:

- Wheezing, a hissing or musical sound
- Rhonchi, a snoring sound
- Crackles (sometimes called rales) are broadly classified as fine (Velcro sound, suggesting interstitial lung disease) or coarse (more suggestive of COPD and congestive heart failure)

- E-to-A changes (patient says "E" and it sounds like "A" when listening with the stethoscope, suggesting consolidated lung or a thin layer of fluid)
- Pleural friction rub (a sound produced by the rubbing together of the two pleural surfaces that occurs with inflammation and sounds like leather squeaking that varies with respiration)

Cardiac Sounds
- Regular or irregular rhythm
- Normal or abnormal S_1 and S_2
- S_3 or S_4 present? (S_4 may be normal, but S_3 usually indicates presence of congestive heart failure)
- Murmurs present?
- Pericardial friction rub (a sound produced by inflammation of the pericardium that resembles leather squeaking and varies with heart beat)

Feel (Palpation)

- Does the chest wall move during inspiration or is it restricted?
- Changes in tactile **fremitus** *(Definition 5)*
- Presence of **pulsus paradoxus** (commonly associated with constrictive pericarditis, but can be seen in pericardial effusions, emphysema, and heart failure) *(Definition 6)*

Testing

5 - Fremitus: Transmission of vibrations of spoken voice to the chest wall. It is often elicited by having patients say "99" in a loud voice and feeling for the vibrations with the hands (the edge of the hand is most sensitive in detecting changes in fremitus). In pneumonia, there is consolidation in the lungs (firm dense lung tissue) that enhances the transmission of the vibrations and increases fremitus. When fluid is in the pleural space between the lungs and the chest wall or when there is thickening of the pleural space from previous infections, fremitus is reduced.

6 - Pulsus paradoxus: A decrease in the size of the pulse or even its momentary disappearance during forced inspiration. When it occurs during quiet respiration, it is pathologic. It is best measured by using a blood pressure cuff and measuring the drop in peak systolic pressure during inspiration.

The history and physical exam will help identify which of the differential diagnoses are most relevant for the patient and will direct what testing will be required. Basic studies that are likely to be helpful include:

- Chest x-ray (posteroanterior [PA] and lateral views). These are important in demonstrating pneumonia, pleural space abnormalities (pleural effusion or pneumothorax), masses, hyperinflation (seen in significant COPD), and signs of interstitial lung disease.
- Spirometry or peak flow. Office spirometry will help assess whether airflow obstruction (such as seen in asthma or COPD) or restriction (such as seen in interstitial lung disease or congestive heart failure) is present. Alternatively, a peak flow meter can be used to determine reduction in airflow, which is useful in assessing asthma.
- Oximetry. Oxygen saturation can be measured to determine if the patient's oxygen status is acceptable (generally should be ≥ 90%) by oximeters that fit on a fingertip or an ear lobe. Alternatively, an arterial blood gas (ABG) may be needed to assess for pO_2 and pCO_2.
- Blood tests. Hemoglobin and hematocrit determine if anemia is present.
- Electrocardiogram (EKG). In patients with suspected cardiac disease, the EKG provides information about ischemia of the heart (as in myocardial infarction) as well as pericarditis and pericardial effusion.

Putting It All Together

A patient complaining of difficulty breathing may have an acute, potentially life-threatening illness that needs immediate attention (hospitalization) or a chronic condition that intermittently causes symptoms and is easily managed as an outpatient. Patients needing hospitalization are often easily identified because they are visibly working hard to breath and appear uncomfortable. Patients with hypoxemia (oxygen saturation < 90% by oximetry) also likely need hospitalization, unless they have a chronic condition for which they already have home oxygen therapy.

Patients with sudden onset of shortness of breath without signs of an asthma attack should prompt a concern for pulmonary embolus. Because the majority of pulmonary emboli arise from blood clots in the legs and pelvis (deep venous thrombosis [DVT]), patients with risk factors for DVT (e.g., being sedentary such as occurs after a recent surgery or on long trips, previous history or family history of blood clots, estrogen-containing medications, obesity) will require specialized testing to exclude the possibility of pulmonary embolus.

Asthma is a common disorder causing dyspnea and occurs in both children and adults (adults are often surprised to learn this fact). The most common trigger of asthma attacks is a viral upper respiratory tract infection, and this etiology is usually apparent from the associated infection symptoms such as fever, cough, nasal congestion, and sputum production. If there are no signs of infection, other asthma triggers such as exercise, allergies, smoking, work environment, pets, and heartburn symptoms (associated gastroesophageal reflux disease) will need to be explored with the patient.

COPD exacerbations are another common cause of dyspnea, especially in older adults. Smoking is the major risk factor for the development of COPD. Thus, COPD should be considered in all patients who are current or ex-smokers, especially in patients older than 40 years. Although most smokers with COPD do not become significantly impaired until they reach their 60s or later, patients who are especially susceptible to the damaging effects of smoking will note symptoms in their late 30s or 40s. Smoking cessation will markedly slow progression of COPD and should be strongly encouraged.

Dyspnea related to cardiac disease is also common in older adults. Patients with cardiac disease may have associated chest tightness or pain, especially when they experience dyspnea on exertion. However, dyspnea secondary to COPD and to cardiac disease may have similar symptoms and be difficult to distinguish on history and exam alone. Because smoking is a risk factor for both COPD and coronary artery disease, both conditions should be considered in older patients with a smoking history.

Many of the other conditions listed in the differential diagnosis may not be immediately apparent on the initial history and physical exam. These conditions become more likely when there is no clear evidence for the more common disorders, such as asthma, COPD, cardiac disease, and pulmonary emboli. Panic attacks are typically associated with several other symptoms in addition to dyspnea, including palpitations (racing of the heart), chest pain, choking or smothering sensation, sweating, faintness, trembling, and feelings of unreality. Dyspnea should generally not be attributed to deconditioning unless basic studies (e.g., chest x-ray, pulmonary function tests) demonstrate no significant abnormalities.

Management

The management of patients with dyspnea will vary based on the most likely etiology of their shortness of breath. Several categories of medications may be appropriate, such as antibiotics for bacterial infections, anti-inflammatory agents and bronchodilators for asthma, bronchodilators for COPD, and diuretics for congestive heart failure. Smoking cessation should be discussed with all patients who are smoking. Other lifestyle changes also may need to be considered, such as reducing exposure to specific allergens in both the home and work environment for patients with asthma or hypersensitivity type reactions. Acutely ill patients with evidence of impending respiratory failure (using accessory muscles to breath, elevated respiratory rate, hypoxemia or increased pCO$_2$, and acidosis on an arterial blood gas) will need immediate attention in the hospital. Patients with suspected chronic illnesses such as asthma and COPD will likely need to be seen in 4–6 weeks after medication(s) have been started in order to assess the effectiveness of the medications and to follow up on smoking cessation *(Consultation and Referral 1)*.

Selected Readings

1. Michelson E, Hollrah S: Evaluation of the patient with shortness of breath: An evidence based approach. Emerg Med Clin North Am 17:221–237, 1999.
2. Morgan WC, Hodge HL: Diagnostic evaluation of dyspnea. Am Fam Physician 57:711–716, 1998.
3. Snider GL: History and physical examination. In Baum, GL, Wolinsky E (eds): Textbook of Pulmonary Diseases, 5th Edition. Boston, Little, Brown, 1994.
4. Thomas DA: Dyspnea. In Juzar A, Summer W, Levitzky M (eds): Pulmonary Pathophysiology. New York, McGraw-Hill, 1999.

1 - Referral should be considered when there is a mass or other abnormality on chest x-ray that has not been previously seen in the patient or is increasing in size. Referral should also be considered if the diagnosis of dyspnea seems unclear and the patient is not responding to initial therapeutic interventions.

29. Dizziness

Brian J. Finley, MD

Synopsis

Dizziness is one of the most elusive and difficult symptoms to evaluate and manage, yet its incidence is second only to fatigue among nonpain symptoms reported to primary care offices. There are two primary reasons why patients present with dizziness as their primary complaint: (1) it interferes with daily activities, and (2) the patient is concerned that he or she might have a serious underlying disease process. In elders, dizziness can lead to falls and significant injuries. A fear of dizziness can cause elderly patients to withdraw from physical activity, social events, and travel, leading to further decline in functional status. Dizziness is a nonspecific symptom that describes a subjective sensation and is impossible to quantify. The first job for a physician in evaluating this complaint is to clarify what the patient means by "dizziness" so that the physical examination, laboratory tests, and treatment options can be directed toward making a specific diagnosis and implementing a focused therapy.

Differential Diagnosis *(Table 1)*

There are many ways to classify the different causes of dizziness. One of the easiest ways is to divide it into **vertiginous causes *(Definition 1)*** and nonvertiginous (NV) causes. Vertigo can be broken down further into **peripheral vertigo** (PV) *(Definition 2)* and **central causes *(Definition 3) (Brain 1)*.** Peripheral vertigo is characterized by:

- Sudden onset
- More severe intensity
- Symptoms that are intermittent and last only a short time
- **Nystagmus *(Definition 4)*** in only one direction (usually horizontorotary)
- Symptoms made worse by a change in position of either the head or body
- Changes in hearing (either hearing loss or **tinnitus** *[Definition 5]*)
- No associated neurologic findings

Examples of this are **benign positional vertigo *(Definition 6)*, labyrinthitis *(Definition 7)*, Meniere's disease *(Definition 8)*,** and **vestibular neuronitis *(Definition 9)*.** These four represent approximately 80–85% of all cases of true vertigo. The central, vertiginous causes of dizziness are more serious and need to be evaluated in a more urgent fashion *(Red Flag 1)*. Either the history or physical exam will yield typical findings that can be used to identify centrally caused vertigo: gradual onset of symptoms, continuous symptoms, all types of nystagmus *(Red Flag 2)*, the presence of associated neurologic symptoms, and no hearing or positional related symptoms. Examples of this are infections of the central nervous system (CNS) (e.g., encephalitis, meningitis, abscess), anything that limits the blood flow to the CNS (e.g., vertebral basilar artery insufficiency, subclavian steal syndrome), cerebellar hemorrhage or infarction, tumors, and multiple sclerosis.

1 - Vertiginous vertigo: The sensation of disorientation in space combined with the sensation of spinning. Patients feel either that they are spinning, called subjective vertigo, or that the environment around them is spinning, called objective vertigo.

2 - Peripheral vertigo: Vertigo caused by conditions of the middle ear (from the ear drum to the oval window) or inner ear (includes the semicircular canals and mastoid areas).

3 - Central vertigo: Vertigo caused by conditions of the eighth nerve or central nervous system.

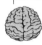
1 - The evaluation of dizziness is based completely on an accurate history and should be in the patient's own words. Ask open-ended questions.

4 - Nystagmus: Rapid, rhythmic, repetitious, involuntary eye movements. There are fast and slow components to the eye movement, and the nystagmus is named by the direction of this fast movement.

Table 1. Classification of Dizziness

Type	Common Description	Example
Vertigo	Spinning, tilting, whirling, toppling, free-falling	Vestibular neuritis, benign positional vertigo, Meniere's disease, brain stem ischemia
Presyncope	Light-headedness, near-faintness, fading out	Orthostatic hypotension, vasovagal near-syncope
Disequilibrium without vertigo	Imbalance only when standing or walking; unsteadiness	Sensory ataxia from diabetic neuropathy, cerebellar ataxia
Cryptogenic dizziness	Chronic rocking, floating, fatigue, wafting, nausea	Postconcussive dizziness, migraine-associated
Psychiatric dizziness	Chronic rocking, floating, fatigue, wafting, nausea	Panic disorder, generalized anxiety, depression, phobias
Physiologic dizziness	Motion sickness, nausea, queasiness, disorientation	Seasickness, carsickness, airsickness, hyperventilation, visual vertigo*

*Visual vertigo is dizziness evoked by seeing objects in motion such as ceiling fans, moving traffic, motion picture scenes, or the motion of people in crowds.

From Goroll AH, May LA, Mulley AG: Primary Care Medicine: Office Evaluation and Management of the Adult Patient, 3rd ed. Philadelphia, Lippincott-Raven, 1995, with permission.

History

"What do you mean when you say you are 'dizzy'?" Encourage the patient to describe the symptom without using the word *dizzy*.

- Spinning sensation or true vertigo
    Peripheral causes—usually benign and identified by associated symptoms
    Central causes—needs immediate attention and more extensive work-up *(Brain 2)*
- Nonvertiginous (usually benign)
    Light-headedness
    Feeling unsteady or unbalanced
    Feeling funny

"When do you notice the 'dizziness'?"

- Only when you move your head or you change positions (peripheral vertigo)
- Intermittent (PV or NV)
- Continuous (more common with central vertigo)

"How long does each episode last?"

- Short and intermittent—benign causes
- Longer and continuous—central causes

"What are the associated symptoms that you notice when you are dizzy?" All of the following are usually associated with different benign causes.

- Nausea, sweating, and fast heartbeat
- Feeling like you are going to pass out or you do pass out
- Headache

5 - Tinnitus: A ringing or funny noise in the ear (usually on the affected side).

6 - Benign positional vertigo: Vertigo usually caused by moving the head rapidly in a certain way and that may be related to a problem with a stone or otolith in one of the semicircular canals.

7 - Labyrinthitis: Inflammation caused by an infection in or near the inner ear. Labyrinthitis can cause vertigo, nystagmus, and hearing loss. There are four different types:
1. Serous: fluid build-up usually due to a viral infection
2. Acute suppurative: caused by bacterial infection
3. Toxic: caused by the toxic effect of medications on hearing apparatus (ototoxicity)
4. Chronic: due to a fistula (an opening) between the middle and inner ear, usually due to barotrauma (a sudden change in pressure in the earz), or cholesteatoma (a benign growth in the outer ear that erodes into the inner ear)

8 - Meniere's disease: Recurrent episodes of vertigo, tinnitus and hearing loss (from injury to the nerve [sensorineural]) due to too much fluid in the inner ear.

9 - Vestibular neuronitis: Intense vertigo (by itself) that usually lasts hours to days and then subsides. There are no other findings.

1 - Central vertigo is caused by conditions of the central nervous system and usually requires additional testing. The patient should probably be admitted to a hospital.

2 - Nystagmus can be horizontal, vertical, or rotary in direction. If it is vertical, always look for a central cause. Peripheral vertigo usually causes vertigo in a horizontorotary direction and is only on one side.

- Palpitations (irregular or extra heartbeat)
- Fever or other signs of infection

"Any other neurologic changes or symptoms?" These are very concerning and need to be investigated urgently, looking for central causes.

- Cranial nerve deficit
- Motor or sensory loss
- Abnormal reflex or abnormal Rinne test (i.e., blind spot, unable to move one eye in a certain direction, muscle weakness or rigidity, paresthesias or numb area, abnormal Romberg)

"Do you feel like you have had any change in your hearing?" Remember that hearing loss or tinnitus is a sign of a **vestibular problem** *(Definition 10)* and is usually associated with peripheral vertigo etiologies.

"Do you take any prescription medications or over-the-counter medications?" A long list of medications is associated with vertigo.

"What do you think might be causing your dizziness?" Try to determine what the patient is most worried about or thinks is causing the symptoms.

Past Medical History and Family History

- Personal history of head trauma *(Red Flag 3)* or heart disease *(Red Flag 4)*
- Family history of dizziness, seizures *(Red Flag 5),* or migraine headaches

Physical Examination

- General observation. Watch the patient walk and change positions (lying down, sitting, standing).
- Vital signs. Check blood pressure and pulse for regularity and **orthostatic changes *(Definition 11)*.**
- Eye exam. Are pupils equal and reactive?
    Is any nystagmus present?
    Do the eyes move together in all directions?
- Ear. Note tympanic membrane appearance and mobility. Any signs of infection? (see Chapter 30).
- Neurologic exam. Include **gross hearing tests *(Definition 12)*, Rinne test *(Definition 13)*,** and **Weber test *(Definition 14)*,** checking that all the cranial nerves are intact and looking for any other neurologic abnormalities.
- Neck exam. Any **bruits**? *(Definition 15)*
- Cardiac exam. Check for ectopy (extra heart beats) or arrhythmia (irregular heartbeat).
- **Romberg test *(Definition 16)***
- **Dix-Hallpike maneuver *(Definition 17)***

Testing

Order these tests only if they are indicated by the history or physical exam (rarely needed or indicated).

- Audiogram—if you notice decreased hearing or the patient complains of decreased hearing or tinnitus

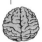
2 - Peripheral causes usually have a sudden onset, last only a few seconds to several weeks, and have horizontorotary nystagmus, and the fast component of the nystagmus is away from the affected side. Eighty-five percent of vertigo is peripheral and is not life-threatening.
Central causes usually have a slow, insidious onset and begin with mild symptoms that progressively get worse. Nystagmus can be in any direction but usually has a vertical component, and there is no relationship between the fast component and the location of the problem. Vertigo is only one of at least a couple of central nervous system symptoms. These can be life-threatening!

10 - Vestibular: Having to do with the hearing apparatus, which includes the bones in the middle ear and the structures in the inner ear.

3 - Dizziness can be caused by any head trauma and is a typical associated symptom of a concussion.

4 - Many heart conditions can cause dizziness.

5 - Asking bystanders about any abnormal movements or loss of consciousness after the patient feels dizzy can be important when looking for a seizure disorder.

11 - Orthostatic hypotension: A drop of 10–15 points in blood pressure or an increase of 10–15 beats in pulse rate, checked after having the patient go from lying to sitting from sitting to standing.

12 - Gross hearing tests: Whisper into one ear ten 2-syllable words (e.g., *baseball, ice cream, hot dog*) while making a sound in the other ear to limit its participation (e.g., crinkling paper). Then have the patient repeat the words.
- < 20% correct—possible retrocochlear lesion
- > 70% correct—intact hearing
- In between—get formal hearing testing (audiogram)

- MRI or CT scan—if there is any concern about central nervous system etiology
- Neurologic consult—if dizziness persists or you find a mixed picture (findings or history suggest several etiologies or are confusing)

Putting It All Together

The vast majority of patients who present with the chief complaint of dizziness have a benign condition. However, the physician must be able to identify the symptoms and signs that indicate a possible central etiology to the vertigo. A comprehensive history and physical exam will do just that. Identifying the exact etiology for the dizziness can be challenging. You can reassure the patient that most of the causes resolve by themselves and that you will give them something to alleviate their discomfort in the interim.

Management

The history and physical examination are geared toward uncovering the serious causes of dizziness. If the cause is thought to be benign, and the symptoms are severe enough to cause illness or disability, you can think about treating the specific symptoms themselves. Meclizine (an antihistamine) is a mild medication effective for treating mild dizziness. For more severe, true vertigo (with accompanying nausea, vomiting, and perspiration), diazepam is often required. Reassure the patient that most dizziness resolves within a couple of days to weeks, and additional testing is unwarranted. Depending on the severity of their symptoms, follow-up in a few days to weeks is appropriate. If symptoms persist or intensify, the physician should consider additional evaluation *(Consultation and Referral 1)*.

Selected Readings

1. Derebery MJ: The diagnosis and treatment of dizziness. Med Clin North Am 83:163–177, 1999.
2. Goldman L, Bennett JC (eds): Cecil Textbook of Medicine, 21st ed. Philadelphia, W.B. Saunders, 2000.
3. Goroll AH, May LA, Mulley AG: Primary Care Medicine: Office Evaluation and Management of the Adult Patient, 3rd ed. Philadelphia, Lippincott-Raven, 1995.
4. Rakel R (ed): Conn's Current Therapy 2000, 52nd ed. Philadelphia, W.B. Saunders, 2000.
5. Rosen P, Barkin R (eds): Emergency Medicine: Concepts and Clinical Practice, 4th ed. St. Louis, Mosby, 1998.
6. Walker JS, Barnes SB: Dizziness. Emerg Med Clin North Am 16:845–875, 1998.

13 - Rinne test: Strike a tuning fork, place it on the mastoid, and then move it to within 1 inch of the external ear.
- Normal—if the patient hears the noise better or longer via the air
- Abnormal—if the patient can hear the noise better or longer via bone conduction. This indicates conductive hearing loss in that ear.

14 - Weber test: Strike a tuning fork and place the vibrating fork on the patient's forehead.
- Normal—if noise is heard equally in both ears
- Abnormal—if the noise is heard predominantly in one ear. This indicates either conductive hearing loss in that ear (problem with eardrum or bony ossicles) or sensorineural hearing loss in the opposite ear (nerve injury or problem).

15 - Romberg test: Have the patient stand with feet together and closed.
- Normal—if he or she can stand there for 30 seconds.
- Abnormal—if he or she begins to fall within 6–10 seconds (usually toward the side of the hearing loss).

16 - Bruits: Musical sounds over arteries during systole (heard with stethoscope). These may indicate plaque build up in the artery.

17 - Dix-Hallpike maneuver: With patient sitting on table, have him turn his head 45° to one side. Then have him lay back with his head hanging over the edge of the table as far as comfortably possible. Watch for nystagmus for about 30 seconds. Repeat with head turned to other side, facing straight ahead.
- If you see nystagmus and it only lasts for 30 seconds, is horizontal or rotary in nature, and decreases with repetition of the test, then the problem is peripheral.
- If you see nystagmus and it lasts for more than 30 seconds, is vertical in nature, occurs every time you do the test, and occurs immediately, then the problem may be central (and potentially more serious).

1 - A neurology consult and possible admission to the hospital may be indicated if there are signs or symptoms of a central cause to the vertigo.

30. Ear Pain and Ear Infections

Fredrick A. McCurdy, MD, PhD, MBA

Synopsis

Ear pain is a common reason to seek medical attention. Ear pain can be due to irritation or infection or it can be produced by irritation at a distant site and represent referred pain. Ear pain can be either acute or chronic. Infection of the middle ear space is referred to as otitis media (OM), whereas infection in the external ear canal is termed *otitis externa* (OE). **Acute otitis media** (AOM) *(Definition 1)* is most frequently associated with a concomitant upper respiratory infection, whereas **acute otitis externa** (AOE) *(Definition 2)* is most frequently associated with swimming.

This chapter will help you find an explanation for ear pain in your patient. Keep in mind that about 50% of cases of AOM are caused by bacteria, whereas virtually all cases of AOE have a bacterial cause. Also remember that AOM and AOE do not cause all ear pain. Specific management decisions will be dictated by the underlying cause.

Differential Diagnosis

- Acute otitis media (AOM)
- Acute otitis externa (AOE)
- **Chronic serous otitis media** (CSOM) *(Definition 3)*
- Referred pain

Referred pain may come from the throat, the temporomandibular joint (TMJ), and cervical lymph nodes. This type of pain arises from regions of the head and neck that are innervated by cranial nerves V, VII, IX, X, and XI, and cervical nerves C2–3 *(Table 1)*. These sources of pain may not be evident at the time of the initial history and physical examination. Thus, the following should also be considered with any patient who presents with ear pain:

- Dental caries
- **Aphthous or herpes stomatitis** *(Definition 4)*
- **Pharyngitis** *(Definition 5)*
- **Cervical lymphadenitis** *(Definition 6)*
- **TMJ disease** *(Definition 7)*
- Head or neck cancer *(Red Flag 1)*

History

Taking a history of ear pain follows the same format as any other history. Ask open-ended questions first, followed by more probing ones to

1 - Acute otitis media (AOM): An infection in the middle ear space that has a fairly rapid onset of 1–2 days. Also called *acute suppurative otitis media.*

2 - Acute otitis externa (AOE): An infection in the external ear canal with a rapid onset of 1–2 days. This is also referred to as "swimmer's ear" because of its association with swimming.

3 - Chronic serous otitis media (CSOM): A condition characterized by persistent fluid in the middle ear space leading to decreased eardrum mobility and a concomitant decrease in hearing acuity. This is a particularly troublesome condition in infants younger than the age of 2, because hearing is decreased and the decreased ability to hear may affect the normal development of speech.

4 - Aphthous stomatitis: Shallow ulcers of the oral mucosa with an overlying grayish-colored membrane usually appearing as a single lesion. There is usually no associate fever. These are commonly called "canker sores."

Herpes stomatitis: Multiple small ulcers, which are exquisitely tender, covering the buccal mucosa, posterior pharynx, and gingiva. The child with herpes is generally quite irritable, with fever ≥ 101.5°F, and refuses fluids or solids by mouth.

5 - Pharyngitis: Irritation of the pharynx, commonly called tonsilitis. The three most common causative agents are group A beta-hemolytic *Streptococcus*, adenovirus, and Epstein-Barr virus.

6 - Cervical lymphadenitis: Swelling with tenderness of the lymph nodes in the anterior cervical region of the neck.

Table 1. Cranial Nerves

Cervical Nerve	Areas Innervated
C1	Blood supply to the head, pituitary gland, scalp, bones of the face, brain, inner and middle ear, sympathetic nervous system.
C2	Eyes, optic nerve, auditory nerve, sinuses, mastoid bones, forehead and tongue
C3	Cheeks, outer ear, face bones, teeth, trifacial nerve
C4	Nose, lips, mouth, and eustachian tube
C5	Vocal cords, neck glands, pharynx
C6	Neck muscles, shoulders, tonsils
C7	Thyroid gland, bursa in the shoulders, the elbows

Adapted from http://www.spinefunction.com/cervical.html.

7 - Temporomandibular joint disease: Pain from TMJ disease is usually localized to the ear or the jaw. Mandibular dysfunction is usually manifested by an inability to open the jaw fully.

1 - Premalignant and malignant lesions of the vocal cords and larynx are most often seen in people who smoke or drink alcohol. Ear pain is a frequent presenting complaint. Most of these cancers are squamous cell carcinomas.

gather sufficient detail. When interviewing a parent of a child, remember to rephrase the questions to refer to the child. Questions to ask a patient with ear pain are:

- "Describe the pain. Is it steady?" (suggests AOM) "Is it aggravated by chewing?" (suggests AOE)
- "Does your ear hurt when it is touched?" (AOE)
- "Have you been irritable or not feeling well?" *(Brain 1)*
- "Have you noticed that you have been pulling at your ear?" (see Brain 1)
- "Are you having trouble sleeping? Is your appetite decreased? Have you been vomiting?"
- "Have you been having a runny nose? A cough? A fever?" AOM is frequently associated with upper respiratory tract infections.
- "Have you been swimming recently? Do you like to put your head beneath the water when you are taking a bath?" (AOE)
- "Could you have placed anything in your ear?" (AOE)
- "Have you had difficulty swallowing recently? Had a sore throat recently? Have you noticed swelling in the glands of the neck?" *(Brain 2)*
- "Have you noticed anything running out of your ear [discharge]? Blood from the ear?" Discharge can result from AOE or from perforation of the tympanic membrane from an AOM.
- "Have you had intense pain in your ear followed by spontaneous pain relief and then a discharge from the ear canal?" Intense pain is frequently associated with AOM with perforated tympanic membrane.
- "Have you noticed any recent discoloration of the teeth? Have there been problems of dental cavities in the past? Been to the dentist recently?" Dental problems can cause referred pain.
- "Do you smoke or use smokeless tobacco?" *(Red Flag 2)*
- "What are your drinking habits?" (see Red Flag 2)

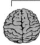

1 - Nonverbal infants or children with ear pain are frequently described by their parents as being irritable or fussy. An infant or child may pull on the infected ear. However, be aware that pulling on one or both ears can be a nonspecific complaint in infants and children and is not a reliable predictor of ear infection.

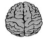

2 - Less common, but just as important, causes of ear pain include a sore in the mouth, a sore throat, and infection of the head and neck causing inflammation of the cervical lymph nodes.

Physical Examination

A careful examination of the entire head and neck region is necessary to search out the possible causes of ear pain.

2 - The use of smokeless tobacco or smoking and drinking increase the risk of head and neck cancer. Patients should be counseled about these risks.

- Before entering the examination room, look at the patient's chart and note the vital signs (especially the patient's temperature) and the chief complaint.
- When you first enter the examination room, note how ill the patient appears. In children, you should also note how active the child is when you first come into the room. Children are normally inquisitive and interact, at some level, with the examiner. Infants and children who do neither should be considered ill until proven otherwise.
- Look at the patient face-on and note if one of the ears is more prominent than the other. Infection of the mastoid air space just behind the ear is called *mastoiditis* and can be a complication of AOM. A patient with mastoiditis will have pain behind the ear along with swelling, redness, and warmth over the mastoid region. The swelling can cause the ear helix on the affected side to be pushed forward, thus causing the ear to appear more prominent.
- Pulling on the external ear helix or pressing on the tragus will often cause pain in AOE. Therefore, this part of the exam should be done very carefully because the severe pain may prevent completion of the rest of the physical examination.
- When examining the ear, first inspect the external ear canal and note if there is any discharge from the canal or redness or swelling. AOE will frequently cause drainage from the canal. Sometimes the patient will notice blood in this discharge.
- The tympanic membrane is normally gray, translucent, and has a light reflex in the lower half *(Figure 1)*.
- In AOM, the tympanic membrane is dull, red or yellow, bulging *(Figure 2)*, and poorly mobile to immobile when doing pneumatic otoscopy (see Testing below). The light reflex is also either diminished or completely absent. An occasional bulla may be present *(Figure 3)*.
- A sign of repeated AOM is **tympanosclerosis *(Definition 8)*** or a **cholesteatoma *(Definition 9)* *(Figure 4)***.
- Examine the nose for nasal discharge.
- Ask the patient to open and close his or her mouth while placing your fingers over the TMJ. Observe for pain, limited ability to open the mouth, or any popping or snapping of the TMJ.
- Examine the mouth and throat.
  1. Look for redness, swelling, or ulcers along the gingiva and buccal mucosa.
  2. Look for ulcers or petechiae on the hard and soft palate.
  3. Look at the tonsils, observing size, presence or absence of redness, and presence or absence of exudate.
  4. Inspect the teeth for any obvious dental caries. Also, look along the gingival margin for any swelling associated with a tooth. This may be a subtle finding for an early dental abscess. Pressing down on each tooth may also cause pain when there is an underlying abscess.
- Palpate the anterior and posterior cervical lymph nodes, noting swelling or tenderness.
- Inspect the skin and run your fingers over the skin of the back and chest looking for any evidence of a skin rash. Streptococcal pharyngitis may have an associated skin rash. Other viral infections of the throat also may produce a skin rash.

8 - Tympanosclerosis: A chalky white deposit in the ear drum.

9 - Cholesteatoma: A yellow, greasy, sac-like mass that contains desquamated epithelial debris. These usually are formed during the healing process after tympanic membrane rupture.

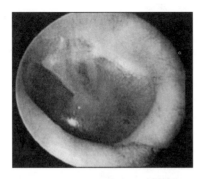

Figure 1: Normal tympanic membrane.
(Courtesy of David McCormick, MD, University of Texas Medical Branch, Galveston, TX. © University of Texas Medical Branch.)

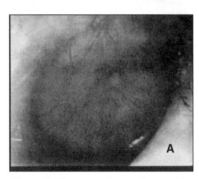
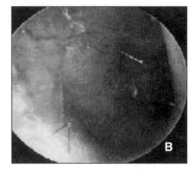

Figure 2: The tympanic membrane with acute otitis media. *A*, Erythema and complete effusion consistent with otitis media. *B*, Erythema and bulging tympanic membrane consistent with otitis media.
(Courtesy of David McCormick, MD, University of Texas Medical Branch, Galveston, TX. © University of Texas Medical Branch.)

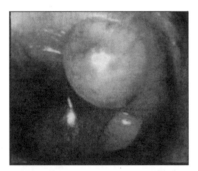

Figure 3: Tympanic membrane bulging with bullae.
(Courtesy of David McCormick, MD, University of Texas Medical Branch, Galveston, TX. © University of Texas Medical Branch.)

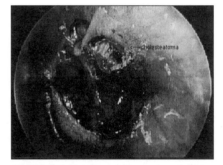

Figure 4: Perforation of the eardrum with destructive cholesteatoma.
(From http://www.earsurgery.org/cholest.html, with permission. © Ear Surgery Information Center.)

Testing

A test commonly done in the office is pneumatic otoscopy. Pneumatic otoscopy should be done in all patients suspected of having AOM because a middle ear effusion must be present for the diagnosis of AOM to be accurate. This procedure is done using an otoscope with a side-port for attaching a piece of flexible tubing along with a mouthpiece or a rubber bulb for introducing air into the external ear canal. The otoscope speculum should have a rubber collar around the tip with which to seal the external ear canal, although sometimes this is possible using a standard speculum without a collar.

Advance the speculum into the external ear canal far enough to occlude the ear canal and force air into the canal by either softly blowing into the rubber tubing or gently squeezing the rubber bulb. Carefully watch the upper half of the eardrum for movement. A normal eardrum will move away when air enters the ear canal and will return to its original position when the air exits. In the patient with AOM, the eardrum will not move. AOM has, by definition, a middle ear effusion.

Tympanometry is also used in many offices (see Chapter 71).

Putting It All Together

Most people who come to the doctor's office with ear pain have either AOM or AOE. At least half of all middle ear infections and all external ear infections are caused by bacteria. These infections have an abrupt onset. Thus, a patient who comes to the office with a complaint of sudden onset of ear pain most likely has an infection in the middle ear or ear canal. If an infectious reason cannot be found after examining the external ear canal and the middle ear, look for reasons that would explain referred pain. You should be alert to identify reasons for referred pain such as pharyngitis, stomatitis, and head or neck cancer, or consider other more lingering conditions such as CSOM. The mnemonic COMPLETES can help you remember all of the important clinical features of AOM *(Table 2)*.

AOE is easily recognized if all the features (ear pain, pain on tragal traction, and purulent discharge in the external ear canal) are present. Confusion comes either when all of these signs and symptoms are not present or when the history is confusing (e.g., ear drainage without a history suggestive of AOM with tympanic membrane perforation). When this occurs, the wisest thing to do is assume that either possibility exists and treat the patient as if both conditions coexist.

Table 2. Acute Otitis Media COMPLETES Exam

C	Color	The normal color for the TM is gray; in AOM the TM is diffusely red or pale yellow.
O	Other	Look at the TM for the presence of other clues such as air-fluid levels, air bubbles, or tympanosclerosis.
M	Mobility	A normal TM should move in response to intermittent changes in air pressure within the external ear canal (pneumatic otoscopy). The presence of AOM should make the TM immobile because of the fluid effusion in the middle ear space.
P	Position	A normal TM is flat, whereas AOM usually causes the TM to bulge outward toward the eye of the examiner.
L	Lighting	Confirm that the otoscope light works before attempting to examine the patient.
E	Entire surface	The entire surface of the TM should be examined, searching for unexpected abnormalities (e.g., cholesteatoma).
T	Translucency	A normal TM is translucent. An opaque TM indicates the presence of a middle ear effusion.
E	External auditory Ear auricle	Before inserting the ear speculum, inspect the ear auricle and the external ear canal andcanal. AOE will produce inflammation of the external auditory canal with purulent discharge.
S	Seal	Achieving a complete pneumatic seal allows the examiner to accurately test for TM mobility using the pneumatic otoscope.

TM = tympanic membrane; AOM = acute otitis media
Adapted from Kalieda PH: The COMPLETES exam for otitis. Contemp Pediatr 14:93–101, 1997.

Management

The management of acute or chronic ear pain is dictated by making the correct diagnosis. AOM is caused by either a virus or bacteria, whereas a bacteria or fungus usually causes AOE. The typical treatment of AOM presumes the cause to be *Streptococcus pneumoniae, Haemophilus influenzae* or *Moraxella catarrhalis*. Oral amoxicillin is the usual antibiotic chosen. However, many patients develop significant resistance to amoxicillin due to the production of the enzyme **ß-lactamase** *(Definition 10)*. This necessitates choosing an antibiotic that is not sensitive to this enzyme, such as amoxicillin and clavulanic acid (Augmentin) or a macrolide. Another problem is that about 50% of all cases of AOM are probably caused by viruses, which have no specific curative agent other than waiting for the infection to spontaneously resolve.

AOE is usually caused by *Pseudomonas aeruginosa, Proteus mirabilis*, streptococci, *Staphylococcus epidermidis*, or fungi. Thus, treatment must be very broad. Topical medications such as a combination of neomycin and polymyxin "eardrops" are commonly prescribed. Topical corticosteroids are also frequently added to help reduce local pain and swelling of the external ear canal. Because of the potential harm that alcohol has on the middle ear space, otic suspensions are preferred in children *(Red Flag 3)*.

For the management of referred ear pain (e.g., pharyngitis, stomatitis), consult the chapter pertaining to the precipitating condition.

10 - ß-Lactamase: An enzyme produced by some bacteria that chemically breaks down penicillin. Thus, these bacteria will be resistant to the effects of penicillin.

3 - Ear discharge may come either from AOE or from AOM with tympanic membrane perforation. Because the TM is not easily visualized in these patients and because alcohol is damaging to middle ear structures, an otic preparation with alcohol (otic solution) should be avoided except when the examiner is certain the tympanic membrane is intact. If eardrops with corticosteroid are chosen for treatment, a suspension (no alcohol) would be preferred.

Selected Readings

1. Arnold JE: The ear. In Behrman RE, Kliegman RM, Arvin AM eds: Nelson's Textbook of Pediatrics, 15th ed. Philadelphia, W.B. Saunders, 1996, pp 1804–1826.
2. Berman S: Otitis media. In Berman S (ed): Pediatric Decision Making. Philadelphia, B.C. Decker, 1991, pp 40–43.
3. Jung TT, Hanson JB: Classification of otitis media and surgical principles. Otolaryngol Clin North Am 32:369–383, 1999.
4. Kaleida PH: The COMPLETES exam for otitis. Contemp Pediatr 14:93–101, 1997.
5. Potsic W: Earache. In Schwartz MW (ed): Pediatric Primary Care: A Problem-Oriented Approach. Chicago, Year Book, 1990, pp 210–213.
6. Simic WJ: Office ENT. Home Study Self-Assessment Program: Monograph, Edition 181. Kansas City, MO, American Academy of Family Physicians, 1994.

31. Elder Abuse

Layne A. Prest, PhD, LMFT • W. David Robinson, PhD, LMFT

Synopsis

Even though an estimated 2 million older adults are mistreated every year, elder abuse is an often overlooked manifestation of the violence that takes place in families in the United States. It is likely, therefore, that primary care providers will come into contact with elders who are being mistreated. Elder abuse takes various forms, including physical abuse, physical neglect, psychological abuse, financial exploitation, and violation of personal rights. Elders may be mistreated by caretakers who are family members, friends or neighbors, community volunteers, or paid paraprofessionals. Therefore, it is recommended that health care providers have a high index of suspicion and routinely screen older patients.

Elder abuse is most often discovered during routine office visits or interviews in the long-term care facility. There are a number of barriers to detection *(Red Flag 1)*, but careful, nonthreatening, and nonjudgmental interviews of both the older patient and the caregiver(s) may provide the basis for assessment and appropriate intervention. The older person and caretakers should be separated during these interviews in order to provide a safe and confidential environment. A plan for ensuring the cessation of the mistreatment and the well being of the patient, including appropriate referrals, are crucial parts of the physician's management plan. Treatment of physical injuries, somatic complaints, and emotional symptoms requires a multidisciplinary approach. The most effective intervention often takes place in a continuity relationship and in concert with the legal and mental health systems in the community *(Brain 1)*.

1 - Elderly patients are at an increased risk for cognitive impairment due to dementia or delirium. Consequently, one of the first steps is to establish whether the patient is competent. In addition to any cognitive impairment from which they might be suffering, being overwhelmed, hesitant, embarrassed, and afraid may discourage elderly patients who are being mistreated from revealing abuse.

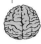

1 - Although the laws may vary from state to state in their reporting procedures, reporting of elder abuse is mandatory. You should familiarize yourself with the reporting requirements and procedures in the jurisdiction in which you are doing your preceptorship. Check with an attorney, the state office on aging, or adult protective services office for details. If you suspect that an elder is being abused or mistreated, you should always share that suspicion with your preceptor.

Differential Diagnosis

The medical differential will depend on the nature of the presenting signs and symptoms. Of course, physical injury should compel the provider to seriously consider abuse as a potential etiological factor (see Physical Examination section for a list of injury-related symptoms). However, most victims of elder abuse do not present acute physical symptoms of abuse in the primary care setting. From a biopsychosocial perspective with a focus on the more psychosocially oriented diagnoses, alternate or coexisting conditions to be considered include:

- Dementia or delirium
- Mood disorders
- Anxiety disorders
- Marital or family dysfunction not involving physical violence
- Substance abuse
- Other psychiatric disorders

History

When mistreatment of an elderly patient is suspected, the health care provider should interview the patient alone in a private setting. The interviewer should use a nonjudgmental manner and avoid blaming the patient for what is happening. Reassure the patient that you are there to help and that, to the greatest extent possible, you will help him or her make decisions about the course of action to be taken. The interview should include questions about the current situation, past history of mistreatment, and the impact of the abuse on the patient. A number of issues put the elder at increased risk and should be investigated *(Brain 2)*. Despite what the patient or caregiver reports, a variety of behavioral signs and symptoms may signal that a problem exists *(Red Flag 2)*.

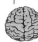

2 - An intergenerational history of violence, substance abuse, poor health, burnout, or other mental health problems in the caregiver(s) put the older person at increased risk. An intergenerational history of violence, substance abuse, physical or cognitive impairment, social isolation, low income, minority status, and low level of education in the older person also make elder abuse more likely.

Opening Questions

Questions about the patient's daily life, including meals, medication, shopping, and social outlets, and interaction with friends or family normalize the issues and should help create a less threatening context.

- "What do you do in a typical day?"
- "Who prepares your meals? How do you get your shopping done?"
- "In a normal week, how often do you get out of the house and see friends and family or have people in to visit you?"

2 - Behavioral signs and symptoms:
- Symptoms of depression, anxiety, or cognitive disturbance, including alterations in mood, activity level, appetite, awareness or alertness, emotional lability, and psychomotor functioning
- Subtle or confusing complaints
- Substance abuse (especially alcohol and prescription medications)
- Delay between onset of injury and presentation for treatment

Questions about the Quality of the Patient-Caregiver Relationship

The relationship between patient and caregiver(s) may vary significantly depending on whether the caregiver is a family member or not. These questions may have to be altered accordingly.

- "How many caregivers do you have?"
- "What is your relationship with each of them?"
- "How do you and the caregivers get along?"
- "Are the caregivers taking good care of you?"
- "Sometimes patients with your types of injuries [complaints] are being hurt by someone. Could it be that this is happening to you?"
- "It is pretty common for family members who are taking care of older people to become frustrated or overwhelmed and take it out on them. Has [your caretaker] been hurting or mistreating you in any way?"
- "We all argue or fight at home, what happens at your house when there are disagreements?"

Questions to Assess the Level of Mistreatment

- "Do you ever feel afraid of, or threatened by, your caregiver(s)?"
- "Do you feel safe at home?"
- "Has your caregiver(s) ever handled you roughly?"
- "Has your caregiver(s) ever confined you so you couldn't leave the room (or house), see friends, or telephone someone when you wanted to?"
- "Has your caregiver(s) ever injured you? To what extent?"
- "Can you describe your concerns about improper care of medical problems [or untreated injuries, poor hygiene, prolonged period before obtaining medical attention, meals, or other care withheld]?

Questions to Ask of the Caregiver(s)

If issues of mistreatment are raised, the caregiver(s) should be interviewed as well. Be careful not to make suggestive comments to or accuse the caregiver(s) based on the patient's report alone, especially if the patient is cognitively impaired.

- "How do you think [the patient] is doing?"
- "Have you seen any improvements or declines in [the patient's] condition lately?"
- "Being a caregiver for an older person can be a tiring, and sometimes thankless, job. How are you doing with the burden of providing this level of care for [patient's name]?"
- "I have noticed that [the patient] is confused [or depressed, anxious, emotional, complaining more, etc]. Do you have any ideas about why that is?"
- "[The patient] has some concerns about how things are going between the two of you. How do you see things? Are you feeling overwhelmed or resentful? Have you found it difficult to control your reactions to some of the things [the patient] does or says?"

Questions to Assess Readiness for Change *(Brain 3)*

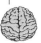

3 - As you interview, it is important to assess whether the patient thinks there is a problem and whether the patient is ready to do something about it. Establish where the patient is in the stages of readiness for change.
- Precontemplation—hasn't considered that there is a problem or that a change is helpful or necessary.
- Contemplation—has wondered whether or not she should leave, call the police, or tell someone else.
- Preparation—is beginning to formulate a plan to change the situation.
- Action—has begun making behavioral or situational changes.
- Follow-up—continued implementation or alteration of plan, despite possible setbacks.

See page 50 for more information.

Thorough, well-documented medical records can provide important evidence should the legal system become involved. These records can actually benefit the patient by providing concrete, objective validation of the injuries or condition from which the patient suffers. It is best to use the patient's own words in recording the chief complaint and description of the abusive event.

Ask of the elderly patient:

- "Have you ever thought that the way you are being treated was wrong?"
- "Have you ever thought that the way you are being treated was affecting your health?"
- "What have you thought you should do about this situation?"
- "Have you ever contacted [local support/social service agency specializing in abuse issues] for help?"

Ask of the caregiver:

- "Do you need some help with [the patient's] care?"
- "Have you ever thought that a change was needed in this situation?"
- "What have you thought you should do about this situation?"
- "Have you ever contacted [local office on aging/elder social services agency] for help?"

Physical Examination

Perform the physical exam as indicated by presenting complaints, signs, and symptoms, but pay particular attention to the following:

- Traumatic alopecia
- Poor oral hygiene
- Hematomas, welts, bite marks, burns, decubitus ulcers
- Fractures or signs of previous fractures

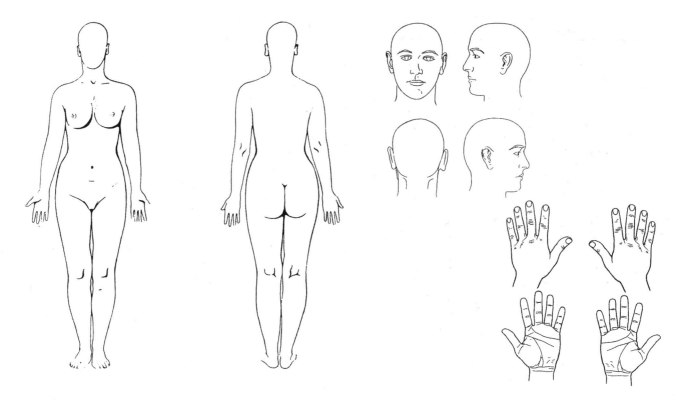

Figure 1: Body chart.
(From Nebraska Medical Association: The Cure Can Begin with You: A Physician's Handbook on Domestic Violence. Lincoln, NE, Nebraska Medical Association, 1995, with permission.)

- No physical evidence of trauma despite subjective complaint by patient
- Poor hygiene, inguinal rash, impaction of feces
- Weight loss, dehydration, unkempt appearance
- Evidence of rape
- Chronic pain, psychogenic pain, pain due to diffuse trauma

The documentation in the medical record should include a complete description of the mistreatment, including type, number, size, location, and resolution of injuries; other complaints; and possible causes and explanations given regarding the injuries or symptoms. Where applicable, the location and nature of the injuries should be recorded on a body chart or drawing *(Figure 1)* and be size proportionate. Many domestic violence experts also recommend that health care providers take 35-mm or Polaroid-type photographs (with permission) of the injuries or the patient's general condition. It is helpful to provide an opinion on whether the explanation of injuries or condition is plausible. Reports of suspected elder mistreatment should be made to the local, county, or state adult protective services office. If the elderly person is a resident of a long-term care facility, a report should be made to the state agency with jurisdiction over these institutions *(Brain 4)*. If the police are called, record the action taken as well as the name, badge number, and phone number of the investigating officer.

Testing

No testing is necessary unless indicated by physical examination or history.

Putting It All Together

More often than not in the primary care setting, the elderly patient who is being mistreated will present somatic complaints or behavioral cues rather than acute injuries. This presentation should raise a red flag for the health care professional. It is important to consider the level of cognitive impairment in an older person, neither relying on them completely as historians nor dismissing their concerns "because they are demented." A careful work-up (history and physical exam) is necessary. Because elder mistreatment is underdetected, it is recommended that all elderly patients be screened. Without change or intervention, elder abuse usually escalates in severity and contributes to the deterioration of the elderly person's overall health.

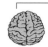

4 - Hotline numbers:
Adult Protective Services: 1-800-652-1999
National Family Violence Hotline:
1-800-799-SAFE
Older Women's League: 1-800-825-3695
Family Violence Prevention Fund:
1-415-252-8900

Management

Appropriate management begins with the initial interaction with the patient. Good interviewing may help the patient and caregiver(s) to begin thinking about their situation more clearly, giving thought to the emotional and physical consequences. Injuries and other somatic complaints should be treated appropriately, but medication (especially pain and psychopharmacologic agents) should not be prescribed without a plan to address the emotional, social, and legal issues involved. Because of the associated acute and chronic stress, patients who are victims of elder abuse frequently experience comorbid conditions. Therefore, the health care professional should be prepared to assess and treat anxiety, depression, and substance abuse as well. Above all, it is important for the health care professional to attempt to provide non-judgmental support and reassurance, resource and referral information, and reasonable follow-up. In every state, and in many counties and cities, there are agencies that provide a variety of services to elderly people, including intervention in cases of mistreatment. You always need to report suspected elder mistreatment, but be familiar with the reporting statutes in your state.

Selected Readings

1. Aravanis SC, Adelmanerrin RD, Brechman R, et al: Diagnostic and treatment guidelines on elder abuse and neglect. Arch Fam Med 2:371–388, 1993.
2. Nebraska Medical Association: The Cure Can Begin with You: A Physician's Handbook on Domestic Violence. Lincoln, NE, Nebraska Medical Association, 1995.
3. Paris BE, Meier DE, Goldstein T, et al: Elder abuse and neglect: How to recognize warning signs and intervene. Geriatrics 50:47–51, 1995.
4. Swagerty DL, Takahashi PY, Evans JM: Elder mistreatment. Am Fam Physician 59:2804–2808, 1999.

32. Failure to Thrive

Laeth Nasir, MBBS • Arwa Nasir, MBBS, MSc

Synopsis

In children, normal growth is a fundamental index of good health. The process of growth in children is measured by documenting the increase in length, weight, and head circumference over time.

The term failure to thrive (FTT) or growth failure is used when children are noted to be not gaining weight as expected or are actually losing weight. FTT is a sign and not a diagnosis, in the same way that fever is a sign of disease that can be due to conditions as diverse as a viral upper respiratory tract infection and cancer. FTT can be most simply defined as those children whose weight falls below the 5th percentile on a standard growth chart or who exhibit the downward crossing of more than one growth percentile. FTT is most commonly seen in children younger than 2 years of age.

FTT is commonly divided into the categories organic failure to thrive (OFTT) and nonorganic failure to thrive (NOFTT). OFTT implies that there is an illness that is causing decreased nutrient intake or absorption. NOFTT usually indicates a subtle and multifactorial cause of decreased nutrient intake and commonly manifests with delayed development, abnormal behavior, and disrupted caregiver–infant interactions. NOFTT accounts for the majority of cases of FTT seen in primary care.

Differential Diagnosis

Organic Failure to Thrive

This includes disorders in any organ system, including:

- Chromosomal disorders
- Disorders of the central nervous system (such as cerebral palsy)
- Chronic inflammatory diseases (such as tuberculosis or rheumatologic disease)
- Renal failure
- Parasitic or malabsorptive diseases of the gastrointestinal tract
- Metabolic and endocrinologic disorders

Nonorganic Failure to Thrive

This category includes:

- Child neglect and abuse
- Infant behavioral problems that make feeding difficult
- Complex social or familial disruptions that result in a loss of the nurturing environment that is necessary to allow normal feeding behavior to occur

Factitious Failure to Thrive (False Failure to Thrive)

These children meet the criteria for diagnosis but do not share the course or outcome of children suffering from FTT. This category may include infants:

- Who are exclusively breast-fed *(Brain 1)*

- Who experienced **intrauterine growth restriction** *(Definition 1)*
- With **familial short stature** *(Definition 2)*
- Suffering from **constitutional growth delay** *(Definition 3)*

History

A complete history, including prenatal and perinatal history, should be taken. A careful past medical history including a full review of systems with particular focus on gastrointestinal symptoms is critical in evaluating these patients. A history of serious illness increases the possibility of OFTT. Patients with NOFTT are frequently noted to have recurrent minor illnesses such as otitis media and recurrent upper respiratory tract illnesses. It is unclear whether the recurrent illnesses are due to malnutrition or neglect. A complete nutritional history is important to determine the adequacy of the diet provided and the environment in which it is consumed.

- "Can you tell me about your pregnancy and delivery?" Birth trauma may lead to FTT.
- "Did you take any medications, recreational drugs, or alcohol during pregnancy?" Fetal alcohol syndrome may lead to FTT.
- "Has your child had any serious or frequently occurring illnesses?"
- "What does your child eat? Is she a picky eater?" *(Brain 2)*
- "Are there any foods that your family does not eat, or that you try to restrict in your child's diet?" *(Brain 3)*
- "Tell me what mealtime is like at your home." Assess the meal time environment and the meal time interactions between child and caregiver.
- "How do you feel that things are going between you and your child?" *(Brain 4)*

Physical Examination

Careful and accurate anthropometric measurements should be performed. A complete physical examination should be carried out. Children with constitutional growth delay, familial short stature, a history of intrauterine growth retardation, or OFTT will usually demonstrate concordant reductions in height, weight, and head circumference measurements. Children with NOFFT will usually exhibit a weight age that is less than height age.

The physician should note:
- General appearance
- Grooming
- Presence of pallor, jaundice, or **syndromic features** *(Definition 4)*
- The infant–caregiver interaction should be observed
- Any signs of child abuse or neglect *(Red Flag 1)*

A formal developmental assessment *(Brain 5)* should be carried out. At some point during the evaluation of FTT, direct observation of the feeding interaction between the caregiver and infant should be made and assessed by a trained observer, such as a home health care nurse or nutritionist.

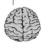

1 - Infants who are breast-fed exclusively may present with a growth pattern that appears to be lagging behind their formula-fed peers. Standard growth charts were developed using measurements from formula-fed infants, and these charts may not be applicable to the population of infants who are breast-fed. Therefore, it is sometimes difficult to make a diagnosis of FTT in the young, exclusively breast-fed infant unless the growth pattern is grossly abnormal. In general, breast-feeding alone is adequate for infant growth up to 4–6 months.

1 - Intrauterine growth restriction: The weight and size of the newborn tends to be a function of maternal size and intrauterine environment, rather than reflecting the neonate's genetic potential. Children who have experienced adverse intrauterine conditions or significantly premature birth may have a protracted "catching up" phase with respect to their peers for a period of time in early life.

2 - Familial short stature: Height limited by genetic potential. These children tend to be of normal birth weight and subsequently experience deceleration of growth, typically before 3 years of age. After this, they grow at constant rates proportional to those children of average height. Their final height is concordant with parental height. Formulas are available to estimate the final adult stature of children based on parental height. This prediction is known as the *target height*, and although it is not highly accurate, it provides an estimate of the growth percentile that the child might be expected to follow.

3 - Constitutional growth delay: A normal variation in the rate of growth. These children are sometimes known as "late bloomers." However, several recent studies have suggested that these children do suffer from some degree of nutrient deprivation and may benefit from dietary modification.

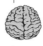

2 - A food diary recorded over 3–7 days is important to assess the adequacy of the diet.

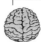

3 - Directly questioning the parent regarding dietary restrictions and excessive intake of high calorie foods with low nutritive value such as sweets or juices is important. A frequently seen nutritional problem is the excessive consumption of juices. This results in a corresponding decrease in protein, fat, and vitamin intake, with subsequent FTT.

Testing

A few basic screening tests to exclude an organic cause of FTT should be performed in all cases. Further testing should be reserved for those patients in whom the history, physical exam, or laboratory testing is suggestive of an organic cause of FTT.

For all patients:

- Complete blood count (CBC)
- Serum electrolytes, blood urea nitrogen (BUN), and creatinine
- Urinalysis and culture **(Brain 6)**
- Stool studies for **Giardia lamblia (Definition 5)**
- Tuberculin skin test

Consider:

- **Radiologic bone age** **(Definition 6)**

Putting It All Together

The majority of patients presenting to the primary care physician with apparent growth failure will have a psychosocial or other subtle cause of FTT or will be experiencing factitious FTT. However, it is critical that those patients with OFTT be identified and treated promptly. Patients with NOFTT need to be identified and intensively treated in a timely manner to limit the negative outcomes seen in children suffering from this condition. Children with NOFTT are more likely than unaffected peers to have persistent deficits in developmental, intellectual, and social maturity.

Management

The physician should remember that attempts to intensify feeding should begin during the evaluation phase of FTT. A high-calorie, high-protein diet is recommended, with sufficient energy provided to allow catch-up growth to occur. Children who are malnourished may suffer from anorexia that will not resolve until refeeding results in an improved state of health. The treatment of patients with NOFTT is usually multidisciplinary, involving intensified feeding, parental education, and ongoing follow-up with nutritionists, mental health professionals, and others. Behavior management and social intervention may be important components of treatment **(Consultation and Referral 1)**.

Remember that most parents feel ashamed of their failure to adequately nurture their child. Occasionally, hospitalization or foster care placement may be necessary to achieve weight gain. Ongoing close follow-up is critical to a favorable outcome.

Selected Readings

1. Gahagan S, Holmes R: A stepwise approach to evaluation of undernutrition and failure to thrive. Pediatr Clin North Am 45:169–187, 1998.
2. Nasir L, Nasir A: Healthy Child Care: Conception to Age Two Years.

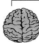

4 - An assessment of the nonfeeding interactions between caregiver and child is important, because difficulties with feeding may stem from other problems the caretaker is having with the child.

4 - Syndromic features: Abnormalities noted on physical examination that may indicate genetic anomaly. Examples of syndromic features include the oblique palpebral fissures, flat nasal bridge, and palmar simian creases suggestive of Down's syndrome.

1 - Signs of child abuse or neglect include unexplained injuries or injuries for which implausible explanations are offered by parents or caretakers. Child neglect may be suspected in children with poor hygiene or neglect of medical conditions or well-child visits.

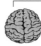

5 - Developmental delay may be a cause of, or be caused by, FTT. The Denver Development Screening Test II is an example of a standardized test that can be administered to accurately evaluate a child's abilities in several developmental areas.

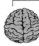

6 - Urinary tract infections, which may be asymptomatic in children, can lead to FTT. A microbiologic culture of urine is necessary to exclude the possibility of occult urinary tract infection in children.

5 - Giardia lamblia: A relatively common parasite that may infect the gastrointestinal tract and lead to malabsorption with relatively few symptoms.

6 - Radiologic bone age: An estimation of skeletal maturity based on a single radiograph of the hand. Skeletal maturity is an accurate measure of chronologic age, but children with certain organic disorders may exhibit an acceleration or delay in skeletal maturity with respect to chronologic age.

1 - Many psychosocial issues including caretaker depression, family violence, and isolation from support systems can contribute to NOFTT. Involvement of skilled professionals to assess the home environment and provide counseling, treatment, and support may be useful in selected cases.

2. Nasir L, Nasir A: Healthy Child Care: Conception to Age Two Years. Monograph, Edition 246: Home Study Self-Assessment Program. Leawood, KS, American Academy of Family Physicians, 1999.
3. Schechter M: Weight loss / failure to thrive. Pediatr Rev 21:238–239, 2000.
4. Schwartz I: Failure to thrive: An old nemesis in the new millennium. Pediatr Rev 8:257–264, 2000.
5. Steward DK, Garvin BJ: Nonorganic failure to thrive: A theoretical approach. J Pediatr Nurs 12:342–347, 1997.

33. Falls in the Elderly

Ed Vandenberg, MD, CMD

Synopsis

Falls in the elderly are a source of significant morbidity and mortality and can have a profound impact on the quality of life. After falling, a majority of patients are fearful of future episodes and report limiting their activities as a consequence. Falls are often caused by multiple factors, including acute illness, medication toxicity, and functional decline. The leading causes and contributing factors include environmental factors, lower extremity weakness, gait or balance dysfunction, visual deficits, and rarely **syncope *(Definition 1)***. Interventions aimed at correction of these contributing factors can lead to a 50% reduction in falls.

The history and physical examination should determine the extent of injury, contributing factors, and rehabilitation potential. Syncope, if considered as a possible cause, requires a careful cardiovascular and pulmonary system evaluation. Patients with new neurologic symptoms will require immediate neurologic evaluation.

1 - Syncope: The sudden, transient loss of consciousness and postural tone followed by spontaneous recovery.

Differential Diagnosis

In the evaluation of geriatric syndromes such as falls, the concept of differential diagnosis and presumption of single cause approach does not serve the elderly patient well. It is rare to have a singular cause of falls in the elderly. Therefore, the pursuit and correction of the multiple causes and contributing factors to the fall give the best result. The initial evaluation should focus on the extent of the injury and the search for contributing factors or causes.

Extent of Injury

- Soft tissue injuries (e.g., bruises, strains)
- Lacerations
- Fractures (hip, femur, humerus, wrist, ribs)
- **Intracranial injury *(Definition 2)***

2 - Intracranial injury: The sequela of a blow to the head such as concussion, subdural hematoma, or intracerebral bleed.

Contributing Factors or Causes

- Acute illness *(Brain 1)*
- Medication toxicities (see History section)
- Functional disabilities
- Environmental factors (e.g., rugs, slick surfaces, stairs, poor lighting, tubs and showers without grab bars, clutter)

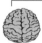

1 - Acute illnesses to consider include, but are not limited to, infections (e.g., urinary, pulmonary); metabolic disorders (e.g., electrolyte disturbance, hypo- or hyperglycemia, hypoxia, hypercarbia); cardiopulmonary disorders (e.g., myocardial infarct, pulmonary embolus, congestive heart failure); CNS diseases (stroke, seizure, meningitis); dehydration; and malnutrition.

History

A good history often requires consulting a collaborative source such as a spouse, family member, friend, nursing home personnel, or anyone who may have witnessed the event or has been in frequent contact with the patient over the last few weeks.

"Tell me about your fall."

- Situation (e.g., location, time of day)
- Activity
- Loss of consciousness

"What was hurt?" Identify areas of body injured.

"Why do you think you fell?" Patient's attribution may provide clues about environment, acute illnesses, or physical disabilities.

"Did you pass out? Do you remember falling?" Consider syncope **(Brain 2).**

"Did you have symptoms immediately before it happened?"

- Spinning sensation? Vertigo might suggest central nervous system (CNS) or middle ear disease as a possible cause.
- Aura (visual or olfactory sensation)? (seizure as possible cause)
- Light-headed when standing? (orthostatic hypotension as possible cause)
- Nausea or vomiting? (acute illness-triggered hypotension as possible cause)
- Pain? (pain-triggered hypotension or **vasovagal** episode) **(Definition 3)**

"Have you been ill recently or since the fall?"

- Fever? (possible infection)
- Nausea vomiting or diarrhea? (may suggest dehydration or metabolic disorder)
- Confused? (consider **delirium [Definition 4]** and **dementia [Definition 5]**)
- Chest pain, dyspnea, palpitations, edema? (assessing cardiopulmonary status)
- Depressed mood? (depression creates carelessness, slowed responses)
- Losing weight? (consider malnutrition)
- Unilateral motor or sensory loss? (CNS disease/injury, stroke, subdural)

"Any medication changes?" **(Brain 3)**

"Do you have problems with your ability to function or to do the things you need to do?"

- Vision?
- Memory loss? (consider delirium and dementia)
- Walking, balance, or getting out of a chair? Inquire about the use of assistive devices such as walkers, canes, and grabbers.
- Urinary incontinence? (may cause hurried trips to toilet and may result in slick surfaces)

"Tell me about where you live." **(Brain 4)**

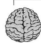

2 - The causes of syncope can be remembered by the mnemonic PASS OUT:

P **P**ressure (hypotensive causes)
A **A**rrhythmia (cardiac)
S **S**ugar (hypoglycemia)
S **S**eizures

O **O**utput (cardiac), **O**xygen (hypoxia)
U **U**nusual (psychiatric, hyperventilation)
T **T**ransient ischemic attacks (and other CNS causes)

3 - **Vasovagal (neurocardiogenic):** Hypotension (usually < 90 mmHg systolic) or bradycardia (usually at least < 60 bpm) that is sufficiently profound to produce cerebral ischemia and loss of neural function.

4 - **Delirium:** Acute onset of altered level of consciousness (primarily inattention) and cognitive changes (e.g., memory problems, disorientation, language difficulties) with a fluctuating course. Usually has a medical cause.

5 - **Dementia:** Two or more acquired deficits in cognitive domains that occur in the absence of acute confusion, that cause dysfunction and have no other medical cause. Cognitive domains include memory, orientation, language, praxis (learned skilled movements), constructions, and executive control (complex decision making).

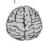

3 - Medications can cause or contribute to falls by slowing cognitive processes (e.g., sedatives, hypnotics, opioids, alcohol, antipsychotic, and medication with anticholinergic properties contained in decongestants and cold medicines) and by lowering blood pressure (e.g., antihypertensives, antianginals, diuretics, vasodilators and antiparkinsonian medications).

4 - If the home environment is suspected as contributing to the fall(s), explore such issues as steps, lighting, and floor coverings (e.g., loose rugs, slippery surfaces). It is helpful to know who else is in the home or who lives nearby and can offer help to the patient. A home safety evaluation by visiting nurse or occupational therapist is often very useful.

Physical Examination

- General. Assess alertness, attention, and appearance.
- Vital signs and orthostatic blood pressures **(Brain 5)**
- HEENT. Use the Hallpike maneuver (see Chapter 29) to assess **nystagmus (Definition 6).** Check vision.
- Skin. Check for turgor, pallor, bruising, and lacerations.
- Neck. Check range of motion (ROM) Does motion recreate dizziness **(Brain 6)** ? Check for **carotid bruits (Definition 7).**
- Cardiopulmonary **(Brain 7)**
  1. Heart. Check rate, rhythm **(Red Flag 1)**, and murmurs.
  2. Lungs. Rales are indicative of pneumonia or congestive heart failure (CHF). Depressed breath sounds may indicate consolidtions from pneumonia, masses, or effusions.
- Extremities. Check for range of motion of joints (any pain?), deformities (acute or chronic, especially knees or feet), injuries (contusions, swelling), and foot problems **(Brain 8)**.
- Neurologic **(Red Flag 2)**
  Mental status **(Brain 9)**.
  Focal deficits (motor, sensory, coordination)
  Peripheral neuropathy (sensory, motor, proprioceptive)
  Cerebellar (test with finger to nose, heel to knee, Romberg)
  Tremor, rigidity, gait, and balance abnormalities **(Brain 10)**

Testing

Decisions about testing are determined by the extent and type of injury sustained by the patient and considerations of the factors contributing to the fall.

Extent of Injury

X-rays of the skeleton in the areas injured may be necessary to rule out bone injury. This is determined by factors such as amount of pain, deformity, dysfunction of area involved, and force of injury. CT scan of the head is necessary in case of suspected intracranial injury **(Red Flag 3)**.

Contributing Factors

The history and physical exam determine the focus of testing **(Table 1)**.

Putting It All Together

The results of the acute injury evaluation direct the immediate care. However, the synthesis of the data from the cause and contributing factors requires more thought. The philosophy is to correct all the acute factors as quickly as possible and set about assisting the patient with the longer term disabilities as reflected in the Management section. The factors that should not be missed or be delayed in care are:

- Intracranial head injuries
- Fractures, especially hip
- Syncope, especially due to cardiac or pulmonary causes
- Infections

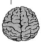

5 - The normal oral temperature range for elderly patients is 35.8–36.8°C (96.4–98.2°F). Orthostatic blood pressure is assessed as follows:

1. Take blood pressure (BP) and pulse after patient has been recumbent for > 5 minutes.
2. Have patient sit up for < 1 minute, then take BP and pulse.
3. Have patient stand and take BP and pulse at 1 and 3 minutes.

A significant change is a drop in systolic BP of ≥ 20 mmHg or increase in heart rate of > 20 bpm with change in position.

6 - Nystagmus: An involuntary rapid movement of the eyeball, which may be horizontal, vertical, and/or rotatory in nature.

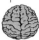

6 - ROM of neck recreating dizziness may indicate that the proprioceptive sensors in the neck are irritated by neck diseases such as arthritis or herniated disc or that ROM stimulates the middle ear or CNS to create vertigo.

7 - Carotid bruits: A blowing sound heard over a blood vessel, due to flow disturbance caused by stenosis, aneurysms, or benign flow disturbance.

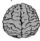

7 - The acute cardiac evaluation is done to rule out arrhythmia, heart failure, and myocardial infarct. The acute pulmonary evaluation is done to rule out pneumonia, pulmonary embolus, and exacerbations of chronic lung disease.

1 - Rate and rhythm abnormalities of significance that need urgent intervention:

Rate	Possible Causes
120–180 bpm	Infection, anemia, hypotension, ventricular tachycardia
>180 bpm	Supraventricular tachycardia, ventricular tachycardia
Irregular rhythm	Atrial fibrillation, ventricular arrhythmia

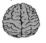

8 - Foot problems that can impair gait and balance include bunions, poorly fitting shoes, ulcerations, tender calluses, and toe deformities.

Table 1. Testing Following a Fall in the Elderly

Illness or Disability	Test/Evaluation
Acute Illness	
Infection	Urine analysis, CBC, chest x-ray
Metabolic/dehydration	Blood glucose, electrolytes, renal and liver function
Cardiac/pulmonary	EKG, chest x-ray, oxygen saturation
Mental status changes	DELIRIUM evaluation *(Brain 11)*
Functional Disability	
Vision	Ophthalmology referral
Memory loss	Neurologic assessment by neurologist, geriatrician, or geropsychiatrist *(Consultation and Referral 1)*
Gait and balance problems	Physical therapy *(Consultation and Referral 2)*; may need neurologist *(Consultation and Referral 3)*
Walking or getting out of a chair	Joint evaluation
Urinary incontinence	Urinalysis (to rule out infection as a cause of incontinence)

CBC = complete blood cell count; EKG = electrocardiogram.

Table 2. Get Up and Go Test

Ask the patient to	What it tests
Rise from the chair without using his or her arms	Leg strength
Walk 10 feet, turn, and return to chair	Observe balance, stride, turning ability, and speed
Sit, without using arms	Vision, coordination, and leg strength

Management

The management is often in two stages: acute and long term. The acute phase focuses on care of the acute injury (e.g., laceration repair, care of musculoskeletal or CNS injuries when present) and any acute illness contributing to falls (e.g., treatment of infections with antibiotics and correction of dehydration). Medication toxicities are addressed by discontinuing the offending medication, reducing medications, or substituting with less toxic medication. The extent of the acute problems and the amount of home support determine whether care ultimately will be provided in a hospital, skilled nursing facility, or the patient's home residence. Safe and appropriate home-based care is generally preferred because hospitalization poses its own risks and complications.

Follow-up treatment of acute problems and the management of functional disabilities are best done longitudinally and may require the assistance of other health care professionals. Physical therapists can assist with the evaluation and management of gait and balance problems. Occupational therapists can provide advice about possible assistive devices. Podiatrists can help with foot problems and deformities affecting walk and balance. Vision problems may require evaluation and intervention by an ophthalmologist. Environmental factors can be assessed by a visiting nurse or occupational therapist. The primary care physician integrates the input of these various professionals to develop a plan of action that best meets the needs of the individual patient.

2 - Any new neurologic symptoms (e.g., motor weakness, sensory loss, vision loss or speech disturbance) may indicate a subdural hematoma or intracerebral bleed requiring emergent neurosurgical care.

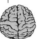

9 - Screen memory with recall of three items after 3 minutes. Give the patient three items to recall and tell him you will ask him to repeat them in 3 minutes. Say, for example, "apple, table, penny." Have the patient repeat the words until he gets all three, then retest after 3 minutes. If the patient does not remember all three items, perform a full Mini Mental Status Exam.
Screen for delirium by noting fluctuating mental status with cognitive impairment in the history. Test attention span by asking the patient to spell the word *world* forward and backward. Problems with attention cause an inability to spell backward, while still being able to spell forward.

10 - Screen gait and balance with the Romberg test and Get Up and Go Test (Table 2).

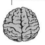

3 - Suspicion of intracranial injury should be based on abnormalities from the history (syncope, seizure, or head injury with loss of consciousness or neurologic symptoms) or the physical exam (significant injury of the cranium, new abnormalities on neurologic exam, or mental status changes). When there is a head injury of significance, the neck should be immobilized until neck injury can be ruled out by exam or x-ray.

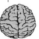

11 - The delirium evaluation can be guided by the mnemonic DELIRIUMS:
D **D**rugs
E **E**motional (e.g., depression, psychoses)
L **L**ow oxygen states (e.g., myocardial infarct, pulmonary embolus, CHF, anemia)
I **I**nfection
R **R**etention of urine or feces
I **I**ctal states (i.e., seizure or fit)
U **U**ndernutrition or **u**nderhydration
M **M**etabolic
S **S**ubdural (to include other acute CNS processes)

Selected Readings

1. Alexander NB: Falls and gait disturbances. In Cobbs EL, Duthie EH, Murphy JB (eds): Geriatrics Review Syllabus: A Core Curriculum in Geriatric Medicine, 4th ed. Dubuque, IA, Kendall Hunt, 1999, pp 145–149.
2. Kane RL, Ouslander JG, Abrass IB: Instability and falls. In Essentials of Clinical Geriatrics, 4th ed. New York, McGraw-Hill, 1999, pp 231–255.
3. Tinetti ME, Baker DI, McAvay G, et al: A multifactoral intervention to reduce the risk of falling among elderly people living in the community. N Engl J Med 331:13, 1994.
4. Yoshikawa TT, Cobbs EL, Brunnel-Smith K, Rubenstein LZ: Falls. In Practical Ambulatory Geriatrics, 2nd ed. St. Louis, Mosby, 1998, pp 262–270.

1 - The evaluation of memory loss in the absence of delirium may require the expertise of a neurologist, geriatrician, or geropsychiatrist to diagnose and treat the patient and educate patients and families on course and prognosis.

2 - Gait and balance disorders have many causes. A physical therapist (PT) can evaluate and prescribe exercises and techniques to compensate even while the evaluation is going on. A common cause (e.g., disuse atrophy) can be corrected with an exercise program prescribed by a PT.

3 - Gait and balance disorders sometimes require the expertise of a neurologist to accurately diagnose and treat more complex problems, such as atypical Parkinson's disease, multiple sclerosis, or atypical strokes.

34. Fatigue

Bruce C. Gebhardt, MD

Synopsis

Fatigue (malaise, lassitude, tiredness, low energy, exhaustion) is a common problem and may result from a multitude of diseases. Acute fatigue is present for 6 months or less, whereas chronic fatigue lasts longer. Fatigue may result from organic diseases (e.g., hypothyroidism), psychiatric illnesses (e.g., depression), physiologic stress (e.g., the expected reaction to life, such as studying for medical school exams), or chronic fatigue syndrome (an etiologic mystery).

A detailed history should include a thorough description of when the fatigue started, what aggravates or ameliorates the fatigue, and other symptoms such as fever, night sweats, and weight change. Symptoms of depression, such as anhedonia or tearfulness, are important to elicit. The social history should focus on habits, family life cycle stage, and stressors. It is vital to understand how the fatigue affects the patient's daily functioning and to determine what the patient fears is causing the problem.

The physical examination must be thorough. Focus particularly on the patient's affect, temperature, weight, skin, conjunctiva, thyroid, lymph nodes, heart and lung auscultation, liver, spleen, and extremities.

Laboratory testing usually consists of a complete blood cell count (CBC), assessment of renal and hepatic function, erythrocyte sedimentation rate (ESR), thyroid-stimulating hormone (TSH), and urinalysis. Treatment depends on etiology. Organic causes are treated with specific therapies. Patients with physiologic fatigue can be advised about lifestyle changes (restructuring work hours, exercise, improving diet). Psychiatric disease can be treated pharmacologically or with counseling. Chronic fatigue syndrome remains a treatment challenge.

Differential Diagnosis

Name a disease, and fatigue is likely to be a symptom. However, the rule of "common things occur commonly" does apply and allows you to plan an orderly evaluation. Certain symptoms should increase your concern of a serious medical problem *(Red Flag 1)*.

 1 - Symptoms that indicate a serious disease-causing fatigue, night sweats, weight loss, fever, and enlarging lymph nodes.

Organic Diseases

Approximately 20–45% of patients will have an organic etiology *(Brain 1)*. Organic diseases that may present as fatigue include:

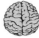 **1 -** An organic disease likely will be accompanied by other symptoms (such as pain) and physical exam findings (such as lymphadenopathy) that point you in the right diagnostic direction.

- Anemia—secondary to menstruation, peptic ulcer disease, or hematologic diseases
- Obesity
- Infections—e.g., HIV, mononucleosis, or viral hepatitis
- Endocrine disorders—e.g., diabetes or hypothyroidism
- Cancer (almost any type)
- Pregnancy (very common)
- Connective tissue diseases—e.g., lupus
- Sleep apnea
- Neuromuscular diseases—e.g., myasthenia gravis
- Congestive heart failure (CHF)

- Iatrogenic—from medications (antihistamines or beta-blockers), herbs, or supplements

Psychiatric Disease

Psychiatric disease is the etiology of 40–45% of cases of fatigue.

- Depression (most common)
- Anxiety
- **Somatoform** disorders *(Definition 1)*
- As with organic disease, patients will have other signs and symptoms consistent with a psychiatric illness *(Brain 2)*

1 - Somatoform: Mental or emotional pain that manifests itself as physical pain or complaints.

2 - The fatigue associated with psychiatric illness and life stressors is usually insidious in onset.

Lifestyle

A thorough social history usually identifies lifestyle issues contributing to fatigue. It takes creativity and sensitivity to help patients cure themselves in these cases. Common examples of lifestyle causing fatigue include:

- Working mothers
- New parents
- People working long or varied shifts
- Sleep deprivation

Chronic Fatigue Syndrome

Chronic fatigue syndrome (CFS) accounts for most patients who have no other diagnosis. Today the Centers for Disease Control and Prevention (CDC) has specific criteria to diagnose CFS *(Table 1)*. Several etiologic theories exist, but for now, no specific cause is known. CFS usually has a very abrupt onset.

Table 1. CDC Definition for Chronic Fatigue Syndrome

A patient must have both major criteria plus at least eight minor criteria or two physical criteria plus six minor criteria.

Major Criteria
1. Chronic or relapsing fatigue for > 6 months that does not resolve with bed rest and reduces usual daily activity by at least 50%.
2. Other causes have been ruled out.

Minor Criteria
1. Mild fever or chills
2. Sore throat
3. Lymph node pain in cervical or axillary chains
4. Myalgias (sore muscles)
5. Prolonged, generalized fatigue (> 24 hours) following previously tolerated levels of exercise
6. New, generalized headache
7. Migratory, noninflammatory arthralgia (joint pain without heat or swelling that moves from joint to joint)
8. Neuropsychologic symptoms (e.g., forgetfulness, photophobia [eye pain secondary to light], difficulty concentrating)
9. Sleep disturbance (too much or too little)
10. Symptoms are acute or subacute (they start abruptly) in onset

Physical Criteria
1. Low-grade fever
2. Nonexudative pharyngitis (a red, sore throat without white "spots" or pus)
3. Palpable or tender lymph nodes < 2 cm in size (see above for location)

Adapted from Epstein K: The chronically fatigued patient. Med Clin North Am 79:315–327, 1995.

History

"How did this fatigue start?"

- Abrupt (as for CFS)
- Insidious (as for depression)

"How long have you felt tired?"

- Acute (e.g., from early pregnancy)
- Chronic (CFS)

"When do you notice the fatigue?"

- Pervasive (hypothyroidism, anemia)
- Exertional (heart failure)
- Muscle fatigue with use (myasthenia gravis)
- Before or during work (job stress or chemical exposure)

"What helps or worsens the fatigue?"

- Does sleep refresh the patient (lifestyle) or not (depression, sleep apnea)?

"Are there other symptoms you notice along with the fatigue?"

- Fever (infection)
- Pharyngitis (mononucleosis, CFS)
- Weight loss (cancer)
- Swollen lymph nodes (infection, lymphoma)
- Melena (peptic ulcer)
- Night sweats (lymphoma, infection)
- Amenorrhea (pregnancy)
- Menorrhagia (anemia)
- Edema (congestive heart failure [CHF])
- Snoring (sleep apnea)
- Cough (CHF, HIV)
- Weight gain (hypothyroidism, obesity)
- Urinary changes (polyurea with diabetes)

"Do you have any other medical problems?"

- Has the patient had fatigue before?
- Has the patient had any of the problems listed above? (This can make your job easy!)

"Tell me more about yourself."

- Life cycle stage—newborn child (see sleep patterns!), empty nest, fear of dying
- Habits—drugs, alcohol, tobacco, caffeine
- Sleep patterns
- Occupation—long hours, changing shifts, chemical exposures, stress
- Marital status and happiness—Does a relationship cause or alleviate stress?
- Exercise—Is the patient able to? Does it help or worsen the fatigue?
- Sexual history—risk for HIV

"What do you think is causing this tiredness? What do you feel will make it better?" *(Brain 3)*

- What does the patient think (or fear!) is causing this problem?
- Does the patient have specific ideas about how to treat the problem?

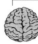 **3 -** It is vital to find out the patient's health belief model.
- What does the patient think (fear) is causing the fatigue?
- What does he or she think will cure it?
- How does the fatigue interfere with daily functioning?

Physical Examination

General Appearance

- Flat affect (depression)
- Body habitus (obesity)

Vital Signs

- Temperature elevation (infection)
- Heart rate and rhythm (fast in hyperthyroidism; slow with beta-blockers; irregular with atrial fibrillation)
- Weight change (ideally the medical record has previous weight for comparison)
- Respiratory rate (increased in CHF or occult pneumocystic infection with HIV)
- Blood pressure (high may indicate secondary heart disease or renal disease)

Skin

- Abnormal nevi (melanoma)
- Texture changes (thyroid disease)
- Jaundice (hepatitis)

HEENT

- Conjunctiva (pale in anemia, icteric in hepatitis)
- Oral pharynx (large, inflamed tonsils with exudate in mononucleosis; thrush in immunodeficiency)

Neck

- Thyroid (goiter)
- Thickness or excess fat (may point to sleep apnea)
- Masses (head and neck cancers)

Lymph

- Enlarged nodes (cancer or infections)

Lungs

- Rales (CHF)
- Wheezes (asthma or CHF)

Cardiac

- Murmurs (aortic stenosis or endocardititis)

Abdomen

- Enlarged liver (hepatitis from alcohol, virus, or cancer)
- Splenomegaly (leukemia or lymphoma)
- Masses (cancer)
- Enlarged kidneys (renal failure)
- Enlarged uterus (pregnancy)
- Rectal to test for occult blood (colon cancer or ulcer)

Genital

- Testicular masses *(Brain 4)*
- Pelvic exam (cancer, pregnancy)

Breast

- Masses (cancer)

Neuromuscular

- Weakness (if initially strong and then weakens quickly, think myasthenia gravis)
- Muscle wasting

Extremities

- Edema (CHF, hypothyroidism)

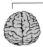

4 - Testicular cancer is the most common cancer among men ages 15–35.

Testing

- CBC
    Hemoglobin will be low if anemia
    White blood cell count will be high if infection
    Platelets can be high in any disease state or low in bone marrow cancers
- Renal panel
    Creatine (kidney function)
    Glucose (high in diabetes)
- Electrolytes—sodium, potassium, calcium (may be abnormal in endocrine diseases such as Cushing's disease or renal disease)
- Liver enzymes (elevated with liver damage from alcohol or viral hepatitis)
- ESR *(Brain 5)*
- Urinalysis
    Protein in the urine may indicate renal disease
    Glucose suggests diabetes
- Pregnancy test (never forget to test for pregnancy)
- Mononucleosis (especially in teens and young adults)
- HIV. You must ask about risk factors (see Chapter 40).
- Others—depends on patient risk factors, such as foreign travel

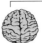

5 - ESR measures inflammation. Think of it as a big fishing net. If you cast a fishing net, you will get fish if there are any, but you don't know what kind you will get. If no fish are present, the net will be empty. If the sed rate is high, it may mean there is an inflammatory process going on (infection, cancer, connective tissue disease), but it will not identify a specific disease. A normal ESR makes you more comfortable that no inflammatory disease is present. Platelets (mentioned above) work this way as well.

Putting It All Together

The history and physical exam are the cornerstone of making a diagnosis when a patient presents with fatigue. The physician must be thorough and sure that nothing is overlooked.

Fatigue is categorized as acute (present < 1–6 months) or chronic. If an organic disease is present, the patient likely will have some other signs or symptoms pointing to a primary etiology (with fatigue being a symptom of that disease). Common reasons include anemia, sleep apnea, and hypothyroidism. A limited screening or confirming lab test set should be sufficient to allay or confirm patient and physician concerns of underlying organic disease. Patient-specific tests are ordered as needed (for example, pregnancy or mono tests). Organic disease is found in 20–45% of cases.

If no organic disease is found, psychiatric disease should be considered. Depression can be screened for with specific history taking or screening tools (see Chapter 14). Anxiety and somatoform disorders can be diagnosed in a similar way.

Physiologic fatigue (due to life stress) is diagnosed by the exclusion of organic and psychiatric disease and a history that is compatible with this etiology. Psychiatric or physiologic etiologies are found in 40–45% of cases. Fatigue in these cases is usually insidious in onset.

CFS is diagnosed by excluding organic disease and finding the presence of CDC-defined characteristics. The fatigue is usually abrupt in onset and, as the name implies, chronic. This syndrome can be extremely debilitating and wreak havoc on a family. Patients often cannot work or enjoy life. No etiology is known. No lab tests are available to diagnose CFS. The course is usually waxing and waning symptoms, and some patients recover.

Management

For the patient, fatigue can be anxiety-provoking and significantly impact daily functioning. Often, the patient fears that a serious disease is causing the problem. For the physician, the complaint of fatigue also can be anxiety-provoking. The differential diagnosis is virtually limitless, and physicians often fear "I'm missing some rare disease."

If an organic disease is found (e.g., hypothyroidism), specific therapy is instituted. Some patients may need further testing or referral to a specialist (e.g., an older patient with iron-deficiency anemia needs a colonoscopy done by a gastroenterologist to rule out colon cancer).

Depression and anxiety may be treated with medication or psychotherapy. Referral to a psychiatrist may be needed.

Physiologic causes can be more difficult to deal with. Patients must believe this is the problem. Even when they do, changing lifestyle is one of the most difficult things for people to do. Working with patients on tobacco, alcohol, or caffeine cessation is time consuming, but very rewarding if they succeed. Some life issues cannot be changed for financial reasons (a factory worker mandated to work 10-hour shifts 6 days a week) or other reasons (a breast-feeding mom). Often the knowledge that no organic disease exists is treatment enough.

CFS is also difficult for doctors to treat. There is no cure, but antidepressant medication and support groups may help. It is sometimes a chicken–egg problem: did depression cause the fatigue or result from the chronic fatigue? Patients with CFS are often adamant that it is not depression. The key is to be extremely supportive and avoid the "it's all in the patient's head" label. Many CFS patients use alternative therapies. The physician must be patient and remember: first, do no harm.

Selected Readings

1. Epstein KR: The chronically fatigued patient. Med Clin North Am 79:315–327, 1995.

2. Hartz AJ, Kuhn EM, Bentler SE, Levine PH: London Richard prognostic factors for persons with idiopathic chronic fatigue. Arch Fam Med 8:495–501, 1999.
3. Mathews DA, Manu P, Lane TJ: Evaluation and management of patients with chronic fatigue. Am J Med Sci 302:269–277, 1991.
4. Ridsdale L: Chronic fatigue in family practice. J Fam Practice 29:486–488, 1989.
5. Ruffin MT, Cohen M: Evaluation and management of fatigue. Am Fam Physician 50:625–634, 1994.
6. Solberg LI: Lassitude: A primary care evaluation. JAMA 251:3272–3276, 1984.

35. Fever in Adults

Arvind Modawal, MD, MPH, MRCGP, DTMH

Synopsis

Fever is the human body's response to pyrogens (substances that cause fever) as a result of an external or internal disease or state. Fever is one of the important vital signs used in clinical assessment. Body temperature is on average 37°C and varies up to 1.5°C throughout the day. Many elders will have a lower baseline temperature. Fever usually results from self-limiting viral infections. Fever must be differentiated from **hyperthermia** *(Definition 1)*, which is often due to environmental factors. Causes of fever can range from trivial to serious illness. Therefore, considerable astuteness is required to obtain a detailed review of systems, history, and physical examination. Laboratory investigations should be individualized based on the history and physical examination, but often will include a complete blood count (CBC), liver and renal assessment, chest x-ray, urinalysis, and cultures of the urine and blood. Recurrent or prolonged fever and **fever of unknown origin** *(Definition 2)* require further investigation. Symptomatic treatment with the use of a fan, cold sponging, and acetaminophen may be helpful. Fluid replacement and judicious antimicrobial therapy are used for definitive treatment.

Differential Diagnosis *(Brain 1)*

See *Table 1*.

History

- "How long have you had fever or high temperature?"
- "Do you have any chills or rigor?" Presence of chills and rigors due to readjustment of heat regulation and central thermostatic mechanisms occur transiently during early phases of the pyrexial illness.
- "Do you have headache, pain, difficulty with bright light, or discomfort anywhere in the body?" *(Red Flag 1)*
- "Do you have a rash on the body?" (see Red Flag 1)
- "Have you had any surgical procedure or instrumentation recently?" (increased risk of infective endocarditis) *(Red Flag 2)*
- "What treatment or antibiotics, if any, have you taken so far?" *or* "Do you take any medications?" *(Red Flag 3)*
- "What kind of hobbies and interests do you have?" Inquire specifically about hiking, camping, and game hunting (risk for tick bites and Lyme disease) *(Brain 2)*
- "What are your dietary practices and habits?" For example, eating raw or poorly cooked meat or consuming unpasteurized milk or cheese increases the risk for zoonosis.

1 - Hyperthermia: Rise in body temperature due to environmental factors (hot climate, lack of air-conditioning, excessive exposure to the sun).

2 - Fever of unknown origin (FUO): Prolonged fever (usually > 8 days) without a definitive diagnosis after routine testing and requiring more extensive investigations.

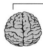

1 - Special features of the types of fever do not always point to a specific diagnosis but may be worth noting in prolonged fever. The classical types are **continued** (1°C change in 24-hour period, but at no time touching normal), **remittent** (> 2°C change over 24-hour period), **intermittent** (present only for several hours during the day), **quotidian** (daily), **quartan** (every 2 days), and **tertian** (on alternate days). Because of early and frequent use of antibiotics, these classical forms of fever are not often seen these days; hence they are of little use for specific diagnosis.

1 - Fever with or without rash, photophobia, headache, neck stiffness, or rigidity suggests **meningitis** and requires a lumbar puncture for cerebrospinal fluid (CSF) analysis.

2 - Fever associated with changing cardiac murmur and prior history of cardiac disease and recent surgical procedure or instrumentation requires consideration of diagnosis of **infective endocarditis** and blood cultures for confirmation.

Table 1. Differential Diagnosis of Fever

Cause	Incidence	Examples
Fever of unknown origin	25%	
Infectious	23%	Abscesses, TB, granulomas, parasites (malaria), pneumonia, salmonella (typhoid), brucellosis, cardiac (infective endocarditis), CNS (meningitis, viruses including HIV)
Multisystem diseases	22%	Rheumatoid arthritis, systemic lupus erythematosus, polyarteritis nodosa, acute rheumatic fever, Still's disease, giant cell arteritis, inflammatory bowel disease
Miscellaneous	14%	Sarcoidosis, familial Mediterranean fever, factitious fever
Malignancy	7%	Lymphomas and leukemia, certain primary neoplasm
Drug-related	3%	Drug reaction (serum sickness), neuroleptic malignant syndrome, malignant hyperthermia

Adapted from Knockaert DC, Dujardin KS, Bobbaers HJ: Long-term follow-up of patients with undiagnosed fever of unknown origin. Arch Intern Med 152:51–55, 1992.

3 - The patient may be at risk of drug-induced fever or serum sickness. Recent history of use of centrally acting medication or anesthetic agent may precipitate **malignant hyperthermia** or **neuroleptic malignant syndrome** in susceptible individuals.

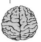

2 - Fever with rash and history of a tick bite or outdoor activity raises the possibility of Lyme disease (caused by *Borrelia burgdorferi*) or Rocky Mountain spotted fever (caused by *Rickettsia rickettsii* infection).

- "Do you have household pets?" (presence of zoonosis)
- "What are your sexual orientation and practices?" (risk for sexually transmitted disease [STD]) *(Brain 3)*
- "Do you smoke, use tobacco, recreational drugs, or alcohol in excess?" (aspiration pneumonia a possibility)
- "Have you had an animal, tick, or insect bite?"
- "Did you receive blood or blood product transfusions?" (hepatitis B and C)
- "Do you have diabetes, renal or liver disease, or history of jaundice?" (or other conditions that may alter immunity to infections)
- "What is the status of your immunizations?"
- "Do you have any drug allergies or hypersensitivity?"
- "Is there any history of recent international or tropical travel?" *(Brain 4)*
- "Have you experienced any weight loss, night sweats, or recurrent fever?" (suggests malignancy, lymphoma, or chronic infections such as tuberculosis [TB])
- "Is there a family history of TB, other febrile or infectious diseases, arthritis or autoimmune disease, or familial condition?" Ethnic origin may point toward predisposition to certain illness.

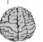

3 - Fever with monoarticular joint involvement and history of STD, especially in women, suggests gonococcal septicemia.

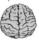

4 - Acute malaria (transmitted by mosquito) has to be excluded if fever appears during travel or *on return*. Because of the speed of travel these days, awareness of diseases existing in far-off places may help in diagnosis of pyrexia during or after international travel.

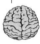

5 - Patients with cardiovascular collapse, coma patients, and the elderly should have their temperature taken rectally with a low-reading thermometer to exclude "accidental hypothermia." Hypothermia recorded during the course of a day in a patient with fever may occur because of severe infections in the elderly patient with organ failure and patients on glucocorticoids.

Physical Examination

- Vital signs, in particular, get a frequent and accurate recording of temperature with the use of a low-reading thermometer, if required *(Brain 5)*. How the body temperature is recorded (oral, axilla, or rectal) is important *(Brain 6)*. Temperature may be altered or masked due to use of steroids, antipyretics, and antibiotics (see Brain 1).
- Skin and oral mucosa for presence of rash and dehydration
- Enlargement of lymph nodes (presence of chronic infections or lymphoma)

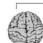

6 - The average normal oral body temperature is about 37°C (range 1– 1½°C) with slight diurnal variations. These ranges apply to 95% of the population (within 2 standard deviations) measured in mid-morning. Temperature of mouth, rectum, or vagina is at least half a degree higher than that of the groin or axilla. Rectal temperatures are considered more reliable than oral temperatures, particularly in mouth-breathers and tachypneic patients. Elderly persons will often have a lower normal body temperature.

- Nails and fingers for clues to etiology of other conditions (splinter hemorrhages, fingernail clubbing)
- Eyes, ears, nose, and throat to look for focus of infection (enlarged tonsils, red tympanic membrane [eardrum], tenderness over sinuses)
- Cardiac examination for presence of murmurs and pericardial rub (see Red Flag 2)
- Chest for pleural rub, crackles, and wheeze (pleurisy or effusion, pneumonia)
- Abdomen including rectal, genital, and pelvic examination for tenderness, distention, guarding, and mass lesions (intra-abdominal abscess, cholecystitis, appendicitis)
- Nervous system for presence of neck rigidity or stiffness and photophobia (see Red Flag 1)
- Confusion (delirium) in elderly *(Red Flag 4)*
- Musculoskeletal system for presence of joint pain and effusion (suggesting rheumatic fever, pyogenic arthritis, rheumatoid disease or autoimmune disease) (see Brain 3)

 4 - Consider the possibility of infections of the urinary tract or pneumonia. Fever may be slow to rise and may not be the first symptom of infections.

Fever with rash merits special attention as it may give clues to a diagnosis and point toward life-threatening serious illness. The following characteristics of the rash should be noted:

- Site of onset
- Distribution of rash
- Rate of propagation
- Central (body trunk) or peripheral (extremities) distribution
- Centrally distributed maculopapular rashes usually suggest viral or rickettsial diseases, drug reaction, or autoimmune diseases.
- Peripheral eruptions on the extremities (with palpable purpuric spots) should be actively sought because these may occur in life-threatening meningococcemia (see Red Flag 1), disseminated gonococcal infection (see Brain 3), and bacterial endocarditis (see Red Flag 2). Lesions of erythema multiforme are often bilateral and symmetric.
- Note presence of macules, papules, plaques, nodules, urticaria, vesicles, bullae, pustules, and purpura, especially palpable purpura.

Testing

Laboratory testing is usually not indicated for simple viral upper respiratory tract infection associated with fever. However, if the history and examination suggest other causes, further investigation is advised. Fairly routine investigations listed below suffice in most individuals.

- CBC with a differential count
- Basic metabolic biochemistry panel with renal and liver function
- Chest x-ray
- Urinanalysis
- Blood and urine cultures

When suggested by the history and physical exam, a wider range of laboratory investigations, such as peripheral blood films, sputum, bone marrow, and cerebrospinal fluid examination, are to be considered to uncover autoimmune diseases and atypical infections. Testing should be individualized on the basis of clinical picture, pattern of fever, history and examination, and knowing what to test for requires clinical acumen and experience in the art of practicing medicine *(Brain 7)*.

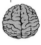 **7 -** The degree of temperature elevation may not correspond to the severity of the illness. Meticulous physical examination and follow-up examinations on subsequent visits are needed, particularly if the diagnosis is unclear on initial examination.

Putting It All Together

It is important to differentiate fever from hyperthermia. Important causes of hyperthermia include environmental factors and drugs, especially neuroleptic agents. Heatstroke due to environmental factors and drug-induced and malignant hyperthermia from neuroleptic agents are important causes of hyperthermia.

Most cases of fever result from short-lived, self-limiting viral infections. However, a clinician should be alert to the possibility of serious underlying infection or disease. A detailed history and examination are required for all cases. Testing should be individualized. Basic blood and chest x-ray investigations should be done in immunocompromised patients, those with cardiac, hepatic, or renal failure, and the elderly. Simple analgesics and the use of sponge baths may lower temperature. Empirical treatment with broad-spectrum antibiotics should be used for patients with possible life-threatening illnesses and should be initiated promptly.

Management

Most cases of fever can be controlled with the use of a fan, ice bags, or cold sponging and the use of antipyretics (e.g., acetaminophen [Tylenol] every 4 hours on a scheduled basis). However, if the fever is prolonged and reaches 41°C, more urgent measures may be required to avoid metabolic disturbances and seizures. Furthermore, fever over 37.8°C in the first trimester of pregnancy may double the risk of fetal neural tube defects.

Fluid replacement to compensate for increased fluid and electrolyte losses will vary depending on the patient. Elderly patients are prone to dehydration during bouts of pyrexial illness. Correction of fluid deficits may clear the delirium (mental confusion). Prompt, speedy, empiric, broad-spectrum antibiotic therapy is indicated for febrile patients with a potential serious infection such as meningitis or septicemia, even before the laboratory confirmation of the source or nature of infection. Atypical infection, such as *Mycoplasma*, responds to erythromycin or macrolides. Amoxicillin, co-trimoxazole, and cephalosporin are useful for mild infections of upper respiratory or urinary tracts. Immunization available against infections (flu, pneumonia, hepatitis A and B, tetanus) must be recommended for prevention. If fever persists and the diagnosis is unclear, referral to an infectious disease specialist may be indicated.

Selected Readings

1. Cunha BA: Fever of unknown origin. Infect Dis Clin North Am 10:111, 1996.
2. Gelfand JA, Dinarello CA: Alterations in body temperature. In Fauci A (ed): Harrison's Principles of Internal Medicine, 14th ed. New York, McGraw-Hill, 1998, pp 84–90.
3. Knockaert DC, Dujardin KS, Bobbaers HJ: Long-term follow-up of patients with undiagnosed fever of unknown origin. Arch Intern Med 152:51–55, 1992.
4. Machowiak PA: Concepts of fever. Arch Intern Med 158:1871, 1998.
5. Magill AJ: Fever in the returned traveler. Infect Dis Clin North Am 12:445, 1998.

36. Fever in Infants and Children

Sheryl Pitner, MD, MPH

Synopsis

Fever is one of the most common reasons that a child is brought to the doctor. Core body temperature (pulmonary arterial temperature) varies 1–1.5°C above or below average of 37°C and follows a **circadian rhythm** *(Definition 1)* that is established by the second year of life. Children have a slightly increased temperature and more pronounced circadian rhythm than adults. Fever occurs when an insult or stimulus increases the anterior hypothalamic heat regulatory set point and the body's temperature rises. Fever must be differentiated from **heat illness** *(Definition 2)*.

1 - Circadian rhythm: A regular recurrence of a cycle set by the biological clock. Temperature has a low point between midnight and 6:00 A.M. and a peak between 5:00 P.M. and 7:00 P.M.

2 - Heat illness: The body temperature exceeds the hypothalamic set point secondary to environmental factors or internal factors that impair the body's heat dissipation ability.

Rectal temperature (36.1–37.8°C) is considered closest to core body temperature and remains the standard measurement. Temperature also may be measured, though less reliably, by oral, axillary, tympanic, and transdermal routes. Both infectious and noninfectious conditions cause fever. Many febrile conditions are diagnosed based on history and physical examination alone (fever with localizing symptoms). If no source of fever is found on exam (fever without localizing symptoms), the differential diagnosis will vary with age, and monitoring for progression of symptoms or laboratory studies may be beneficial. **Fever of unknown origin** *(Definition 3)* requires a more extensive work-up. Most fevers are not harmful and do not require treatment. Therapy should be directed toward the underlying cause.

3 - Fever of unknown origin: Fever that has persisted ≥ 8 days and a focus that has not been found based on the initial work-up (including the history, physical exam, and laboratory and imaging studies).

Differential Diagnosis

The causes of fever include:

- Infection: bacterial and viral
- Inflammatory disease
- Endocrine and metabolic disorders
- Immunologic and rheumatologic disorders
- Malignancy
- Tissue injury
- Vaccines
- Drugs
- Biologic agents
- **Factitious** *(Definition 4)*

4 - Factitious fever: An elevated recorded temperature due to manipulation of the thermometer or to inoculation of the patient with fever-producing substances.

In infants, especially those ≥ 3 months of age, who have fever without localizing signs, one must consider:

- Viral illness
- Sepsis

- Pneumonia
- Meningitis
- Bacteremia
- Urinary tract infection or pyelonephritis
- Osteomyelitis

Fever of unknown origin may be caused by:

- Infectious disease
- Connective tissue disease
- Malignancy

History

At any age, you want to obtain a good history and review of systems for localizing signs and symptoms. Ask the parent or caregiver questions about the fever:

- "When did the fever start? How long did it last?" (chronic versus acute illness)
- "Does the fever follow any pattern?" *(Brain 1)*
- "How did you measure the temperature?" (Rectal measure is the most reliable in infants and young children.)
- "How high was the fever?" The magnitude of fever does not distinguish viral from bacterial causes, but bacterial infection is more likely at temperatures ≥ 41°C.
- "Did the fever respond to medication? What medication and how much was given?"

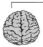

1 - A few causes of fever, such as systemic juvenile rheumatoid arthritis (JRA) and malaria, have a pattern that if present may help make the diagnosis. Systemic JRA has a daily or twice daily spike to ≥ 102°F (38.9°C) and rapidly returns to normal.

Determine any contributing or complicating factors:

- Travel (exposure to indigenous infectious agents via food, water, animals, people, ticks)
- Contacts with sick individuals
- Immunocompromising condition (e.g., treatment for malignancy, chronic steroid use, AIDS,)
- Chronic disease (e.g., sickle cell disease, nephrotic syndrome)
- Immunization status

Questions for parents of infants 3 months of age or younger *(Red Flag 1)*:

- "Is your baby sleepier than usual or not waking to feed?"
- "Is your baby fussier than usual?"
- "Is your baby feeding as usual?" (i.e., the same amount over the usual amount of time)
- "Does your baby have an unusual cry?"

1 - Any deviation from normal behavior may be a sign of serious illness, such as sepsis, pneumonia, pyelonephritis, meningitis, bacteremia, or osteomyelitis.

Note other important symptoms:

- Rash
- Headache
- Pain
- Other associated symptoms

Physical Examination

The physical exam should be driven by symptoms obtained from the history and review of symptoms. If there are no localizing symptoms by history, a complete physical exam should be performed (especially in infants). Below are specific reminders for parts of the physical exam.

- Vital signs *(Brain 2)*
- General appearance. Is the child alert and interactive, or lethargic and ill in appearance?
- Skin. Petechial rash is suggestive of *Neisseria meningitidis* infection.
- Interaction with the parent/caregiver and environment. Altered responsiveness could be a sign of intracranial involvement.
- Tympanic membranes. Immobile, opaque, and bulging TM is a sign of middle ear infection or otitis media (see Chapter 30).
- Pharynx *(Red Flag 2)*
- Lungs. Crackles and decreased breath sounds could indicate pneumonia; wheezing usually indicates asthma or bronchiolitis *(Brain 3).*
- Abdomen. Right lower quadrant tenderness is a sign of appendicitis, check for rebound tenderness) *(Red Flag 3).*
- Joints. Swelling, redness, and warmth suggest infection.
- Extremities. Point tenderness may suggest bone infection or neoplasm.
- Check Kernig's and Brudzinski's signs for meningeal irritation *(Brain 4).*

Examination specific to the infant:
- Palpate the fontanel(s) and suture lines. Bulging of the fontanel and widening suture lines may result from increased intracranial pressure *(Red Flag 4).*
- Examine the umbilical cord site or stump in the newborn *(Red Flag 5).*

Testing

Most conditions are diagnosable by history and physical exam, but confirmatory tests may be needed. Children younger than 3 months without a focus of infection require a more extensive work-up because of the increased possibility of serious disease. Practice guidelines suggest a complete blood count (CBC) with differential, blood culture, urinalysis, urine culture, cerebrospinal fluid studies and culture, and stool white blood count (if diarrhea is present).

In older infants, testing should be based on history and exam findings. Urinary tract infections and occult bacteremia are easily missed, so a urine and blood culture in infants without a known viral illness or localizing physical finding may be prudent.

Putting It All Together

The most common cause of fever still remains a viral illness. However, caution must be taken when the source of the fever cannot be found from the history and physical exam, especially in young infants. Fever

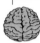
2 - Fever may produce tachycardia and tachypnea, so these signs should be interpreted carefully. Tachypnea may be a sign of respiratory disease, and tachycardia may be a sign of several things, including dehydration, sepsis, and heart disease. Antipyretics may be given, and the heart rate and respiratory rate can be monitored for changes as the fever decreases.

2 - A child with fever and respiratory distress—drooling (unable to swallow secretions), forward posture, difficulty breathing—may have epiglottitis and should never be examined orally with a tongue blade to prevent further narrowing and complete obstruction of the airway. The child should be taken immediately to the operating room to be examined under anesthesia by someone capable of intubating the child (otolaryngologist).

3 - Crackles may not always be heard in newborns with pneumonia.

3 - Rebound tenderness and pain with release of pressure can be a sign of inflammation of the peritoneal lining and perforation of the gut.

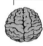
4 - Kernig's and Brudzinski's signs are not reliable in children younger than 2 years of age.

4 - Increased intracranial pressure could be a sign of meningitis.

5 - An infection of the umbilical stump (omphalitis) results in erythema, edema, and drainage of the umbilicus. It requires hospitalization and IV antibiotics to prevent spread to the fascia, portal vessels, liver, or peritoneum, which often leads to sepsis.

without localizing symptoms is more common in children younger than 5 years of age (peak 6–24 months), and laboratory evaluation may be needed. The extent of the evaluation will depend on the age of the infant and the infant's physical appearance and temperament (Is the child alert and interactive versus lethargic?).

It is important to listen to parental concerns and not discount them. Parents may report findings that are not present while the child is in the office. For example, a 5-week-old infant who has been very fussy and febrile at home but is afebrile and quiet in the office still requires a work-up for fever. After obtaining the history and physical exam, develop a plan of action and relay this to the parent and patient. Infants younger than 3 months of age who appear ill require laboratory studies, and the first dose of antibiotics should be started in a very short period of time to prevent sequelae from bacterial disease. It is important to communicate the significance of this to the parents and to address their concerns and emotions.

Management

Not all fevers need to be treated. The potential benefits of fever include retarded growth of pathogens, enhancement of neutrophil migration and production of superoxides, promotion of T-cell proliferation, and increased release and activation of interferon. Adversely, fever increases the body's metabolic demand: increased oxygen consumption, carbon dioxide production, water loss, and caloric need.

Treatment of fever provides symptomatic relief only, and the underlying condition should be treated if possible. Aspirin, acetaminophen, and ibuprofen all act to inhibit cyclooxygenase (prostaglandin E_2 synthesis), and doses are calculated based on weight *(Treatment 1)*. To decrease the risk of **Reye's syndrome *(Definition 5)***, aspirin should not be given to anyone 19 years of age or younger, especially with viral illnesses. A sponge bath with water (lukewarm) can help lower the body temperature temporarily and is often used by parents in conjunction with medication when a child has a high temperature. Alcohol is absorbed through the skin and should never be used for sponge baths.

1 - Acetaminophen dose: 10–15 mg/kg/dose every 4 hours as needed for fever. Ibuprofen dose: 10 mg/kg/dose every 6 hours as needed for fever.

5 - Reye's syndrome: A syndrome of acute encephalopathy and fatty degeneration of the liver.

Selected Readings

1. Adam HM: Fever and host responses. Pediatr Rev 17:330–331, 1996.
2. Grossman M: Fever. In Rudolph AM, Hoffman JIE, Rudolph CD (eds): Rudolph's Pediatrics, 20th ed. Stamford, CT, Appleton & Lange, 1996.
3. Lorin MI: Fever: Pathogenesis and treatment. In Feigin RD, Cherry JD (eds): Textbook of Pediatric and Infectious Diseases, 4th ed. Philadelphia, W.B. Saunders, 1998.
4. Powell KR: Fever and fever without a focus. In Behrman RE, Kliegman RM, Jenson HB (eds.): Nelson Textbook of Pediatrics, 16th ed. Philadelphia, W.B. Saunders, 2000.

37. Fractures

Paul W. Esposito, MD • Patrick Morgan, BS, BA

Synopsis

Bones may fracture because of acute injury, repetitive minor trauma, or weakening by a pathologic process. Grossly deformed bones following significant trauma are easily diagnosed as fractures. Other fractures, however, such as stress fractures or incomplete fractures, may demonstrate little, if any, swelling or deformity. Stress fractures occur when an individual performs repetitive activities in excess of the body's ability to remodel and strengthen the bone after mechanical stress of the activity. An individual with metabolic bone disease, such as rickets or severe osteoporosis, may sustain fractures more easily. Fracture after seemingly trivial injury may indicate a pathologic fracture *(Table 1)* *(Red Flag 1)*. Careful history of both the mechanism of injury and the patient's occupation or avocation is important in determining the type of injury and can often predict the fracture pattern.

1 - When abnormal bone gives way, this is referred to as a pathologic fracture. Fractures that occur spontaneously or after trivial injury must be regarded as a pathologic fracture until proven otherwise. Older patients should be asked about previous illnesses or operations. A malignant tumor, even in the distant past, may be the source of a metastastic lesion. A history of gastrectomy, intestinal malabsorption, or prolonged drug therapy (especially corticosteroids) may suggest a metabolic bone disorder. In children, rickets and osteogenesis imperfecta are frequently diagnosed following an injury secondary to trivial trauma (see Table 1).

Table 1. Common Causes of Pathologic Fractures

- Congenital (e.g., osteogenesis imperfecta)
- Fibrous dysplasia
- Infection (e.g., osteomyelitis)
- Metabolic (e.g., osteomalacia, osteoporosis, Paget's disease)
- Benign tumors (e.g., bone cysts, enchondroma)
- Malignant tumors (e.g., primary bone tumor, myeloma, metastatic disease)

Careful vascular and neurologic exams are vital whenever a fracture is sustained *(Red Flag 2)*. Most patients, especially those sustaining long bone fractures, will require a complete physical examination. Keep in mind that high-energy fractures are often associated with visceral and spinal injuries. Once the physical examination is complete, proper radiographs should be obtained in both the anteroposterior (AP) and lateral planes and should include the joints proximal and distal to the site of injury. Splinting the fracture in a position of comfort without manipulating the extremity whenever possible prevents further injury, decreases bleeding, and remarkably improves the patient's comfort.

2 - A pulseless, painful extremity requires immediate emergency care.

Differential Diagnosis

- Fracture
- Bone tumor
- Sprained or torn ligaments
- **Avulsed tendons**, or **avulsion fracture** *(Definition 1)*
- **Contusion** *(Definition 2)*
- Metabolic disease

1 - Avulsion: A tearing away by forcible separation. Avulsion of a tendon may occur at the musculotendinous junction or the bone–tendon interface, or it may produce an avulsion fracture where a small piece of bone is torn away with the tendon.

2 - Contusion: A mechanical injury resulting in structural disruption and hemorrhage within muscle beneath unbroken skin. It is often caused by a direct blow and will usually result in ecchymosis (bruise).

History

- "Did you have an accident? What happened exactly?" Establishing the mechanism of injury helps establish possible fracture patterns and offers clues to other injuries.
- "Can you feel your arm [or leg] below where it hurts?" Nerves can be damaged by laceration, traction, pressure, or prolonged ischemia. After any injury, patients should be questioned about numbness, any change of feeling, or weakness.
- "Does your back, chest, or abdomen hurt?" Evaluate the patient for any comorbidities sustained at the time of injury. The rule is to treat the patient, not simply the part most obviously injured.
- "What do you do for a living? What do you like to do for fun?" The differential diagnosis you formulate for wrist pain might be very different for a karate instructor than a person who works all day at a keyboard. Knowing what stresses your patient places on his or her limbs and joints is important in establishing both the mechanism and nature of the injury *(Table 2)*.

Table 2. Sport-Specific Stress Fractures

Sport	Common Injury
Running	Tibia, navicular, fibula, hip or femur
Marching	Second metatarsal
Golfing	Rib
Bowling	Ulna
Weight lifting	Rib, clavicle
Gymnastics	Foot, acromion, distal radius, spine (pars interarticularis)
Basketball	Fibula, foot (fifth metatarsal, navicular), proximal tibia
Football	Metatarsals
Dancing	Metatarsals, midshaft tibia
Rowing	Rib

Adapted from Orthopaedic Knowledge Update 1999. Rosemont, IL, American Academy of Orthopaedic Surgeons, 1999.

Physical Examination

- General observations. Is the patient comfortable or screaming in pain?
- Vital signs
- Head and neck exam. Note any abnormalities, neck tenderness, or limited motion.
- Screening examination of the heart, lungs, and abdomen
- Extremity exam. Note the following:
  1. Swelling. Are the muscle compartments soft or tense? Evaluate for **compartment syndrome (Definition 3), (Red Flag 3), (Consultation and Referral 1).**
  2. Skeletal instability
  3. Location of tenderness
  4. Skin integrity. Is this an **open fracture**? *(Definition 4).*
  5. Motor and sensory function: Examination of the neurologic integrity of the limb begins with evaluation of sensation to light touch. Test all peripheral nerves in region of injury and distal to it.

3 - Compartment syndrome: Fractures to the arm or leg can give rise to severe ischemia even if there is no damage to a major vessel. Bleeding or edema can increase the pressure within one of the osteofascial compartments. If this increase in the compartment's pressure exceeds capillary filling pressure, it can lead to a cycle of muscle ischemia, further edema, greater pressure, and thus more profound ischemia. Necrosis of the muscle and nerve results. Though nerve is capable of regeneration, necrotic muscle is replaced by inelastic fibrous tissue (Volkmann's ischemic contracture). Similar events may be caused by the swelling of a limb within a tightly applied splint or cast. The hallmark of a compartment syndrome is severe pain even with normal pulses and capillary filling.

3 - The following may indicate an evolving compartment syndrome:
- Pain at rest and/or rapidly increasing pain out of proportion to the injury
- Paresthesias (tingling, burning, numbness) distal to the injury site
- Soft tissue tenseness
- Pain with passive motion of joint distal to the compartment

1 - The involved compartment in an evolving compartment syndrome must be decompressed promptly by surgical fasciotomy. Concomitant fracture stabilization and vascular repair may also be necessary.

6. Passive and active range of motion of joints proximal and distal to| the injury. Evaluate for dislocation.
7. Note if motion is painful or if there is crepitation (a crunching sound or feeling) *(Red Flag 4)*.
8. In children, tenderness and swelling over a physis almost always means a fracture through the growth plate, even if x-rays read as normal *(Consultation and Referral 2)*.

Testing

- AP and lateral radiographs of all injured bones and joints
- Inspect for fracture lines (Figure 1)
  Transverse: direct blow
  Spiral or oblique: torsion
  Comminuted: more than two fragments
  Segmental: fracture in more than two places
  Greenstick: a fracture through only one side of the cortex that generally occurs in children, usually markedly angulated
- Bone scan or magnetic resonance imaging (MRI) may be necessary to diagnose stress fractures.

 4 - Open fracture: Fracture causing skin to be punctured either inside out, by a fragment of fractured bone, or outside in at the time of injury exposing the fracture to the outside.

 4 - An audible or palpable crepitation or crunching typically means dislocation or fracture.

 2 - Pediatric patients present a challenge when reading radiographs. Pediatric patients with growth plate injuries may have normal-appearing x-rays. Therefore, if a physis (growth plate) is tender, it must be treated as a growth cartilage fracture regardless of the x-ray appearance. Also, young bone may bow or buckle without any obvious fracture line. These patients should be evaluated by a pediatric orthopedist or by a general orthopedist who has experience with pediatric patients.

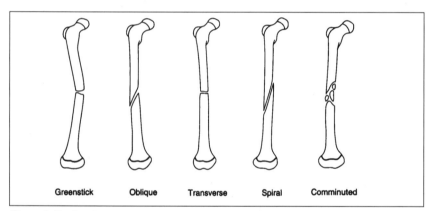

Figure 1: Fracture types.
(From Staheli L: Fundamentals of Pediatric Orthopedics, 2nd ed. Philadelphia, Lippincott-Raven, 1998, with permission.)

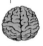 **1 -** Patients with chronic pain related to repetitive activities can have stress fractures or stress reaction not seen on standard x-rays.

Putting It All Together

Stress injuries typically can be treated with activity modification. A careful history is necessary, because some injuries are more common in specific circumstances. For example, women who run long distances on a regular basis are more prone to pubic rami and femoral neck fractures than other patients. If not treated aggressively, femoral neck stress fractures become complete fractures, a condition that can lead to avascular necrosis of the hip, which can lead to collapse and deformity of the head of the femur *(Brain 1)*.

In the patient with an acute high-energy injury, it is vital to examine carefully the whole patient and not be distracted by the obvious deformity. For example, fracturing the femur requires a tremendous amount of energy. Because such injuries are often sustained in accidents involving motor vehicles, the femur fracture is often associated with serious intra-abdominal or intrathoracic injuries. However, even an isolated femur fracture may result in significant blood loss and shock.

All fractures should be immobilized to prevent further injury, even prior to obtaining x-rays. Once the x-rays are obtained, more permanent casting or splinting should be undertaken. In some cases, operative treatment may be necessary to rigidly stabilize the fracture and allow healing and early mobilization of the limb. Operative treatment is done on an urgent basis for patients with multiple fractures.

Acute compartment syndrome occurs frequently with fractures when the pressure within the muscle compartment exceeds the capillary filling pressure. It must be recognized early to prevent ischemic contracture and loss of the entire musculature of the compartment. Tight bandages, splints, or casts should be removed immediately when the cardinal signs of pain out of proportion to injury, paresthesias, tense soft tissues, and pain on passive motion of the distal joint become evident. Prompt surgical release of the fascial compartment is necessary to save the patient's extremity. Neurologic and circulatory involvement requires immediate medical referral and potentially immediate surgical treatment.

Management

Initial treatment of all fractures should include splinting in the position of deformity unless there is a circulatory abnormality, in which case careful reduction must be performed emergently. Open wounds should be dressed with a sterile bandage prior to splinting. Elevation above the level of the heart is mandatory to diminish swelling. Ice also helps decrease pain and swelling but should never be applied directly to skin.

Recognizing the mechanism of injury and close physical examination allow for proper treatment. The type of fracture determines duration of casting and the need for operative treatment. Immobilization of the fracture fragments in proper anatomic alignment will greatly increase the patient's level of comfort. Analgesics may be necessary in the initial postinjury period and postoperatively if the fracture requires surgical treatment.

Always evaluate closely for associated injuries, because the most obviously deformed fracture may not be the injury with the most potential for morbidity *(Red Flag 5)*.

 5 - Unconscious patients should be presumed to have a neck or spine injury and must be protected from motion until it is certain they did not sustain a spinal fracture or spinal cord injury.

Selected Readings

1. Beaty JH: Orthopaedic Knowledge Update 6. Rosemont, IL, American Academy of Orthopaedic Surgeons, 1999.
2. Salter RB, Harris WR: Injuries involving the epiphyseal plate. J Bone Joint Surg 45A:587, 1963.
3. Snider RK (ed): Essentials of Musculoskeletal Care. Rosemont, IL, American Academy of Orthopaedic Surgeons-American Academy of Pediatrics, 1997.
4. Staheli LT: Fundamentals of Pediatric Orthopaedics. New York, Raven Press, 1992.

38. Genitourinary and Vaginal Complaints in Children

Amy E. Lacroix, MD

Synopsis

Genitourinary and vaginal complaints in children are common. The prevalence of urinary tract infections (UTI) varies with age, and UTIs are more common in school-aged girls. **Vulvovaginitis (Definition 1)** may occur in up to 75% of girls during childhood or adolescence. Genitourinary and vaginal complaints may include painful urination (dysuria), blood in urine (hematuria), local skin rashes, a swollen penis, scrotal masses or swelling, vaginal discharge, and vaginal bleeding. Boys with **balanitis** or **posthitis (Definition 2)** commonly present with complaints secondary to **phimosis** or **paraphimosis (Definition 3)**. Other causes of urinary complaints include vaginal foreign bodies and kidney stones. More serious causes of these symptoms include **pyelonephritis (Definition 4)**, **postinfectious nephritis (Definition 5)**, or sexual abuse. History taking should be directed at exclusion of these causes. In boys with a swollen scrotum, an **incarcerated hernia (Definition 6)** or **testicular torsion (Definition 7)** must be ruled out. A careful history of the patient should note presence of urinary symptoms, preceding trauma, and constitutional symptoms such as fever, nausea, vomiting, decreased physical activity, or decreased appetite. A complete physical examination of the urinary and genital system is necessary in all patients to help identify these conditions. Confirmation of diagnoses with appropriate laboratory testing may include a urinalysis and urine culture or a culture of vaginal secretions. Referral is indicated in cases of suspected sexual abuse. Hospitalization is usually necessary for children with suspected pyelonephritis. Children with postinfectious nephritis may require hospitalization or close clinical observation. Boys with a scrotal mass may require immediate surgery. Most common urinary and vaginal complaints can be managed successfully in the outpatient setting.

Differential Diagnosis

Children who present with dysuria or hematuria may be diagnosed with the following conditions:

- Lower urinary tract infection
- Vulvovaginitis (specific or nonspecific)
- Balanitis or posthitis
- **Labial fusion (Definition 8)**
- **Hemorrhagic cystitis (Definition 9)**
- Urinary stones
- Pyelonephritis **(Red Flag 1)**
- Postinfectious nephritis

 1 - Vulvovaginitis: Inflammation of the female vulva (labia majora, labia minora, mons pubis, vestibule of the vagina, and vaginal orifice) or vagina, which may be accompanied by a vaginal discharge.

 2 - Balanitis: Inflammation of the glans penis. **Posthitis:** Inflammation of the prepuce of the penis.

 3 - Phimosis: The inability to retract the foreskin at an age when the foreskin should be retractable (over the glans penis) in children. Ninety percent of uncircumcised boys aged 3 years old have a retractable foreskin. This condition may be inflammatory or congenital. **Paraphimosis:** A condition in which a phimotic prepuce is retracted behind the corona of the glans and cannot be reduced. This is a painful condition that is commonly ameliorated with lubrication and traction under mild sedation.

 4 - Pyelonephritis: Inflammation of the kidney and renal pelvis in children, primarily caused by bacterial infection.

 5 - Postinfectious nephritis: Inflammation of the kidney secondary to deposition of immune complexes and activation of complement. A history of recent infection with a sore throat or virus is common. Patients often present with painless hematuria. Urine is often grossly bloody, and urinalysis often is positive for both blood cells and protein with a negative urine culture (i.e., no evidence of infection). Complications that are most concerning are hypertension and prolonged proteinuria with decreased renal function.

In girls who present with vaginal bleeding or discharge before the age of puberty, the following must be considered:

- Vulvovaginitis (specific or nonspecific)
- Vaginal foreign body
- Sexual abuse *(Red Flag 2)*
- Trauma
- Premature puberty
- Vaginal tumor (rare)

In boys who present with a mass or swelling of the scrotum, the following must be considered:

- Inguinal hernia *(Red Flag 3)*
- **Hydrocele** *(Definition 10)*
- **Varicocele** *(Definition 11)*
- **Epididymitis** *(Definition 12)*
- Testicular torsion (see Red Flag 3)
- Hematoma secondary to trauma

History

Depending on the age of the child, questions can be directed to the child or to the parent or caregiver. In children with complaints of pain with urination:

- "Does it hurt when you pee [or potty]?" and "Where does is hurt?"
- "Does it itch?"
- "Do you [or does your child] have a rash?"
- "Is there swelling present? If so, where?"
- "What does the urine look like?"
- "Is there blood in the urine?" or "Is there blood on the toilet paper?"
- "Does your child have fever, vomiting, abdominal pain, or back pain?" (see Red Flag 1)

In children with blood in the urine but without painful urination, the above questions are appropriate, plus:

- "Has your child had a recent sore throat, skin wound, or other infection?"
- "Do you have a family history of kidney stones?"

In girls with complaints of vaginal discharge or bleeding:

- "Does your child have a rash?"
- "Has there been any trauma to the area?" (e.g., slipped and fell onto a fence post or bicycle bar, straddling it)
- "Are you concerned about the possibility of someone harming or abusing your child?"
- "Is your child developing signs of puberty, such as pubic hair or hair under the arms?"

In boys with complaints of an enlarged scrotum, the following questions are appropriate:

- "Does the swelling go up and down, or is it consistent?"
- "Does anything make it worse?" (e.g., crying or straining to have a bowel movement)

6 - Inguinal hernia: Entrapment of a loop of intestine into the inguinal ring and canal, often into the scrotal sac. This often can be reduced (pushed back) into the abdomen through the inguinal canal by applying manual pressure on the hernia with the patient relaxed or sedated.

Incarcerated hernia: An intestinal hernia that cannot be manually reduced and is a surgical emergency.

7 - Testicular torsion: Twisting of the testicle on its pedicle (the spermatic cord), which results in interruption of the blood supply to the testicle and subsequent necrosis or atrophy of the testicle if not immediately corrected surgically.

8 - Labial fusion: Adherence of the opposing sides of the epithelium of the labia minora, which may partially or completely occlude the vaginal and urethral openings and predispose to urinary infection by means of obstruction of urinary outflow. This condition is often due to poor hygiene.

9 - Hemorrhagic cystitis: Inflammation of the bladder that is often accompanied by grossly bloody, heme-positive urine, urinary frequency, urinary urgency, and dysuria. The causes include bacterial infection, drug reactions, and viral infections and should be treated as bacterial infection until proven otherwise.

1 - Signs of acute pyelonephritis include fever, chills, abdominal pain, vomiting, and flank pain in the costovertebral angle (CVA) of the affected side. Patients may or may not present with signs of lower urinary tract infection, which include urinary frequency, urinary urgency, or dysuria.

2 - If parents have serious concerns about child abuse as a cause of a genitourinary complaint, they should always be taken seriously. The child and parent should be interviewed by someone experienced with child abuse and neglect. A thorough genitourinary exam should be performed by the examining physician with careful documentation of all findings. Cultures for gonorrhea and chlamydia should be obtained. The patient should be referred to a child abuse specialist for colposcopy if any abnormal findings (unexplained abrasions, contusions, or lacerations) are identified on screening exam.

- "Is there any redness?"
- "Is it painful?"

Physical Examination

General Observations

- Is the child acting distressed, uncomfortable, crying, fussy, frightened?

Vital Signs

Check:

- Fever
- Blood pressure
- Tachycardia (high heart rate)

Abdominal Exam

Genital Exam

This is most frequently performed with the child supine in frog-leg position (*Figure 1*):

- In girls, inspect skin, external genitalia, labia, urethra, and hymen.
- In boys, inspect skin, penis, scrotum, and urethra.
  1. A scrotal mass that is reducible (able to be pushed back through the inguinal canal) is usually a hernia.
  2. Transillumination with a light may help to discern a mass (hernia, tumor) from fluid (hydrocele).
  3. Note any tenderness on palpation of the scrotum.
- Look for erythema, rashes, and edema (common)
- The presence of abrasions, contusions, or lacerations is suspicious for trauma or abuse (see Red Flag 2).
- Palpate the back for CVA tenderness.

Testing

- Urinalysis with microscopic exam of urine *and* urine culture:
  1. In children who are not toilet-trained, a catheterized specimen must be obtained. A clean-catch specimen (obtained after cleaning the genital area thoroughly) may be obtained in older children with parental assistance.
  2. A urine culture should be obtained on all children suspected of having urinary tract infection. A urinalysis alone is not sufficient.
  3. A urinalysis suspicious for infection may test positive for any of the following: red blood cells, white blood cells, leukocyte esterase, protein, or nitrates. However, these do not have to be present to have infection. Microscopic exam of centrifuged urine that is infected will commonly show many bacteria and white blood cells.
- Culture of vaginal secretions (vulvovaginitis)
- Potassium hydroxide prep (KOH) for suspected yeast rash or vaginitis
- Other testing is necessary in patients suspected of having pyelonephritis, genital trauma secondary to abuse, or postinfectious nephritis.

 3 - In boys, if the patient has a tender or painful scrotal mass that is non-reducible, it is vitally important to exclude either an incarcerated hernia or testicular torsion. Both of these are surgical emergencies and must be corrected at once to prevent either bowel (hernia) or testicular necrosis. Ultrasound examination of the scrotum can be helpful in identifying the mass as either bowel or testicle and facilitating rapid surgical correction of these conditions.

 10 - Hydrocele: A collection of peritoneal fluid in the tunica vaginalis of the testicle or along the spermatic cord, within the scrotal sac.

 11 - Varicocele: A swelling of the veins of the spermatic cord, which is accompanied by pain, and may appear bluish through the skin of the scrotum.

 12 - Epididymitis: An inflammation of the epididymis of the testes. This is most commonly caused by infection (viral or bacterial, often by *Chlamydia* in sexually active persons) or by trauma. It is often accompanied by extreme tenderness to palpation.

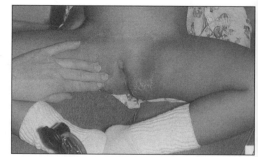

Figure 1: Child in frog-leg position for genitourinary exam.
(From Zitelli BJ, Davis HW (eds): Atlas of Pediatric Physical Diagnosis, 2nd ed. New York, Gower Medical Publishing, 1992, with permission.)

- Ultrasound examination of the scrotum may help differentiate testicular torsion and incarcerated hernia from other more benign causes.

Putting It All Together

Genitourinary and vaginal complaints are common in prepubertal children. They are most commonly related to nonspecific vulvovaginitis or lower UTI. The history should be targeted at obtaining symptoms and duration and ruling out serious medical conditions that need prompt attention, referral, or hospitalization. A complete genitourinary exam is essential, often diagnostic, and is standard in children with urinary or vaginal complaints. UTI can be confirmed by urinalysis and urine culture. Pyelonephritis, postinfectious nephritis, testicular torsion, incarcerated hernia, and possible sexual or physical abuse can often be ruled out with history, physical exam, and results from a clean urinalysis specimen. If any of these are suspected, further testing and close follow-up, including hospitalization, may be warranted.

Management

Urinary and vaginal complaints are managed with specific regard to diagnosis. Urinary infections are commonly treated empirically based on common pathogens *(Table 1)*, and treatment should always be confirmed by sensitivity of the organism obtained from urine culture. Vulvovaginitis may be treated symptomatically with improved voiding practices *(Table 2)* or may be treated specifically based on culture of vaginal secretions or KOH prep. Labial fusion is treated with topical estrogen application. Balanitis and posthitis may be managed conservatively with good hygiene. Many of these common problems can be prevented with attention to appropriate voiding, clothing choices, and hygiene. Hernias are managed by surgical reduction, and testicular torsion is considered a surgical emergency. Children with pyelonephritis often require hospitalization and treatment with IV antibiotics. Children with suspected sexual abuse require referral to a specialist in child abuse for procurement of appropriate specimens and colposcopy (magnified visualization of the genital structures). Children with suspected postinfectious nephritis require close follow-up with attention to altered renal function or hypertension.

Table 1. Common Urinary Pathogens and Their Sensitivity to Antibiotics

Bacterial Pathogen	Microbiologic Identification	Common Antibiotic Sensitivity
Escherichia coli	Gram-negative rod, enteric	TMP-SMX, nitrofurantoin
Klebsiella pneumoniae	Gram-negative rod, enteric	TMP-SMX
Proteus mirabilis	Gram-negative pleomorphic rod, enteric	TMP-SMX, nitrofurantoin
Enterococcus	Gram-positive cocci, enteric	Ampicillin

TMP-SMX = trimethoprim-sulfamethoxazole.

Table 2. Common Problems with Pediatric Urinary Hygiene and Their Solutions

Problem	Solution
Bubble bath use: common skin irritant	Eliminate bubbles in the tub
Nylon panty use for girls: poor air circulation	Use cotton panties
Poor wiping technique in girls	Always wipe front to back
Poor self-cleaning in boys	Always retract foreskin as much as comfortably possible, and cleanse the glans when bathing
Back-wash of urine into vagina in obese females	Spread legs wide apart when emptying bladder
Parent/guardian hesitant or nervous about cleaning genital area appropriately	Teach parent/guardian appropriate cleaning technique of genitals during early infancy
Frequent masturbation	Setting up rules for masturbating (e.g., not in public, only at bedtime)
Frequent application of antibiotics may predispose to yeast infections	Avoid unnecessary antibiotics

Selected Readings

1. Dorland's Illustrated Medical Dictionary, 28th ed. Philadelphia, W.B. Saunders, 1994.
2. Emans SJ: Vulvovaginal problems in the prepubertal child. In Emans SJ, Laufer MR, Goldstein DP (eds): Pediatric and Adolescent Gynecology, 4th ed. Philadelphia, Lippincott-Raven, 1998.
3. Farrington PF: Pediatric vulvovaginitis. Clin Obstet Gynecol 40:135–140, 1997.
4. Gonzalez R: Urologic disorders in infants and children. In Nelson WE (ed): Nelson Textbook of Pediatrics, 15th ed. Philadelphia, W.B. Saunders, 1996.
5. Sanfilippo JS: Gynecologic problems of childhood. In Nelson WE (ed): Nelson Textbook of Pediatrics, 15th ed. Philadelphia, W.B. Saunders 1996.
6. Skoog SJ: Benign and malignant pediatric scrotal masses. Pediatr Clin North Am 44:1229–1250, 1997.
7. Zitelli BJ, Davis HW, (eds): Atlas of Pediatric Physical Diagnosis, 2nd ed. New York, Gower Medical Publishing, 1992.

39. Headache

Dennis P. Goeschel, MD

Synopsis

Although headaches are a common reason for office visits to a primary care physician, most patients treat headaches themselves. Those who do see a physician can be a diagnostic and therapeutic challenge. A thorough history and physical examination will determine the cause in a majority of patients. Most patients will not need testing, especially if their exam is negative. Blood and x-ray testing is reserved for those with histories and exams that suggest serious underlying disorders *(Red Flag 1)*. Although the causes of headaches in the majority of patients are benign, it is important to rule out serious disorders such as hemorrhage or hematoma, temporal arteritis, meningitis, and transient ischemic attack.

Management is directed toward treating any underlying disorder, avoiding provocative factors, and symptomatic treatment in nonserious cases. Patient education and close follow-up until symptoms improve are effective long-term measures.

> **1 -** Indications for CT or MRI scanning include "worst ever headache," decreased mental status, stiff neck, abnormal neurologic exam, worsening of symptoms, new onset of headaches lasting > 2 months in patient ages 40–60, new onset in patient with cancer, and headaches triggered by cough or coitus.

Differential Diagnosis *(Table 1)*

- Tension (or muscle contraction) headache
- Migraine. Migraines are commonly described as vascular headaches. The physiologic event seems to be constriction of cerebral blood vessels, with release of certain neuroactive substances.
- Headaches caused by drugs or other substances. Examples include medications, foods, hormones, withdrawal from caffeine.
- Infections. These can include infections of the scalp, head and neck, and the central nervous system itself. Generalized infections such as infectious mononucleosis and influenza can have associated headaches.
- Intracranial pathology. Space-occupying lesions cause pain as they enlarge within a closed space. Examples include tumors, blood and blood clots from trauma or hemorrhage, and certain vascular malformations. Transient lack of oxygen from reduced blood flow also can cause headaches.
- Temporal arteritis. This is an inflammation of the temporal artery of the scalp.
- Psychological disorders. Depression and anxiety are often associated with headaches, usually musculoskeletal in nature. **Malingering** *(Definition 1)* can also be a cause of reported headaches.

> **1 - Malingering:** Feigning illness for one or more of the following reasons: to arouse sympathy, escape work, obtain medication, or receive compensation.

Table 1. Headache Types and Treatment

Headache Type	History	Physical Exam	Testing	Treatment
Tension (muscle contraction)	Occipital, nuchal or temporal. Location: may be "bandlike." Worse as day goes on	Tender scalp or neck muscles, Neurologic exam normal	None necessary	Stress reduction, ice, heat, massage, over-the-counter meds, or NSAIDs
Migraine (vascular)	Unilateral or generalized. Often family history. May be throbbing. Triggered by caffeine, stress. Relief with sleep	Usually normal	Usually none necessary	Similar to tension. In addition, ergotamines, midrin, and many classes of medications for prophylaxis
Infectious	Nuchal "stiff neck." Prior sore throat or respiratory symptoms, fever, visual complaints, nausea and vomiting	Positive for Kernig and/or Brudzinski signs. Fever, possible rashes. Acutely ill appearance. Possibly abnormal mentation	CBC, CT scan, lumber puncture	Hospitalize. Treat infection with appropriate antibiotics.
Subarachnoid hemorrhage	"Worse headache ever." Stiff neck, visual complaints. Nausea and/or vomiting	Meningeal irritation. Possible neurologic and mental abnormalities. Kernig/Brudzinski	CBC, coagulation studies, CT scan, lumbar puncture	Hospitalize. Neurosurgery consultation
Intracranial pathology	Progressive, worsening. May be worse in mornings. May be associated with changes in gait, mentation, vision, speech, or strength	May be normal or a wide variety neurologic abnormalities can be found	CT or MRI testing	Neurosurgeon referral

CBC = complete blood count; CT = computed tomography; MRI = magnetic resonance imaging; ESR = erythrocyte sedimentation rate; NSAIDs = nonsteroidal anti-inflammatory drugs.

History

The history of present illness should include location, character and severity, duration, and temporal associations of the headache. Provocative and palliative features, including a history of trauma, should be determined, as well as any associated physical symptoms. Some past medical, social, and family history and a review of systems are also necessary. As always, begin with an open-ended question such as "Tell me about your headache." Then, follow up with more specific questions depending on the additional information you need.

Location

- "Where does your head hurt?"
- "Where does the pain start?"

Unilateral headaches can be seen with migraines, temporal arteritis (inflammation of the temporal artery), cluster headaches, and various other inflammatory or infectious conditions. Occipital and nuchal headaches can be associated with tension headaches or more serious conditions such as meningitis or subarachnoid bleeding. Generalized headaches can be seen with systemic infections or advanced muscle tension.

Character and Severity

- "Can you describe how this feels?"
- "How does it rate on a scale of 1 to 10, with 10 being the worst?"

"Band-like" or "squeezing" are often used to describe tension headaches. Throbbing may be associated with vascular headaches. The "worst headache I have ever had" may describe a subarachnoid hemorrhage *(Red Flag 2)*.

Temporal Associations (Timing)

- "Is there a time of day when the headache is better or worse?"
- "Does it get worse as the day goes on?"

- "How long have you had headaches?"
- "How long does the headache last?"

Determine whether the headache occurs more frequently or severely at a particular time of day. Morning headaches can be associated with migraines, sinus problems, intracranial lesions, and hypertension. Tension headaches often get worse as the day progresses. One to two days can be common for migraines. Days to weeks may suggest chronic tension. Worsening headaches over days and weeks may be caused by intracranial problems.

Provocative Factors (What Makes It Worse?)

- "What brings the headache on?"
- "What things make it worse?"

If a headache can be provoked, a diagnosis often can be made. Timing relative to eating, dosing of medications, or menstrual periods should be determined. Is there a relationship to physical or emotional stress? Has there been recent trauma or symptoms of infection, for example?

Palliative Factors (What Makes It Better?)

- "What can you do to make the headache better?"

Rest and sleep often make migraines better. Do over-the-counter medications or massage help? Is it better on weekends, when the stress from work or school is less?

Associated Symptoms

- "Do you feel ill in any other way when you have headaches?"

These questions will help decide the severity of the condition and will aid in the decision to do testing. Associated neurologic symptoms, such as difficulties with vision, speech, coordination, and mentation, must be determined. Other symptoms suggesting scalp, jaw, sinus, or upper respiratory involvement should be pursued.

Other History

- "Is there a history in your family of headaches?"
- "Have you hit your head or sustained an injury to your head?"

Determine whether the patient has a past history of headaches. Many patients with migraines have a family history of migraines. Does the social history reveal exposures to caffeine, alcohol, tobacco, or other drugs? Obtain a review of systems for evidence of infection (fever, chills, sweats) or weight loss. Determine whether the patient has suffered trauma to the head.

Functional Impact and Patient Attributions

- "What effect does your headache have on things you need to do or want to do?" It is important to assess the extent to which the patient's headache interferes with activities of daily living.
- "What ideas have you had about what might be causing these headaches? What worries you most about these headaches?" By discovering what the patient is most worried about, the clinician is in a better position to offer targeted education and reassurance.

2 - Subarachnoid hemorrhage. Bleeding into the space beneath the arachnoid membrane.

Physical Examination

The majority of patients with headache will have a normal physical examination. However, in evaluating the headache patient, particular attention should be paid to the following:

- Vital signs. Patients with extremely high blood pressure or uncontrolled hypertension are more prone to intracranial and subarachnoid hemorrhage. An elevated temperature can be found in temporal arteritis, subarachnoid hemorrhage, encephalitis, and meningitis.
- General appearance. How sick does the patient look? Is the patient in distress?
- Skin. Evidence of rashes or cyanosis may suggest severe infection or critical illness.
- HEENT. Look for scalp tenderness or tender temporal artery. It is important to look for signs of infection (ears, nose, throat; palpate sinuses). Inflammation of the temporomandibular joint (TMJ) or tenderness over the muscles of mastication can suggest TMJ syndrome.
- Neck. Tenderness of the neck muscles is seen with muscle tension headaches.
- Positive Kernig's and Brudzinski's signs *(Figure 1)* are signs of meningeal irritation and may indicate meningitis or subarachnoid hemorrhage *(Brain 1)*.
- Neurologic. A general exam should be done. This should include testing cranial nerves and doing a funduscopic exam to check for papilledema. The exam should include cerebral and cerebellar testing, as well as mental status evaluation.

Testing

In general, testing is usually not necessary. If testing is necessary, the following are the most common:

- Cerebrospinal fluid (CSF). This is done by means of a lumbar puncture (spinal tap). A computed tomography (CT) scan or magnetic resonance of the head is usually done first to rule out significant intracranial pathology or increased pressure. CSF is tested for infection and the presence of blood in the patient with acute headache.
- Erythrocyte sedimentation rate (ESR). This test is quite elevated in temporal arteritis.
- Computed axial tomography (CAT) scan. This is used (as is MRI) to scan the head for evidence of trauma, bleeding, and tumor. Indications for head scanning include "worst ever headache," decreased alertness or cognition, stiff neck, abnormal neurologic findings, worsening of symptoms or condition, new onset of headache > 2 months in patient aged 40–60, new onset in patient with history of cancer, and headache triggered by cough or coitus.
- Electroencephalography. Although often ordered, in general, an EEG is not useful in evaluation of the headache patient.

Putting It All Together

Most patients with headaches do not have a serious underlying problem. For these patients, a thorough history and physical exam will

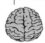
1 - A positive Kernig's sign may also occur with a herniated disk or tumors of the cauda equina (see Chapter 16).

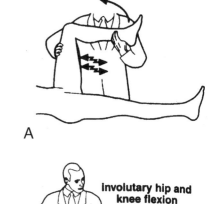

A

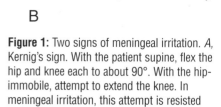

involutary hip and knee flexion

B

Figure 1: Two signs of meningeal irritation. *A,* Kernig's sign. With the patient supine, flex the hip and knee each to about 90°. With the hip-immobile, attempt to extend the knee. In meningeal irritation, this attempt is resisted and causes pain in the hamstring muscles.

B, Brudzinski's sign. Place the patient supine and hold the thorax down on the bed. Attempt to flex the neck. In meningeal irritation, this maneuver causes involuntary flexion of the hips.

(From DeGowin RL: Diagnostic Examination, 7th ed. New York, McGraw-Hill, 2000, with permission.)

determine the severity of the condition. The critical point is determining which patient has a serious underlying disorder. Although most patients do not need testing, it is important to remember the findings for which testing is necessary. Important in the history are complaints of worsening headaches over days or weeks, trauma, associated neurologic symptoms, and "worst headache ever." Physical findings of trauma, severe infection, temporal artery inflammation, or neurologic dysfunction need to be addressed with further testing and possibly consultation. CT or MRI scanning of the head is indicated to evaluate head trauma, central nervous system infection, hemorrhage, and space-occupying lesions.

Management

Most patients with headaches treat themselves with over-the-counter medications. The key is to treat the underlying disorder if an identifiable cause can be found. Headaches caused by infection and inflammation will resolve when the underlying problem is corrected. Serious problems will be treated in a hospital setting, usually in consultation with neurologists and neurosurgeons.

For most patients, the headache will be either muscle tension or migraine in nature. The first step in these patients is to identify and avoid any precipitating factors. Stress reduction, massage, ice and heat to affected muscle groups, physical therapy, and relaxation techniques may be useful. Patient education about headaches is important.

Acetaminophen, aspirin, nonsteroidal anti-inflammatories (NSAIDs), muscle relaxants, and "triptans" are first-line choices for therapy. Opioid analgesics may be used acutely, but the clinician must be alerted to patients who are "drug seeking" or prone to addiction.

Close follow-up by telephone or office visits should be done until the problem improves or the symptoms are stable. Occasionally, the patient will not be reassured easily, and testing will need to be done for peace of mind. Research shows that headache patients do better when they feel their physicians take their concerns seriously.

Selected Readings

1. Barker LR, Burton JR, Zieve PD: Principles of Ambulatory Medicine, 5th ed. Baltimore, Williams & Wilkins, 1999.
2. Coutin IB, Glass SF: Recognizing uncommon headache syndromes. Am Fam Physician 54:2247–2252, 1996 [published erratum appears in Am Fam Physician 55:1586, 1997].
3. Rudolph AM, Kamei RK, Sagan P: Rudolph's Fundamentals of Pediatrics, 2nd ed. Stamford, CT, Appleton & Lange, 1998.
4. Silberstein SD, Lipton RB, Goadsby PJ: Headache in Clinical Practice. Oxford, UK, Isis Medical Media, 1998.

40. HIV

William Henry Hay, MD

Synopsis

Since its emergence in the early 1980s, human immunodeficiency virus (HIV) has become one of the most socially significant illnesses in the world. Although the rate of death from acquired immunodeficiency syndrome (AIDS) *(Definition 1)* in the United States has been declining in recent years, there has been no significant decrease in the rate of new cases of HIV. Consequently, efforts must be maintained to prevent and detect new cases of HIV.

Those at highest risk for this disease include gay and bisexual men, injection drug users, hemophiliacs, and the regular sexual partners of persons in these categories. However, the spread of HIV among heterosexuals, including adolescents and women of childbearing age, has been rapid. African-Americans and Latinos are at particular risk. In the developing world, heterosexual sex is the main route of transmission.

The history and physical examination are meant to assess both the physical and biopsychosocial impact of this illness. Testing is vital in assessing the stage of the illness and determining the course of therapy.

1 - Acquired immunodeficiency syndrome (AIDS): HIV infection that has progressed either to development of an indicator condition (one of many specified infections or tumors, such as pneumonia and Kaposi's sarcoma) or to a CD₄ count ≤ 200.

History

- Take sexual history to assess risk (see Chapter 56).
- "Have you ever, even once, used injectable drugs?"
- "Have you had any infections or other disorders that may have been related to HIV?"
- "What symptoms are you experiencing?" *(Table 1)*
  - Fever, chills, or night sweats
  - Weight loss or change in appetite
  - Changes in vision
  - Sores or white film in the mouth
  - Cough or shortness of breath
  - Nausea, vomiting, swallowing difficulties, abdominal pain, or diarrhea
  - Genital sores, itching, or discharge
  - Swelling or lumps in the neck, axillae, or groin
  - Headache, seizures, balance problems, or numbness or burning in the extremities
  - Depression, anxiety, insomnia, or problems with concentration or memory
- If the patient is known to have HIV:
  - "How have you been coping with your illness?" *(Brain 1)*
  - "Have you told anyone about your infection? How have they reacted?"

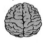

1 - It is important to assess the psychosocial and functional impact HIV has had on the patient. These effects will impact the patient's quality of life and affect his or her ability to follow the often complicated treatment regimens.

Table 1. Conditions Suggesting AIDS

- Candidiasis, of esophagus, trachea, bronchi, or lungs (oral also common)
- Cervical cancer, invasive
- Coccidioidomycosis, extrapulmonary
- Cryptococcosis, extrapulmonary
- Cryptosporidiosis with diarrhea > 1 month
- Cytomegalovirus of any organ other than liver, spleen, or lymph nodes; most commonly eye and esophagus
- Herpes simplex with mucocutaneous ulcer > 1 month or bronchitis, pneumonitis, esophagitis
- Histoplasmosis, extrapulmonary
- HIV-associated dementia
- HIV wasting syndrome
- Isoporosis with diarrhea, > 1 month
- Kaposi's sarcoma
- Lymphoma, Burkitt's
- *Mycobacterium avium*, disseminated
- *Mycobacterium tuberculosis*
- Nocardiosis
- *Pneumocystis carinii* pneumonia
- Recurrent bacterial pneumonia
- Progressive multifocal leukoencephalopathy
- *Salmonella* septicemia, recurrent
- Strongyloidosis, extraintestinal
- Toxoplasmosis of internal organ (primarily the brain)

> Impact on patient's relationships with family and significant others
> Impact on ability to care for self
> Impact on job and social activities
> Mood disorder or substance use
> "What sort of difficulties have you had with taking your medications?
> What side effects have you encountered?"

- "What have you heard about HIV or AIDS? What do you expect from treatment?"
- "What are your major concerns about HIV? What do you expect from treatment?"

Physical Examination

- General observation (e.g., pale, wasting)
- Vital signs including temperature and weight
- Funduscopic exam
- Neck, axillary, or inguinal lymphadenopathy
- Lung exam
- Heart exam
- Abdomen exam for tenderness, masses, or organomegaly
- Genital and rectal exam
- Muscle exam for weakness or atrophy
- Neurologic exam
- Skin for rashes or nodules

Testing

- **HIV serology** is used to detect HIV infection. It consists of an enzyme immunoabsorbant assay; a repeatedly positive assay is confirmed by a Western blot test. The sensitivity and specificity of this combined assay is > 99.9%. Remember, and make the patient aware, that it may take up to 6 months after acquiring the infection for the test to become positive but that the patient will still be contagious during that period.

Many patients are concerned about the confidentiality of their test. The option of confidential or anonymous testing should be offered to these patients. (This can be accomplished by sending the blood sample identified by a number rather than the patient's name. Unfortunately this usually will mean that the patient will need to pay for the test him or herself). Alternately, many public health departments offer anonymous testing.

- **CD4 count** measures the class of lymphocytes attacked by the virus. A count < 350 cells/mm³ is considered an indication for treatment and most opportunistic infections occur at counts < 200 cells/mm³.
- **Viral load** measures levels of viral RNA particles in the blood. This serves as a measure of disease activity, risk of disease progression, and treatment effectiveness *(Brain 2)*.

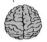

2 - Additional tests usually done on a newly diagnosed patient with HIV include a complete blood count (CBC), serum chemistry panel, syphilis serology, chest x-ray, PPD skin testing, anergy testing, Pap smear, serology for hepatitis B and hepatitis C viruses, toxoplasmosis, and cytomegalovirus.

Putting It All Together

It is important to maintain a high index of suspicion to decide who needs to be tested for HIV. Assess each patient's individual risk and not just those in high-risk groups. Those at risk who test negative should be counseled to take steps to lower their risk of contracting HIV.

The physician must be alert for the wide variety of complications or opportunistic infections that result from both HIV and its treatment.

HIV is a complex condition that impacts all areas of the patient's life. Therefore, the physician needs to assess the biopsychosocial impact of this disease as well as the physical manifestations of the illness.

Management

It is best to have the patient return to the office for the results of HIV testing. If the results are negative, an explanation of the meaning and limitations of the screening tests should be given, along with counseling on how to prevent acquisition of HIV in the future (see Chapter 56). If the testing is positive, the patient will need support as well as recommendations for the next steps in his or her care. The patient's reaction to the diagnosis must be assessed, including risk of suicide. The physician also should assess what social and psychological support the patient may have or need to cope with this news. Close follow-up is mandatory. Counsel the patient to always engage in safer sex practices *(Consultation and Referral 1)*.

2 - Referral depends on the physician's knowledge level and comfort with the care of patients with HIV. Some primary care physicians will care for the HIV patient themselves, whereas others prefer to refer these patients to specialists in infectious diseases. Consultation should always be considered for patients who respond poorly to treatment or develop serious complications. It is still the primary care physician's responsibility to provide comprehensive preventive care to the patient.

Some controversy exists, but it is generally recommended to begin antiviral therapy when the CD4 count is ≤ 350, although viral load is also a factor. Current guidelines recommend using at least three antiretroviral drugs to minimize the occurrence of drug resistance. These regimens can be very complicated, involving multiple daily doses of several antiretroviral drugs plus any drugs the patient needs to prevent or treat opportunistic infections. Further, many of these medications have multiple severe side effects and interactions that may affect other drugs in the regimen. Unfortunately, missed doses can lead to the development of drug resistance, so careful monitoring of compliance is required.

Selected Readings

1. Bartlett JG, Gallant JE: Medical Management of HIV Infection, 2001–2002. Baltimore, The Johns Hopkins University, Department of Infectious Disease, 2001. Available at http://www.hopkins-aids.edu/publications/book/book_toc.html. Accessed April 7, 2002.
2. Goldschmidt RH, Dong BJ: Treatment of AIDS and HIV-related conditions—2001. J Am Board Fam Pract 14:283–309, 2001. Available at http://www.familypractice.com/journal/abfpjournal_frame.htm?main=/journal/2001/v14.n04/1404.08/1404.08.htm.
3. HIV/AIDS Treatment Information Service: Treatment Guidelines. Available at http://hivatis.org/trtgdlns.html. Accessed April 7, 2002.

41. Hypertension

James H. Stageman, MD

Synopsis

Approximately 50 million adult Americans have hypertension (high blood pressure). Although hypertension is generally divided into two categories, **systolic hypertension** and **diastolic hypertension** *(Definition 1)*, many patients will have both. Because of its prevalence, hypertension is a major public health concern. It is a major contributor to **myocardial infarctions, cerebrovascular accidents** *(Definition 2)*, renal failure, eye disease, peripheral vascular disease, and other problems. Every organ system in the body requires an adequate blood supply to function properly, so no organ system is immune from the deleterious effects of hypertension. Rarely are any symptoms associated with mild (stage 1) or even moderate (stage 2) hypertension *(Table 1)*. As the disease slowly progresses, patients start to exhibit symptoms associated with end organ failure. Occasionally, patients may have a rapidly developing "crisis" with blood pressure readings that are significantly elevated above their normal baselines. Therefore, the clinician must distinguish between low-grade elevations (preventing long-term complications) and significant elevations above baseline **(accelerated** or **malignant hypertension *[Definition 3]***) and whether there is a **hypertensive urgency** or **emergency** *(Definition 4)* (preventing short-term disasters).

Finally, in evaluating blood pressure, the physician needs to be aware of the cause. In many cases, there is no immediately identifiable cause. These cases are referred to as *primary* (or essential) *hypertension*. Occasionally, a disease process will cause an elevation in blood pressure, called *secondary hypertension*, and blood pressure will be improved when the underlying disease process is corrected. It is important to remember that hypertension often begins in childhood.

Most patients with hypertension will not require an extensive evaluation to determine the cause. Numerous medications are available to treat hypertensive patients, and there is rarely a reason that you cannot have a patient obtain the blood pressure goal outlined by the Sixth Report of the Joint National Committee on Prevention, Detection, Evaluation, and Treatment of High Blood Pressure (JNC VI) guidelines.

1 - Systolic hypertension: Blood pressure is elevated during the contraction or ejection phase of the left ventricle. The top number noted when you take a blood pressure (i.e., <u>160</u>/80).

Diastolic hypertension: Blood pressure is elevated during the relaxation or filling phase of the left ventricle. The bottom blood pressure number (i.e., 130/<u>100</u>).

2 - Myocardial infarction (MI): Loss of arterial blood flow to a portion of the heart resulting in cell death (heart attack).

Cerebrovascular accident (CVA): Same as MI except involving the brain (stroke).

3 - Accelerated hypertension: A substantial increase over the baseline.

Malignant hypertension: Same as accelerated but with papilledema, which is a swelling of the optic disc often associated with increased intracranial pressure.

4 - Hypertensive urgency: A substantial increase over the baseline without evidence of end organ injury (in this definition, papilledema is not necessarily considered evidence of end organ injury).

Hypertensive emergency: Same as urgency plus evidence of end-organ injury.

Differential Diagnosis

Common Conditions Associated with and Causes of Primary Hypertension

- Genetic basis
- Smoking
- Substance abuse (e.g., alcoholism)

Table 1. Classification of Blood Pressure for Adults Age 18 and Older*

Category	Systolic (mmHg)		Diastolic (mmHg)
Optimal†	< 120	and	< 80
Normal	< 130	and	< 85
High-normal	130–139	or	85–89
Hypertension‡			
Stage 1	140–159	or	90–99
Stage 2	160–179	or	100–109
Stage 3	≥ 180	or	≥ 110

* Not taking antihypertensive drugs and not acutely ill. When systolic and diastolic blood pressures fall into different categories, the higher category should be selected to classify the individual's blood pressure status. For example, 160/92 mmHg should be classified as stage 2 hypertension, and 174/120 mmHg should be classified as stage 3 hypertension. Isolated systolic hypertension is defined as SBP of 140 mmHg or greater and DBP below 90 mmHg and staged appropriately (e.g., 170/82 mmHg is defined as stage 2 isolated systolic hypertension). In addition to classifying stages of hypertension on the basis of average blood pressure levels, clinicians should specify presence or absence of target organ disease and additional risk factors. This specificity is important for risk classification and treatment.

† Optimal blood pressure with respect to cardiovascular risk is below 120/80 mmHg. However, unusually low readings should be evaluated for clinical significance.

‡ Based on the average of two or more readings taken at each of two or more visits after an initial screening.

From The Sixth Report of the Joint National Committee on Prevention, Detection, Evaluation, and Treatment of High Blood Pressure. Arch Intern Med 157:2413–2446, 1997. NIH publication no. 99-4080.

- Obesity
- Stress
- Medication-induced (e.g., oral contraceptives, stimulants such as caffeine, decongestants, and certain herbs such as ephedra)
- Pregnancy

Common Situations That Can Cause the Blood Pressure to Be Temporarily or Falsely Elevated

- Poor technique: using a cuff that is too small for the arm or not having the cuff at the level of the heart
- "White coat hypertension": seen in patients who become anxious when visiting the doctor

Long-Term Consequences Associated with Untreated Hypertension

Cardiovascular
- Left ventricular hypertrophy (LVH; enlargement of the left ventricle)
- Congestive heart failure
- **Atherosclerosis** *(Definition 5)*
- Angina pectoris (chest pain because the heart muscle is not receiving enough oxygen): usually due to the combination of atherosclerosis and associated coronary spasm
- Nose bleeds
- Menorrhagia (excessive menstrual flow)

5 - Atherosclerosis: Deposition of fatty plaque in the artery.

Central Nervous System
Stroke can be caused by hemorrhage or thrombosis (blockage of artery).

Eyes
- Arteriovenous compression due to **arteriosclerosis** *(Definition 6)*
- Retinal hemorrhages and exudates
- Papilledema

6 - Arteriosclerosis: Loss of elasticity, thickening, and hardening of the arteries.

Kidneys
Arteriolar nephrosclerosis can result in increased urination, dilute urine, increased night time urination, blood or protein in urine, or nitrogen retention.

Dangerous Complications Associated with Hypertensive Crisis

- Encephalopathy (any disease of the brain). Can be manifested by:
  Headache
  Vision problems
  Nausea or vomiting
  Seizure
  Stupor
  Coma
- Intracranial hemorrhage (bleeding into the cerebrum or occurring within the cranium)
- Aortic dissection (splitting forces causing the layers of the aorta to separate from each other)
- Rapidly progressive renal failure
- Cardiac arrhythmias
- Congestive heart failure
- Myocardial infarction
- Cerebrovascular accident (CVA)

History

When evaluating a patient for newly diagnosed hypertension, the medical history should include:

- Known duration and levels of elevated blood pressure
- Patient history of symptoms of coronary artery disease (CAD), heart failure, cerebrovascular disease, peripheral vascular disease, renal disease, diabetes mellitus, dyslipidemia, other comorbid conditions, gout, or sexual dysfunction
- Family history of high blood pressure, premature CAD, stroke, diabetes, dyslipidemia, or renal disease
- Symptoms suggesting causes of hypertension (e.g., paroxysms of hypertension accompanied by headache, palpitations, pallor, and perspiration suggest pheochromocytoma)
- History of recent changes in weight, leisure-time physical activity, and smoking or other tobacco use
- Dietary assessment, including intake of sodium, alcohol, saturated fat, and caffeine
- History of all prescribed and over-the-counter (OTC) medications, herbal remedies, and illicit drugs, some of which may raise blood pressure or interfere with the effectiveness of antihypertensive drugs *(Brain 1)*
- Effectiveness and adverse effects of previous antihypertensive therapy
- Psychosocial and environmental factors (e.g., family situation,

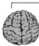

1 - Drugs that can increase blood pressure:
- Sympathomimetics
- Nasal decongestants
- Appetite suppressants
- Cocaine, amphetamines, and other illicit drugs
- Caffeine
- Oral contraceptives
- Adrenal steroids (mineralocorticoids and derivatives, anabolic)
- Licorice (as may be found in chewing tobacco)
- Immunosuppressive agents (cyclosporine, tacrolimus)
- Erythropoietin
- Antidepressants (monoamine oxidase [MAO] inhibitors)
- Nonsteroidal anti-inflammatory drugs (NSAIDs)

employment status and working conditions, educational level) that may influence hypertension control

If the patient is well known and has been previously evaluated or treated for hypertension, it may be appropriate to focus the history:

- Review the history of the problems with hypertension, including any past evaluations and management strategies
- Review the present crisis (if applicable)
- Determine what medications the patient is taking. Include *all* medicines, because one of them may be contributing to the present problem.
- Verify dosage and frequency. It is not unusual for a hypertensive crisis to be precipitated because a patient did not take prescribed antihypertensive medication correctly.
- In reviewing medications, be sure to include OTCs such as decongestants and herbal products because they may contribute to blood pressure problems.
- If dealing with a crisis, determine whether the patient is having any difficulty with:
    - Vision or amaurosis fugax (intermittent loss of sight related to carotid artery disease)
    - Headaches, nausea, vomiting—could indicate encephalopathy
    - Dizziness or transient ischemic attacks (TIA; stroke-like symptoms that resolve in < 24 hours)
    - Chest pain—could indicate angina, dissection
    - Dyspnea (shortness of breath)—pulmonary edema or congestive heart failure
    - Orthopnea (shortness of breath lying down)—congestive heart failure
    - Palpitations (heart rhythm)
    - Edema (swelling)
        - Legs, dependent edema—congestive heart failure
        - Total body—toxemia of pregnancy
    - Right upper quadrant abdominal pain—a swollen liver could mean toxemia of pregnancy or HELLP syndrome (hemolysis, elevated liver enzymes, low platelets), dangerous conditions associated with pregnancy.
    - Painful extremities, especially with exertion—intermittent claudication peripheral vascular disease

Physical Examination

- General observation. Observe behaviors that might indicate a problem as outlined above.
- Vital signs including temperature, with particular emphasis on proper blood pressure technique *(Brain 2)*
- If pressure is elevated, the physical examination should include the following:
    1. Two or more blood pressure measurements separated by 2 minutes with the patient either supine or seated and after standing for at least 2 minutes
    2. Verification in the contralateral arm (if values are different, the higher value should be used)
    3. Measurement of height, weight, and waist circumference *(Brain 3)*
- Funduscopic examination for hypertensive retinopathy (i.e., arteriolar

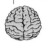

2 - Patient should:
- Rest for 5 minutes before measurement.
- Refrain from smoking or ingesting caffeine for 30 minutes prior to measurement.
- Be seated with feet flat on floor, back and arm supported, arm at heart level.

Clinician should:
- Use the appropriate size cuff for the patient; the bladder should encircle at least 80% of the upper arm.
- Use calibrated mercury manometer.

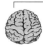

3 - The deposition of excess fat in the upper part of the body (visceral or abdominal), as evidenced by a waist circumference of ≥ 34 inches (85 cm) in women, or ≥ 39 inches (98 cm) in men, has also been associated with the risk of hypertension, dyslipidemia, diabetes, and coronary heart disease mortality (JNC VI).

narrowing, focal arteriolar constrictions, arteriovenous crossing changes, hemorrhages and exudates, disc edema)
- Examination of the neck for carotid bruits, distended veins, or an enlarged thyroid gland
- Examination of the heart for abnormalities in rate and rhythm, increased size, precordial heave, clicks, murmurs, and third and fourth heart sounds
- Examination of the lungs for rales and evidence of bronchospasm
- Examination of the abdomen for bruits, enlarged kidneys, masses, and abnormal aortic pulsation
- Examination of the extremities for diminished or absent peripheral arterial pulsations, bruits, and edema
- Neurologic assessment

Testing

Most cases of hypertension are essential in nature and very little evaluation is required. Routine laboratory tests are recommended before initiating therapy to determine the presence of target organ damage and other risk factors. These routine tests include urinalysis, complete blood cell count (CBC), blood chemistry (potassium, sodium, creatinine, fasting glucose, total cholesterol and high-density lipoprotein [HDL] cholesterol), and 12-lead electrocardiogram.

Occasionally, a patient may present with surprisingly high blood pressure or one that is difficult to control. This situation may represent secondary hypertension. The conditions that cause secondary hypertension are complex and will nearly always require consultation *(Consultation and Referral 1)*.

Putting It All Together

The vast majority of patients with elevated blood pressure, either systolic, diastolic, or both, have essential hypertension and are best treated with lifestyle modifications and should respond to conventional therapy *(Treatment 1)*. However, the physician should be alert to identify:

- That blood pressure readings have been done properly and the diagnosis has been correctly established.
- That patients with substantial increases over their baseline are properly evaluated to determine if the patient has a hypertensive urgency or emergency.
- That patients who are not responding to conventional therapy be reevaluated for possible secondary causes.

Management

Because elevation of blood pressure can occur under normal conditions, the practitioner should hesitate to label a patient as "hypertensive" based on a single reading or on multiple readings during a single visit. If a patient's blood pressure exceeds guidelines, but there isn't a hypertensive urgency or emergency, the patient should be asked to return on several separate occasions to verify prior readings. Once an

1 - Causes of secondary hypertension that require consultation are:
- Renal parenchyma disease
  Glomerulonephritis
  Chronic pyelonephritis
  Interstitial nephropathy
  Diabetic nephropathy
  Polycystic disease
  Obstructive nephropathy
- Renovascular obstructions
- Coarctation of the aorta
- Drugs
  Oral contraceptives
  Steroids
  Thyroid hormones
  Vasopressor drugs
- Cushing's syndrome
- Pheochromocytoma
- Primary aldosteronism

1 - To prevent primary hypertension encourage patients to make healthy lifestyle choices:
- Quit smoking to reduce cardiovascular risk
- Lose weight, if appropriate.
- Restrict sodium intake to no more than 100 mmol per day (2.4 g sodium or 6 g NaCl).
- Limit alcohol intake to no more than 1–2 drinks per day (1/2–1 oz ethanol).
- Get at least 30–45 minutes of aerobic activity on most days.
- Maintain adequate potassium intake— about 90 mmol per day.
- Maintain adequate intakes of calcium and magnesium for general health.

Table 2. Treatment Recommendations

Blood Pressure Stages (mmHg)	Treatment		
	Risk Group A	**Risk Group B**	**Risk Group C**
	No major RFs* No TOD/CCD†	At least 1 major RF, not including diabetes No TOD/CCD	TOD/CCD and/or diabetes, with or without other RFs
High-normal (130–139/85–89)	Lifestyle modification	Lifestyle modification	Drug therapy for those with heart failure, renal insufficiency, or diabetes Lifestyle modification
Stage 1 (140–159/90–99)	Lifestyle modification (up to 12 months)	Lifestyle modification (up to 6 months) For patients with multiple risk factors, consider drugs as initial therapy plus lifestyle modification	Drug therapy Lifestyle modification
Stages 2 and 3 (≥ 160/≥ 100)	Drug therapy Lifestyle modification	Drug therapy Lifestyle modification	Drug therapy Lifestyle modification

* Major risk factors (RFs) include smoking, dyslipidemia, diabetes mellitus, age > 60 years, male gender, postmenopausal women, and family history in women younger than 65 years.
† Target organ damage/clinical cardiovascular diseases (TOD/CCD) include heart diseases (LVH, angina, prior MI, prior CABG, heart failure), stroke or TIA, nephropathy, and peripheral arterial disease.

Adapted from Sixth Report of the Joint National Committee on Prevention, Detection, Evaluation, and Treatment of High Blood Pressure. Arch Intern Med 157:2413–2446, 1997.

Table 3. Classes of Antihypertensive Agents

• Diuretics	• Vasodilators
• Adrenergic inhibitors	• Angiotensin-converting enzyme (ACE) inhibitors
Beta blockers	• Angiotensin II receptor inhibitors
Alpha blockers	• Calcium channel blockers
Centrally acting agents	• Endopeptidase inhibitors

Adapted from The Sixth Report of the Joint National Committee on Prevention, Detection, Evaluation, and Treatment of High Blood Pressure. Arch Intern Med 157:2413–2446, 1997.

average blood pressure for the patient is determined, the JNC VI guidelines should be followed **(Table 2)**.

If the use of medications is indicated for the control of a patient's blood pressure, numerous classes and combinations of medications can be used. In selecting an agent, several factors need to be considered **(Brain 4)**. Classes of oral drugs that are available to use either as a single agent or in combination with other agents are listed in **Table 3**.

Unless there are compelling reasons to use other agents, start with a diuretic or beta blocker **(Table 4)**. Start with a low dose and titrate upward. If no response, try a drug from another class or add a second agent from a different class (diuretic, if not already used). Consider low-dose combinations.

If the patient is having a true hypertensive emergency, hospitalization probably will be required, and you may need to select a parenteral agent to achieve initial control of a patient's blood pressure.

4 - When selecting an antihypertensive agent, consider:
- Age (elderly respond differently than the young)
- Race (whites respond differently than African-Americans)
- Socioeconomic class (what can the patient afford)
- Hemodynamics (cardiac output, peripheral resistance)
- Biochemical information (renin and aldosterone levels)
- Concomitant conditions (e.g., chronic obstructive pulmonary disease [COPD], diabetes, angina)

Table 4. Complicating Factors in Hypertension Drug Therapy

Hypertension Complication	Medication
Uncomplicated	Diuretics, beta blockers
Complicated by:	
Diabetes type 1 (IDDM)	Start with ACE inhibitor if proteinuria is present
Heart failure	Start with ACE inhibitor or diuretic
Myocardial infarction	Beta blocker (non-ISA); ACE inhibitor for LV dysfunction
Isolated systolic hypertension (older patients)	Diuretics (preferred) or calcium antagonists (long-acting DHP)

IDDM = insulin-dependent diabetes mellitus; ACE = angiotensin-converting enzyme; ISA = intrinsic sympathomimetic activity; DHP = dihydropyridine.

When treating elderly patients, special care must be given to prevent lowering the blood pressure too rapidly because their organs (particularly heart, brain, and eyes) may be dependent on the higher pressure to maintain perfusion. A sudden loss of pressure could trigger a myocardial infarction (MI), CVA, visual loss, or orthostatic hypotension. In the latter, a patient's blood pressure may be normal until he or she stands up. Because many blood pressure medications work by interfering with a blood vessel's ability to constrict, the normal compensatory mechanism that maintains circulation to the brain when body position is changed (e.g., lying to standing) is inhibited, and the net result can be that a patient's blood pressure in the brain can become temporarily too low. This situation can result in dizziness or even brief loss of consciousness, fall, and fracture, all of which can be considerably more dangerous than the blood pressure elevation. The admonition in treating elders is always "start low and go slow."

Finally, patients often need encouragement to adhere to the treatment plan *(Brain 5)*.

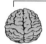

5 - Hypertension basics:
- Encourage lifestyle modifications. Be supportive!
- Educate patient and family about disease. Involve them in measurement and treatment.
- Maintain communication with patient.
- Discuss how to integrate treatment into daily activities.
- Keep care inexpensive and simple.
- Favor once-daily, long-acting formulations.
- Use combination tablets, when needed.
- Consider using generic formulas or larger tablets that can be divided. This may be less expensive.
- Be willing to stop unsuccessful therapy and try a different approach.
- Consider using nurse case management.

Selected Reading

National Institutes of Health, National Heart, Lung, and Blood Institute. The Sixth Report of the Joint National Committee on Prevention, Detection, Evaluation, and Treatment of High Blood Pressure. Bethesda, MD, NIH, 1997, NIH publication no. 98-4080.

42. Memory Problems

Debra E. Mostek, MD • Wendy L. Adams, MD, MPH

Synopsis

Memory problems affect at least 8% of the population over 65 years of age, and the incidence increases with advancing age. Memory problems can be very subtle initially. Commonly, a concerned family member brings the patient in for evaluation, because the patient is unaware or denies that a memory problem exists. Memory impairment is often progressive and leads to significant disability. When memory problems cause difficulty with decision-making or activities of daily living, **dementia** should be suspected *(Definition 1)*. Alzheimer's disease is the most common type of neurodegenerative dementia. Memory problems may also occur with depression, medications, heavy alcohol use, vitamin B_{12} deficiency, and **delirium** *(Definition 2)*.

Most memory problems can be diagnosed through history and physical examination and use of the Mini-Mental Status Exam (MMSE). It is particularly important to obtain collateral history from family or caregivers. Determine the onset and progression of the memory problem. Search for history of head injury, urinary incontinence, and symptoms of depression. On physical examination, focus on the neurologic examination. The object of the investigation is to determine whether a reversible cause or contributing factor of the memory problem is present.

Most treatment is symptomatic; probably less than 1% of patients have a truly reversible dementia. However, correcting reversible causes or contributing factors can greatly improve patients' quality of life. Provide caregivers with community resource information. Patients with an atypical history, inconsistent findings on MMSE, or suspected underlying psychiatric disease should be referred for neuropsychologic testing.

1 - Dementia: A decline of intellectual and memory function, often accompanied by a change in personality or mood. At least one of the following should also be present:

- Impairment of judgment, decision-making and organizational ability
- Reduction of visual-spatial function and difficulty with task performance
- Language difficulties
- Decreased recognition of familiar objects

2 - Delirium: An acute change in mental status with fluctuating levels of awareness and decreased attention span. Some causes of delirium include acute systemic illness, drug side effects, hypoxia, metabolic derangements, infection, and head injury. Delirium may be superimposed on dementia.

Differential Diagnosis

Neurodegenerative Diseases *(Table 1)*

- Alzheimer's dementia
- Vascular dementia
- Mixed dementia
- Parkinson's disease with dementia
- Lewy body dementia
- Frontal lobe dementia
- Huntington's disease

Secondary Dementias *(Definition 3)*

- Pseudodementia due to depression
- Medications causing central nervouse system (CNS) side effects *(Brain 1)*

3 - Secondary dementias: Cognitive impairment that may result from a systemic illness, toxicity, or central nervous system lesion that is potentially reversible with correction of underlying disorder.

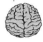

1 - Drugs with CNS toxicity include major tranquilizers, benzodiazepines, nonsteroidal anti-inflammatory drugs (NSAIDs), H_2 blockers, methyldopa, and anticholinergics.

Table 1. Characteristics and Treatment of Neurodegenerative Diseases

Neurodegenerative Diseases	Onset and Progression	Characteristics	Treatment
Alzheimer's dementia	Gradual	Slow progression, language problems early, motor problems later	CI trial in mild to moderate stages
Vascular dementia (multi-infarct dementia)	Stepwise	History of recurrent strokes, asymmetric neurologic exam, gait problems, psychomotor retardation	Aim to prevent further strokes: consider ASA, control lipids and blood pressure, stop smoking
Mixed dementia	Gradual	Stroke superimposed on Alzheimer-type features	CI trial and stroke prevention per vascular dementia
Parkinson's disease	Gradual	30% develop dementia several years after onset of tremor, rigidity, and gait problems	Anti-Parkinson's agents for motor symptoms and trial of CI
Lewy body dementia	Gradual, most common in males aged 65–75 yrs	Fluctuating symptoms, visual hallucinations, syncope, extrapyramidal motor symptoms	CI, avoid major tranquilizers
Frontal lobe dementia	Gradual	Rare incidence, early judgment loss, disinhibition, high MMSE scores early in course	Symptomatic, control agitation and behavioral problems
Huntington's disease	Gradual, onset in midlife	Autosomal dominant, uncoordinated gait, poor judgment	Symptomatic, control agitation and behavioral problems

CI = cholinesterase inhibitor, ASA = aspirin, MMSE = Mini-Mental Status Exam.

- Delirium
- Vitamin B$_{12}$ deficiency
- Normal pressure hydrocephalus (NPH) *(Definition 4)*
- CNS infections
- Endocrinopathies
- CNS mass lesions

History

The patient may not be able to give an accurate history because of his or her memory impairment. Collateral history from family members or associates provides information on the course of the memory decline and the degree of functional impairment.

Questions to Ask the Patient *(Brain 2)*

- "How are your memory problems affecting your daily activities?" (e.g. bathing, shopping, cooking) *(Brain 3)*
- "Tell me about your health and past medical problems." The following may contribute to cognitive impairment:
    Current medications
    Alcohol or sedative use
    Mood disorder
    Thyroid disease symptoms *(Brain 4)*
    Previous stroke
    Head trauma with loss of consciousness
    Headache

4 - Normal pressure hydrocephalus (NPH): A degenerative condition of the central nervous system of unknown etiology that results in impaired absorption of cerebral spinal fluid and is associated with enlargement of the ventricles. This condition frequently first manifests itself by gait problems and urinary incontinence. Later, rapid cognitive impairment occurs. If detected early enough, the symptoms may be improved by a surgical procedure to shunt excess cerebrospinal fluid away.

2 - Questions are focused to determine if there is evidence of functional impairment or secondary causes of memory problems. Occasionally the patient will become quite defensive about his or her memory impairment because of poor insight. In those situations, it is best to focus questions on the physical symptoms present and have a separate interview with your collateral source. Rapid progression of symptoms necessitates immediate brain imaging to rule out CNS lesions.

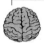

3 - It is important to assess the functional impact of the memory problem.

Questions to Ask the Collateral Source

- "How long has the memory problem been present?"
- "Was the onset sudden or gradual?"
- "Has the impairment progressed?"
- "Have you noted any other associated problems?"
  Gait disturbance
- Behavioral problems (e.g., hiding things, agitation, accusations of theft)
- Hallucinations or delusions
- Snoring or sleep apnea
- "Is there a family history of dementia?"

The clinician should explore these safety issues with the caregiver *(Red Flag 1)*:

- Safety concerns (e.g., leaving the stove on)?
- Getting lost
- Car accidents
- Inability to handle finances
- Falling episodes
- Firearms in the home
- Forgetting medications or taking improperly

Particularly assess for the following red flags *(Red Flag 2):*

- Sudden onset
- Rapid progression
- Urinary incontinence
- Gait impairment
- Headache
- Recent head trauma
- New-onset neurologic impairment

Physical Examination

A careful general examination should be performed for medical conditions that may be contributing to the patient's memory problems (e.g., evidence of hypothyroidism or lung disease causing hypoxia). Vision should be assessed using a handheld Rosenbaum or Jaeger chart. Hearing should be screened with the **whisper test** *(Definition 5)*. A systematic neurologic examination looking for asymmetry of cranial nerves, sensation, strength or deep tendon reflexes is crucial. Inspect muscle tone and look for **cogwheel rigidity** *(Definition 6)*. Assess balance using the Romberg test (see Chapter 29). Evaluate gait by asking patient to ambulate in the hallway and observe posture, stride, and arm swing, and note any dragging of the feet, hesitancy, unsteadiness, and the number of steps necessary to turn around *(Red Flag 3) (Brain 5)*.

Testing

The most popular screening tool to measure cognition is the MMSE *(Table 2).* The MMSE measures the patient's orientation to time and place as well as attention and calculation skills, short-term memory, and

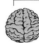
4 - Thyroid disease may cause fatigue, cold or heat intolerance, constipation or diarrhea, change in weight, muscle cramps, skin dryness or increased sweating, change in hair texture and growth, irritability, palpitations, or congestive heart failure.

1 - If significant safety concerns are present, efforts should be directed toward finding an appropriate living situation (e.g., in-home care, assisted living, or nursing home placement) based on the patient's needs and available resources. Referral to a social worker may be helpful.

2 - The presence of these symptoms is suggestive of serious underlying conditions and usually requires brain imaging to rule out cerebrovascular accident (CVA), neoplasm, hydrocephalus, or intracranial bleed.

5 - Whisper Test:
1. Explain to the patient that you are going to check his or her hearing.
2. Stand along the right side of the patient. Reach around the back of the patient's head with your left arm and cover the patient's left ear with your left hand.
3. Whisper three numbers into the patient's right ear from a distance of about 2 feet (or as far away as you can stretch while still keeping the left ear covered). Be sure the patient does not see your lips; some patients are able to lip-read!
4. Ask the patient to repeat the numbers out loud.
5. Repeat the process on the left side.

6 - Cogwheel rigidity: A series of repetitive small "catches" noted when passively moving a joint through its range of motion. Most often tested by passively flexing and extending the elbow or moving the wrist joint through its circular range of motion. The catches are actually due to an underlying tremor.

3 - The physical exam searches for systemic diseases that may be causing memory impairment. Asymmetric neurologic findings may indicate prior stroke or a CNS mass lesion dictating the need for brain imaging.

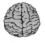
5 - Cogwheel rigidity, shuffling gait, and a "pill-rolling" resting tremor are suggestive of Parkinson-type syndromes.

Table 2. Mini-Mental Status Examination

Task	Instructions	Scoring	Maximum Score
Orientation	"Tell me the date." Have pt supply year, season, date, day, and month.	1 point for each	5
	"Where are we?" Have pt supply state, county, town, hospital, and floor.	1 point for each	5
	Name three objects to the pt. Ask the pt to repeat all three after you.	1 point for each	3
Attention and calculation	Ask the pt to count backward from 100 by 7 (stop after five answers). Alternatively, ask pt to spell the word *world* backward.	1 point for each correct number or letter	5
Recall	Ask the pt to recall the three objects mentioned above.	1 point for each object	3
Language	Show the pt a pencil and your watch. Ask the pt to name them.	1 point for each	2
	Have the pt repeat the following: "no ifs, ands, or buts."	1 point	1
	As you give the pt a plain piece of paper, give this instruction: "Take the paper in your right hand, fold it in half, and put it on the floor."	1 point for each command followed	3
	Show the pt a piece of paper with the following written on it: "Close your eyes."	1 point if pt closes eyes	1
	Ask the pt to write a sentence.	1 point if sentence makes sense and has a subject and a verb.	1
	Ask the pt to copy this design:	1 point	1
			Total: 30

A score of ≥ 26 indicates a low risk of dementia.
pt = patient.

Adapted from Folstein MF, Folstein SE, McHugh PR: Mini-Mental State: A practical method for grading the cognitive state of patients for the clinician, J Psychiatr Res 12:189–198, 1975.

language abilities. This brief, standardized test gives a quick overview of the patient's intellectual functioning. A score less than 26 suggests cognitive impairment, but the educational level of the patient must be taken into account. Formal neuropsychological testing may be required in patients with subtle memory problems, mood disorders, or questionable impairment of judgment.

The neurodegenerative dementias are diagnosed on the basis of the history and physical examination. No laboratory or radiographic testing is currently available for definitive diagnosis. Most clinicians obtain a complete blood cell count (CBC) with differential, thyroid-stimulating hormone (TSH), electrolytes, creatinine, liver function, calcium, vitamin B_{12} level, and erythrocyte sedimentation rate (ESR) to identify any underlying systemic illnesses that may be contributing to the memory impairment. Further testing should be dictated by clinical findings. If there is a history of multiple sex partners, obtain rapid plasmin reagin (RPR) and HIV testing. If history suggests heavy metal exposure (e.g., pesticide exposure, occupational history of mining, glass, or metal manufacturing), perform a heavy metal screen. If **nonconvulsive epilepsy** *(Definition 7)* is suspected, an electroencephalogram (EEG) would be helpful. Cushingoid features on physical exam would dictate further adrenal testing *(Brain 6)*.

7 - Nonconvulsive epilepsy: Abnormal electrical activity within the brain that results in problems with awareness (e.g., staring spells, unresponsiveness), but without any tonic-clonic jerking of muscles typically seen in seizures.

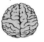

6 - Cushingoid features include central obesity, "moon" face, muscle weakness, and easy bruisability.

Most authorities now recommend a brain imaging study (either CT or MRI of the brain) only when signs and symptoms suggest a potentially treatable cause of the memory impairment (e.g., rapid progression, localizing neurologic exam, gait disturbance and urinary incontinence suggestive of NPH).

Putting It All Together

A patient with excellent verbal skills can "cover up" his or her memory difficulties and appear to have no deficits during superficial conversation. Consequently, collateral informants and the MMSE are essential to the evaluation. Neuropsychological testing is often helpful if there is uncertainty about the diagnosis. When memory impairment is present, the clinician must determine whether a reversible condition exists. Neurodegenerative disorders usually result in gradual loss of memory and cognitive function. Rapid progression of dementia is an ominous sign and should spur a vigorous search for a precipitating cause. The history often provides the most important clues. Both history and physical findings should guide further work up.

Vision or hearing difficulty may cause a patient to misinterpret his or her environment and lead to confusion. Correction of the sensory impairment often improves function, even if there is an irreversible dementia. Treatment of hypothyroidism, when present, may improve both cognition and physical function. Correction of vitamin B_{12} deficiency may also lead to improvement.

If reversible etiologies have been ruled out and the clinical findings point to a neurodegenerative disorder, the type of dementia should be determined. This will help guide subsequent symptomatic treatment (see Table 1).

Management

If a treatable etiology is discovered, appropriate therapy should be initiated. One of the most common causes of reversible memory impairment is CNS toxicity related to medication. Cessation of the offending drug can lead to dramatic improvement. Heavy alcohol use should be stopped. If depression is present, appropriate treatment of the depression (e.g., with selective serotonin reuptake inhibitors) often results in improved function.

The diagnosis of a neurodegenerative dementia can be devastating for the patient and the family. Provide information on available community resources and educational materials. Discuss the necessity of respite for the caregiver *(Brain 7) (Treatment 1)*.

Safety issues must be addressed. If the dementia is impairing driving ability, the patient must be advised to stop driving. Firearms in the household should be removed. For a patient unable to manage safely at home, appropriate alternative living situations should be discussed. Occasionally, severe behavioral problems necessitate psychiatric hospitalization *(Consultation and Referral 1)*.

Four cholinesterase inhibitors (CIs), donepezil (Aricept), rivastigmine (Exelon), galantamine (Reminyl), and tacrine (Cognex), are approved for treatment of mild-to-moderate Alzheimer's disease. Unfortunately, only 20–30% of Alzheimer's disease patients will show improvement with CI therapy.

In summary, the treatment of the neurodegenerative dementias is largely symptomatic. The goal is to improve function and quality of life for the patient if possible and provide caregiver support.

Selected Readings

1. Beers MH, Berkow R: The Merck Manual of Diagnosis and Therapy, 17th ed. Whitehouse Station, NJ, Merck & Company, 1999.
2. Bird TD: Memory loss and dementia. In Fauci AS, Braunwald E, Isselbacher KJ, et al (eds): Harrison's Principles of Internal Medicine, 14th ed. New York, McGraw-Hill, 1998.
3. Cobbs EL, Duthie EH, Murphy JB: Geriatrics Review Syllabus: A Core Curriculum in Geriatric Medicine, 4th ed. Dubuque, IA, Kendall/Hunt Publishing Company, 1999.
4. Knopman D: The differential diagnosis of dementia in the elderly. Mediguide Geriatr Neurol 1:1–7, 1997.
5. Patterson CJS, Gauthier S, Bergman H, et al: The recognition, assessment and management of dementing disorders: conclusions from the Canadian Consensus Conference on Dementia. CMAJ 160:S1–S15, 1999.
6. Richards SS, Hendrie HC: Diagnosis, management, and treatment of Alzheimer's disease: A guide for the internist. Arch Intern Med 159:789–798, 1999.
7. Small GH: Differential diagnosis and early detection of dementia. Am J Geriatr Psychiatry 6:S26–S33, 1998.

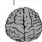

7 - The Alzheimer's Association (1-800-272-3900) provides educational materials and information on support groups available. The Eldercare Locator Service (1-800-677-1116) provides information on how to reach the closest Area Agency on Aging. These agencies provide local community resource information (e.g., home health care agencies, adult day care facilities)

1 - Educate the patient and family about the natural course of the dementia. Give them the phone number of the Alzheimer's Association. Provide the caregiver with information on respite care, adult day care, and other community resources. Treat any contributing factors that may be worsening the patient's function. Correct visual and hearing deficits when possible. A CI may be helpful for Alzheimer's dementia and Lewy body dementia. Vitamin E may be helpful.

1 - Referral for neuropsychologic testing is often helpful for patients whose memory problems are suspected to be related to a mood disorder or those patients with an atypical history or inconsistent MMSE scores. Social work referral may be necessary to arrange a new living situation for patients unable to care for themselves at home. Geriatric psychiatry consultation and hospitalization should be considered for demented patients with suicidal ideation, significant delusions, hallucinations, or severe behavioral problems that cannot be safely managed on an outpatient basis.

43. Menopause

Carol A. LaCroix, MD

Synopsis

Menopause technically means "the cessation of menses." The average age for this event is 51 ± 3 years. The only factor known to alter this is smoking, which hastens menopause. Climacteric refers to the perimenopausal years. The menopause syndrome refers to symptoms that may occur during the climacteric. It is important to help women sort out the causes of physical changes and to identify what interventions are available.

Many of the physical symptoms during the climacteric are due to altered hormone levels. The natural aging process involves waning of ovarian function, which results in decreased estrogen and androgen levels. Approximately 80% of women will experience vasomotor symptoms, which include hot flashes and night sweats. Menstrual irregularities can involve change in length of cycle (more or less frequent) and change in amount of blood flow (heavier or lighter). These symptoms also may occur in pathologic conditions such as thyroid dysfunction, uterine fibroids, ovarian cysts, **endometriosis (Definition 1)**, and pelvic infections. The woman may need guidance as to whether she can still conceive and what she can do about decreased libido. **Dyspareunia (Definition 2)** and bladder infections may increase because of thinning of the mucosa in the vagina and urethra. Mood swings often improve with treatment of the hot flashes that disturb sleep. Frequently, the woman is also dealing with environmental stressors such as moody adolescents, ailing parents, and job demands. Osteoporosis and heart disease accelerate in estrogen-deficient women.

1 - Endometriosis: A pathologic condition in which abnormal growths of tissue, which are histologically similar to the uterine lining, are found outside the uterus.

2 - Dyspareunia: Pain experienced during or after sexual intercourse. It may be due to physical or psychological causes.

Hormone replacement therapy (HRT) is recommended for all menopausal women who do not have contraindications to taking estrogen. Every woman who still has her uterus should also take progesterone to prevent **endometrial hyperplasia (Definition 3)**.

3 - Endometrial hyperplasia: An increase in the number of endometrial cells leading to a thickening of the endometrial lining.

All of the problems mentioned above can be dealt with initially at the primary care level. Interventions will be more successful if the woman feels like she is part of the health care team.

Differential Diagnosis

Normal Aging Phenomena *(Table 1)*

Patients may present with the following worries and complaints:

1 - Rule out pregnancy!

- "My periods have been getting less regular."
- "Can I still get pregnant?"
- "My husband is complaining about my lack of sex drive."
- Amenorrhea *(Red Flag 1)*

Table 1. Normal Aging Phenomena

- The ovary quits producing estradiol.

- Estrone is still produced in the liver and peripheral fat, but it is one-third as potent.

- Atrophy of the vulvae occurs due to decreased estrogen.

- The presence of fewer gonadotropin-sensitive follicles results in lengthening of the follicular phase of the menstrual cycle, anovulatory cycles, and irregular menses.

- LH pulses occur every 10–20 minutes, instead of every 90–120, contributing to hot flashes.

- FSH rises above 40 mIU/mL.

- Androgen levels drop because they were previously made from estrogen. However, the ovary does continue to make some testosterone.

Symptoms Due to Estrogen Deficiency

- Night sweats
- Hot flashes
- Dyspareunia

Symptoms Due to Pathology

- "My periods have been getting heavier, with more clots." Rule out infection, fibroids, ovarian cysts, or endometrial hyperplasia
- "Hot flashes" due to anxiety or environmental stressors
- Weight gain, which may occur from estrogen supplements but is more likely due to diet or decreased physical activity

History

If the woman is still menstruating: "Tell me about your periods."

You may need to ask more specific questions:

- "Have your periods changed since the last exam?"
- "Are your periods regular? Have you skipped any periods?"
- "How long do you bleed? How many days are heavy?"
- "How many days do you have cramps? Do you take anything for the cramps?"

If the woman has stopped having her periods: "Did this occur naturally or did you have an operation?"

If menopause occurred surgically, ask:

- "Why was the hysterectomy done?" *(Brain 1)*
- "Were the ovaries removed as well as the uterus?" *(Red Flag 2)*
- "Are you having any problem with hot flashes or night sweats?" *(Brain 2)*
- "Are you having any trouble with vaginal dryness, pain during intercourse, or decreased sex drive?"
- "Are you having any trouble with mood swings (or irritability)?" *(Brain 3)*
- "How well are you sleeping?"
- "Tell me about your home life. Who lives at home? Do you feel safe at home?"

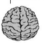

1 - If the surgery was done for cancer, yearly follow-up is needed. If the hysterectomy was done for heavy bleeding or infection, the Pap is no longer necessary, but a bimanual exam should be done yearly if the ovaries are still present. If both ovaries were removed, the woman needs HRT (if there are no contraindications).

2 - Beware of the term "total abdominal hysterectomy." It does not necessarily mean the ovaries were removed!

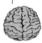

2 - Vasomotor symptoms generally begin early in the climacteric. Eighty percent of women experience these for over 1 year, but less than 25% struggle for more than 5 years. Women often experience the night sweats before the hot flashes become disruptive during the day. The typical hot flash involves a sudden sensation of warmth and flushed skin, involving the face and upper chest. It may also be accompanied by sweating, palpitations, nausea, dizziness, or headache. The episode lasts for only a few minutes and is totally unrelated to the woman's activity at that time. Hot flashes should be addressed because they can be embarrassing. Night sweats disturb the woman's sleep. These also may disturb any bed partner because the woman suddenly does not want any bedcovers and she may have to get up to change clothing that has become drenched with sweat.

- "Tell me about your job. Do you enjoy it?"

If the woman is a potential candidate for HRT, ask:

- "What have you heard about hormone replacement therapy?" *(Brain 4)*
- "Have you ever been treated with hormones?"
- "If so, any problems with the medications?" *(Brain 5)*
- "Which medications, vitamins, and herbal supplements have you already tried?" *(Red Flag 3)*

Physical Examination

All of the following should be done at least yearly. It is recommended that the weight and blood pressure be checked at every visit to monitor any trends. If the woman has not had a general physical in the past year, also examine HEENT, skin, heart, and lungs looking for nongynecologic health problems.

- Weight
- Height. Screen for osteoporosis.
- Blood pressure
- Breast exam
- Pelvic
- Rectal
- Varicose veins. If present, do they cause pain or ankle edema?

Testing

Mammogram

Mammogram should be performed yearly from age 40 to 65. Encourage each woman to continue every 1–2 years thereafter as long as she is physically and mentally able and she can afford it.

Pap Test

If the uterus is present, the Pap should be done every year until there have been three consecutive normal ones and then at least every 3 years until age 65. A Pap should be done more frequently in women who have changed sexual partners. Consider performing the Pap yearly while on HRT because it may detect endometrial hyperplasia. If the uterus was removed because of cervical cancer, the Pap should probably be done yearly. If the uterus was removed for any other reason (such as bleeding, infection), the Pap is *not* necessary. The bimanual exam should be done yearly if the ovaries are still present.

Hemoccult

This can be done at the time of the rectal, if stool is present. A more accurate screen is three specimens collected on different days. If any abnormality is found, rule out false positives and then evaluate the colon.

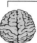

3 - It is important to figure out whether the woman is experiencing sleep disturbances due to hot flashes, anxiety or depression, or both.

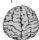

4 - If appropriate, discuss risks versus benefits of HRT. Generally, the small risks of gallstones or cancer of the uterus or breast are far outweighed by the benefits of an improved sense of well being and the prevention of osteoporosis. Fortunately, the woman can be monitored closely for the potential risks.

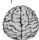

5 - Obese women will produce some estrogen from the peripheral fat, which may contribute to postmenopausal bleeding. Women often become frustrated with weight gain on estrogen supplements. However, the weight gain is usually accompanied by decreased physical activity.

3 - Patients often will not volunteer information about vitamins and herbs for fear that the health care provider will scoff at them. An open, nonjudgmental attitude will elicit more complete information.

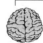

6 - Complaints of hot flashes, night sweats, change in frequency of menses, and change in amount of flow are possible symptoms of the perimenopausal syndrome. When the woman has an FSH over 40 mIU/ml in conjunction with these symptoms, she is postmenopausal.

Follicle-Stimulating Hormone (FSH) and Luteinizing Hormone (LH)

FSH and LH can be drawn if there is a question from the woman's history as to whether she is menopausal *(Brain 6)*.

Endometrial Biopsy

Should be performed when there is unexplained vaginal bleeding on HRT. Some physicians routinely do this prior to initiating HRT.

Bone Density Screening by Dual Photon Absorptiometry

This may be done in perimenopausal women who are at risk for osteoporosis. Risk factors include:

- Lack of estrogen replacement after menopause
- Caucasian or Asian race
- Family history of osteoporosis
- Prolonged treatment with glucocorticoids
- Excessive use of alcohol, caffeine, and nicotine
- Diet that includes less than 1000–1500 mg of calcium per day
- Minimal physical activity

Putting It All Together

4 - Menorrhagia: Excessive amount of menstrual flow.

Metrorrhagia: Excessive time of flow. A helpful way to remember which is which is that metrorrhagia and time both have the letter t.

The climacteric is a time of multiple physical changes for a woman. The goals for the physician are to:

- Identify problems related to the changes, such as meno- or metrorrhagia, and hot flashes *(Definition 4).*
- Provide education about symptoms, causes, and natural course.
- Recommend suitable therapies (hormone replacement therapy, vitamin supplements, regular exercise, medications for osteoporosis, heart disease, and depression).

Management

Because women have the potential to live almost half of their lives after menopause, they should be encouraged to take supplements that will preserve their quality of life. Hormone replacement therapy, calcium and vitamin D supplements, and antioxidants help prevent osteoporosis and heart disease.

If the woman is a candidate for HRT, address any concerns and emphasize the potential benefits. HRT should be offered when the woman begins to have disruptive vasomotor symptoms, even if she is still menstruating. Otherwise, HRT should be recommended when there have been no menses for 6–12 months.

Multiple forms of estrogens and progestins are available, some made by pharmaceutical companies and others obtained from herbal sources. Estrogen should be taken continuously. If the woman still has her uterus, she should also take a progestin to prevent endometrial cancer. This can be dosed continuously or cyclically.

Estrogen supplementation will definitely help women struggling with hot flashes and vaginal dryness. Mood swings often improve when sleep is improved by reduction in hot flashes. Many women are dealing with their climacteric at the same time that they are dealing with teenagers in the family, ailing parents, and a job outside the home. They need to be encouraged to take time for themselves (so they can continue to care for everybody else!). Regular exercise helps maintain strong bones and reduces stress. Antidepressant medication or counseling may also be helpful.

Selected Readings

1. American College of Obstetricians and Gynecologists: ACOG educational bulletin: Osteoporosis. Int J Gynaecol Obstet 62:193–201, 1998.
2. Ott K: Osteoporosis and bone densitometry. Radiol Technol 70:129–148, 1998.
3. Pinkerton JV, Santen R: Alternatives to the use of estrogen in postmenopausal women. Endocr Rev 20:308–320, 1999.
4. Shoupe D: Hormone replacement therapy: Reassessing the risks and benefits. Hospital Pract (Off Ed) 34:97–103, 1999.
5. Slott J, et al (eds): Danforth's Obstetrics and Gynecology. New York, JB Lippincott, 1994.

44. Nutrition Problems

Cynthia L. Van Riper, MS, RD, CDE

Synopsis

Good nutrition is a cornerstone for overall health. At a basic level, an adequate and balanced intake of macro- and micronutrients can prevent nutrient deficiency disorders and malnutrition. Moreover, a healthy diet, in combination with physical activity, can help maintain normal body weight, lower risks for chronic diseases such as cardiovascular disease, diabetes, and hypertension, and contribute to positive outcomes for medical and surgical interventions.

In an affluent society, classic nutrient deficiency disorders are rare except in high-risk groups *(Red Flag 1)*. Instead, obesity and the overconsumption of calories and other dietary constituents are a major concern for a growing proportion of the U.S. population.

 1 - High-risk groups include infants and very young children; the elderly; individuals with severe disabilities or chronic diseases that impair their ability to ingest, digest, or absorb nutrients; homeless individuals and those living in extreme poverty; and individuals who are dependent on others for basic needs and are thus vulnerable to neglect and abuse.

Differential Diagnosis

- Obesity
- Overweight
- Excess visceral (intra-abdominal) fat
- Disordered eating and unhealthy eating behaviors
    Restrictive dieting
    Overeating, binge eating
    Use of harmful weight-control behaviors (e.g., self-induced vomiting, excessive exercise or fasting)
    Anorexia nervosa *(Table 1)*
    Bulimia nervosa *(Table 2)*

History

Body Weight

- "What is your usual body weight?"
- "What was your highest adult weight?"
- "What was your lowest adult weight?"
- "Have you had any recent changes in your weight?"
- "Over what period of time?"
- "What do you think may have caused or contributed to these weight changes?" Weight gain may be associated with illness or injury that limits physical activity, smoking cessation, use of medications, depression, or stressful life events. For women, pregnancies may be associated with weight gain.

Table 1. Diagnostic Criteria for Anorexia Nervosa

- Refusal to maintain body weight at or above a minimally normal weight for age and height (e.g., weight loss leading to maintenance of body weight < 85% of that expected; or failure to make expected weight gain during period of growth, leading to body weight < 85% of that expected).
- Intense fear of gaining weight or becoming fat, even though underweight.
- Disturbance in the way in which one's body weight or shape is experienced, undue influence of body weight or shape on self-evaluation, or denial of the seriousness of the current low body weight.
- In postmenarchal females, amenorrhea (i.e., the absence of at least three consecutive menstrual cycles). A woman is considered to have amenorrhea if her periods occur only following hormone administration (e.g., estrogen).

Specify type:
- Restricting type: During the current episode of anorexia nervosa, the person has not regularly engaged in binge-eating or purging behavior (i.e., self-induced vomiting or the misuse of laxatives, diuretics, or enemas).
- Binge eating or purging type: During the current episode of anorexia nervosa, the person has regularly engaged in binge-eating or purging behaviors (i.e., self-induced vomiting or the misuse of laxatives, diuretics, or enemas).

Adapted from American Psychiatric Association: Diagnostic and Statistical Manual of Mental Disorders, 4th ed., revision. Washington, DC, APA, 1994.

Table 2. Diagnostic Criteria for Bulimia Nervosa

- Recurrent episodes of binge eating. An episode of binge eating is characterized by both of the following:
  1. Eating, in a discrete period of time (e.g., within any 2-hour period), an amount of food that is definitely larger than most people would eat during a similar period of time and under similar circumstances.
  2. Lack of control over eating during the episode (e.g., feeling that one cannot stop eating or control what or how much one is eating).
- Recurrent, inappropriate compensatory behavior in order to prevent weight gain, such as self-induced vomiting, misuse of laxatives, diuretics, enemas, or other medications; fasting; or excessive exercise.
- The binge eating and inappropriate compensatory behaviors both occur, on average, at least twice a week for 3 months.
- Self-evaluation is unduly influenced by body shape and weight.
- The disturbance does not occur exclusively during episodes of anorexia nervosa.

Specify type:
- Purging type: During the current episode of bulimia nervosa, the person has regularly engaged in self-induced vomiting or the misuse of laxatives, diuretics, or enemas.
  2. Nonpurging type: During the current episode of bulimia nervosa, the person has used other inappropriate behaviors such as fasting or excessive exercise but has not regularly engaged in self-induced vomiting or the misuse of laxatives, diuretics, or enemas.

Adapted from American Psychiatric Association: Diagnostic and Statistical Manual of Mental Disorders, 4th ed., revision. Washington, DC, APA, 1994.

- "Have you noticed any other changes in your health or physical state along with these weight changes?" *(Red Flag 2)*
- "Do you have any concerns about your weight?" Even though a person may be overweight by clinical standards, he or she may not be personally concerned about it. A person who is not concerned about his or her weight is not likely to be motivated to engage in weight loss strategies. If there are no other risk factors or comorbidities associated with the elevated body weight and the individual is otherwise healthy, treatment may not be indicated. If there are other risk factors and comorbidities present, an initial step in treatment may be

2 - Unintentional weight loss of more than 10% of usual adult body weight may be an early symptom of an underlying illness and requires a thorough investigation.

preventing further weight gain and beginning to educate the patient on the health risks associated with his or her current weight status and the potential benefits to be expected with even a modest weight loss. Conversely, a person with a normal body weight by clinical standards who is attempting to lose weight or expresses significant dissatisfaction with his or her current body shape and weight may have or be at risk for an eating disorder.

Current/Past Weight Loss Efforts

- "Are you currently trying to lose weight?"
- "Have you tried to lose weight in the past?"
- "What are you doing or what have you done to try to lose weight? (e.g., dieting, exercise, medication, alternative therapy such as hypnosis)
- "How well do you think this (these) method(s) are currently working? Or, why do you think this (these) method(s) did or did not work in the past?"

Dietary History

Accurate quantitative information on energy (calorie) intake is difficult to obtain, but questions can be directed to identify usual eating habits, food and beverage choices, and abnormal eating behaviors. A thorough dietary assessment can be provided by a registered dietitian (see Consultation and Referral 1).

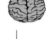 **1 -** Often people with chaotic schedules or no consistency in mealtimes have difficulty making dietary adjustments needed for treatment of obesity, diabetes, or other lifestyle-related disorders. Individuals who skip meals or eat only once or twice a day may be using this as a dieting technique but may still be consuming a significant number of calories. Binge eaters often do not have regular meals but, instead, snack throughout the day.

- "Tell me about your usual daily schedule: what time you get up, what time you usually go to bed, and usual times for eating. How consistent is this schedule from day to day?" *(Brain 1)*

Table 3. Calorie Content of Common Beverages

Beverage	Calories/Fluid Ounce
Fruit juices	
Grapefruit juice	12
Orange or apple juice	14–15
Grape or pineapple juice	18–19
Dairy	
Nonfat skim milk	11
1% milk	13
2%	15
Whole	19
Soft drinks	
Gingerale	10
Colas, cherry cola (e.g., Dr. Pepper), lemon-lime (e.g., 7-Up, Sprite), root beer	12–13
Fruit-flavored sodas, (e.g., Mellow Yello, Mountain Dew)	15
Creme sodas	16
Alcohol*	
Beer	12–13
Light beer	8–11
Wine	20–21
80 proof vodka	65
86 proof whiskey	70
90 proof gin	73

*Standard servings of beer, wine, and spirits (e.g., a 12-ounce can of beer, a 5-ounce glass of wine, and a cocktail with 1.5 ounces of 80-proof spirits) all contain the same amount of absolute alcohol. Beer, wine, and liquor have the same affect if a person drinks them in a standard size serving and at the same rate.

Table 4. Ten-Question Drinking History

Category	Question
Beer	How many times per week do you drink beer?
	How many cans each time?
	Every drink more?
Wine	How many times per week do you drink wine?
	How many glasses each time?
	Ever drink more?
Liquor	How many times per week do you drink hard liquor?
	How many drinks each time?
	Ever drink more?
General	Has your drinking changed during the past year?

Adapted from Rossett HL, Weiner L, Edelin KC: Treatment experience with pregnant women drinkers. JAMA 249:2029–2033, 1983.

- "What do you usually have to drink with your meals? What do you usually drink between meals?" *(Brain 2)*
- "How often do you eat meals away from home? Where do you usually go for meals away from home?" *(Brain 3)*
- "Who in your household is primarily responsible for preparing meals? Who in your household is primarily responsible for grocery shopping?" *(Brain 4)*
- Information about alcohol consumption may be obtained using screening tools such as the 10-Question Drinking History *(Table 4)* or the four-item CAGE questionnaire (see Chapter 59).

Abnormal Eating Behaviors

The following direct questions may be useful in identifying behaviors associated with eating disorders:

- "Have you ever consumed an excessive amount of food in a short period of time?"
- "Have you ever made yourself vomit?"
- "Have you ever used laxatives, enemas, diuretics, or other medications (including herbal and over-the-counter weight-loss aids) to keep you from gaining weight or to help you lose weight?"
- "Have you ever fasted (gone without food entirely) for a full day or more to keep you from gaining weight or to help you lose weight?" (Fasting may be a part of cultural or religious practices.)

Physical Activity *(Red Flag 3)*

- "What are some of your usual daily activities?" (e.g., housework, gardening, child care, watching television)
- "What type of physical activity does your job require?"
- "What do you do for recreation?"
- "Do you currently engage in any physical activities as a way to improve your health and fitness level? Have you done this in the past?"
- "If you are currently engaging in physical fitness activities, describe your fitness program. How often (how many times a week) do you engage in your fitness program? How long do your fitness sessions usually last? Do you ever miss a session? If yes, how often do you miss sessions?"

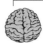

2 - Besides providing fluids, beverage choices can have a significant impact on both total calorie and nutrient intake. Some beverages, such as fruit juices and milk, provide vitamins, minerals, or protein, along with calories and fluid. Other beverages provide mostly calories and fluid. Beverages are generally consumed to satisfy thirst, which is independent of hunger. Over the past several decades, consumption of water (calorie-free) as a means to alleviate thirst has diminished in favor of soft drinks, juices, and other flavored drinks. Beverages can be a source of excess calories that, over time, can contribute to obesity *(Table 3)*.

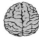

3 - A pattern of frequent meals away from home can result in a higher intake of calories, fat, and salt compared to home-prepared meals where the person may have more control over food preparation. Suggestions for healthy restaurant eating can be found at http://www.diabetes.org/nutrition. Calorie and nutrition information for popular fast food chains can be found at http://www.fastfood-facts.com. Individual fast food chains often publish calorie and nutrition information for their menu items and make this available to customers on request.

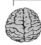

4 - If an individual does not have responsibility for food procurement or preparation, changing eating habits may be difficult without support and active involvement from other family members. A situation where special low-calorie meals are prepared for one family member and the rest of the family continue to consume high-fat, high-calorie meals does not bode well for long-term success, either.

3 - Strenuous exercise (i.e., exercising for more than an hour just to keep from gaining weight) after an episode of binge eating is a behavior associated with bulimia nervosa.

- "What are some things that keep you from being more active?"
- "What are some things that support you in being physically active?"

Health History

- Disease or risk factors associated with obesity *(Red Flag 4)*
- Family history of obesity *(Brain 5)*
- Menstrual periods. Amenorrhea for three consecutive cycles may be associated with a very low body weight and is a part of the diagnostic criteria for anorexia nervosa.

Physical Examination

Anthropometric Data

- Body mass index (BMI) (see Chapter 9)
- **Waist circumference** *(Definition 1)*

Blood Pressure

There is a close correlation between obesity and elevated blood pressure (see Chapter 4 on Hypertension).

Physical Signs Associated with Eating Disorders

Signs associated with very low body weight include:

- Bradycardia
- Hypothermia, cold intolerance
- Loss of muscle mass
- Amenorrhea[2,6]

Signs associated with self-induced vomiting include:

- Demineralization of tooth enamel
- Abnormal dentition
- Swelling of the parotid and submandibular glands
- Abrasions on the dorsum of the hand (caused by scraping against the incisors during attempts at vomiting)[2,6]

Behavioral or Psychiatric Assessment

Individuals with suspected eating disorders or serious emotional and psychological barriers to adopting healthier eating behaviors should be evaluated by a trained mental health professional (e.g., a psychiatrist, psychologist, or clinical social worker).

Testing

Blood Lipids

The National Cholesterol Education Program (NCEP) recommends that all adults over the age of 20 have their cholesterol checked at least once every 5 years. *Table 5* lists targeted and high-risk cholesterol levels.

Glucose Tolerance

New guidelines suggest that everyone over the age of 45 should be tested for diabetes every 3 years. People at high risk for diabetes

4 - Diseases or risk factors associated with obesity that pose a high absolute risk for subsequent mortality include:

- Established coronary heart disease
- Other atherosclerotic diseases
- Type 2 diabetes
- Sleep apnea
- 3 or more of the following:
  1. Hypertension
  2. Cigarette smoking
  3. High LDL cholesterol
  4. Impaired fasting glucose level
  5. Family history of early cardiovascular disease
  6. Age (male ≥ 45 years; female ≥ 55 years).

Factors that increase risk, but are not life-threatening include osteoarthritis, gallstones, stress incontinence, gynecologic abnormalities (e.g., amenorrhea and menorrhagia).

5 - In addition to strong evidence of a genetic component to obesity, family members tend to share similar food choices, eating habits, and physical activity preferences. From a treatment standpoint, it can be difficult for an individual, within a family unit, to make significant lifestyle changes without support and cooperation from other family members.

1 - Waist circumference: Excess abdominal fat is an independent risk factor for diseases such as coronary heart disease and diabetes. *Waist circumference* (measured above the iliac crests and below the lowest rib margin) is an indicator of abdominal fat. It is particularly useful for individuals who are classified as normal or overweight by BMI. According to the National Institutes of Health, high-risk waist circumference in women is > 35 inches and in men is > 40 inches.

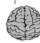

6 - Risk factors for diabetes:

- Age > 40 years
- Overweight
- Family history of diabetes
- History of having diabetes during a pregnancy (gestational diabetes)
- History of giving birth to an infant weighing over 9 pounds
- African, Asian, Hispanic, or Native American

Table 5. Classification of Blood Lipid Levels

	Desirable	Borderline High Risk*	High Risk
Total cholesterol	≤ 200 mg/dl	200–239 mg/dl	≥ 240 mg/dl
HDL cholesterol	> 45 mg/dl	35–45 mg/dl	< 35 mg/dl
LDL cholesterol	< 130 mg/dl	130–159 mg/dl	≥ 160 mg/dl

*Risk increases with the presence of other risk factors such as cigarette smoking, hypertension, diabetes, family history of premature cardiovascular disease, and age (≥ 45 years for men, ≥ 55 years for women).

should be tested at younger ages *(Brain 6)*.

Other Tests

Health history or physical examination may suggest other testing to rule out other causes of obesity (e.g., thyroid or endocrine problems) or to evaluate potential complications of obesity (e.g., sleep study for suspected sleep apnea). For individuals with suspected eating disorders, evaluation of serum electrolytes, serum glucose levels, and complete blood count may be indicated.

Putting It All Together

The prevalence of overweight and obesity is increasing at an alarming rate among the U.S. population. Although genetics play a role in obesity, the dramatic increases in prevalence are more likely due to changing lifestyles in the latter part of the 20th century (e.g., decreasing physical activity, changing food supply, and eating habits). Obesity increases an individual's risk of having high blood pressure, heart disease, diabetes, and other health problems.

Paradoxically, as more of the population becomes obese, the social stigma of obesity is also increasing. For vulnerable individuals, this may lead to engaging in extreme or abnormal behaviors to control body weight. Although eating disorders are associated with adolescent girls or young women, they can develop in older individuals and are seen increasingly in boys and men. Individuals with these disorders may fail to recognize the health consequences and may not seek medical treatment until the eating disorder is well established. They also may be reluctant to disclose abnormal behaviors such as binge eating or self-induced vomiting. Excessive concern about body shape and body weight and a distorted perception of their own body weight or shape are characteristic of patients with these disorders.

Management

Obesity

Treatment of obesity should be tailored to the individual and focused on achieving and maintaining a healthier body weight. For some individuals, prevention of further weight increases may be a reasonable goal. In others, a modest weight loss of even 5–10%, which can be maintained over time, can have a beneficial effect on comorbidities such as diabetes, blood pressure, dyslipidemia, and cardiovascular disease.

Weight loss is achieved by creating a calorie or energy deficit. As a general rule, it takes a calorie deficit of 500 calories per day to produce a weight loss of 1 pound per week. This deficit can be created by reducing calorie intake or increasing physical activity (energy output) or a combination of both.

A person is more likely to make and sustain changes in their food choices when their general preferences are taken into account and when they are provided education about food composition, labeling, preparation, and portion size. A registered dietitian can evaluate a person's usual diet, provide nutrition education, and assist him or her in the process of dietary adjustment to reduce calorie intake *(Consultation and Referral 1)*.

There are no quick-fix weight loss strategies *(Treatment 1)*. Although dietary fats are a major source of calories, simply reducing fat intake without lowering caloric intake will not produce weight loss. Likewise, the consumption or avoidance of particular foods or groups of foods will not promote weight loss unless total calorie intake is reduced. Diets that are significantly different from a person's usual food choices are difficult to maintain for long periods of time. When the person returns to his or her usual meals, any weight lost is usually regained. Very low calorie diets (< 800 calories a day) produce a larger initial weight loss but are difficult to maintain for a long period of time and are associated with a higher rate of weight regain.

Physical activity increases energy expenditure and can help create a calorie deficit needed for weight loss. More importantly, it can help prevent weight regain. The benefits of physical activity go beyond weight loss and maintenance. It helps preserve lean body mass and can reduce risk for diabetes and coronary heart disease beyond that attributable to weight loss alone. Reviewing activities of daily living can reveal opportunities for incorporating greater physical activity throughout the day (e.g., by walking greater distances, taking the stairs instead of the elevator). An exercise program can be developed based on the person's preferences and physical abilities, but it will only be effective if the person engages in it regularly.

For persons with suspected eating disorders, serious emotional and psychological barriers to adopting healthier eating behaviors, or difficulty establishing and maintaining healthy eating and activity behaviors, a referral to a trained mental health professional (e.g., a psychiatrist, psychologist, or clinical social worker) may be beneficial.

Drug Therapy

Pharmocotherapy may be helpful for some high-risk patients (BMI ≥ 30 or BMI ≥ 27 with concomitant risk factors or diseases such as hypertension, hyperlipidemia, diabetes, sleep apnea) who have difficulty achieving and maintaining weight loss with diet, physical activity, and behavior therapy approaches. Weight-loss drugs should be used only in the context of a treatment program that offers diet therapy, physical activity, and behavior therapy.

1 - Registered dietitians (RDs) are health care professionals who provide medical nutrition therapy and preventive nutrition counseling. Their training in food and nutrition includes completion of at least a bachelor's degree in nutrition, completion of an accredited practice or training program, passing a registration exam demonstrating their knowledge in food and nutrition, and ongoing professional training and education in food and nutrition. Medical nutrition therapy from an RD includes a complete assessment of overall nutritional status, medical data, and diet history, followed by a personalized course of treatment. (Source: http://www.eatright.org)

1 - A safe and effective weight management plan:
- Includes a variety of foods from all five major food groups in the Food Guide Pyramid and provides at least the minimum number of servings recommended from each food group to provide an adequate amount of essential nutrients.
- Includes appealing foods a person will enjoy eating the rest of his or her life, not just a few weeks or months.
- Includes foods available at the supermarket where the person usually shops.
- Allows a person to eat favorite foods in moderation.
- Recommends changes in eating habits that fit the person's lifestyle and budget.
- Includes regular physical activity.

Suggested Readings

1. American Dietetic Association: Position of the American Dietetic Association: Nutrition intervention in the treatment of anorexia nervosa, bulimia nervosa, and eating disorders not otherwise specified (EDNOS). J Am Diet Assoc 101:810–819, 2001. Available at http://www.eatright.org.
2. Becker AE, Grinspoon SK, Klibanski A, Herzog D: Eating disorders. N Engl J Med 340:1092–1098, 1999.
3. Collazo-Clavell ML: Safe and effective management of the obese patient. Mayo Clin Proc 74:1255–1260, 1999.
4. Krauss ML, Eckel RH, Howard B, et al: AHA Dietary Guidelines Revision 2000: A statement for healthcare professionals from the Nutrition Committee of the American Heart Association. Circulation 102:2284–2299, 2000.
5. National Association for the Study of Obesity (NAASO), National Heart, Lung, and Blood Institute (NHLBI): Practical Guide to the Identification, Evaluation, and Treatment of Overweight and Obesity in Adults. Bethesda, MD, NHLBI, 2000. Available at http://www.nhlbi.nih.gov/guidelines/obesity/practgde.htm.
6. Story M, Holt K, Sofka D (eds): Bright Futures in Practice: Nutrition. Arlington, VA, National Center for Education in Maternal and Child Health, 2000. Available at http://www.brightfutures.org.

Web Sites

U.S. Government sites with nutrition information: http://www.nutrition.gov.

American Dietetic Association site: http://www.eatright.org

American Diabetes Association: http://www.diabetes.org

American Heart Association: http://www.americanheart.org

Shape Up America!: http://www.shapeup.org

45. Occupational and Environmental Medicine, Workers' Compensation, and Disability Evaluation

Mary Wampler, MD, MPH

Synopsis

Occupational and environmental medicine is a broad field that includes a number of different disciplines, including musculoskeletal medicine, toxicology, and internal medicine. The physician also needs to have knowledge of workers' compensation, disability systems, and regulatory programs and legislation, including the Department of Transportation and the Americans with Disabilities Act. An occupational and environmental history is important in the assessment of all patients. In less than 15 minutes, enough information can be obtained to determine if the occupation or environment is involved in an illness or injury. If occupational or environmental hazards can be identified in the history, future injury or exposure to the patient and others can be prevented. Knowledge of workers' compensation allows the physician to assist an injured or ill worker to get back to work promptly and safely. Certain specialty examinations are commonly requested. It is important to help match the workers' capabilities with job demands and appropriately assess for disability.

Occupational History

This information should be included in the history for *all* patients.

Ask about the patient's occupation:

- "What do you do?"
- "How long have you been doing this job?"
- "Describe your work and your exposures there." If there is a question about a particular exposure causing illness, request a **material safety data sheet** *(Definition 1)*.
- "Under what circumstances do you use protective equipment (such as gloves or a respirator?"
- Ask about other employment.
- Have the patient list previous full-time positions in chronologic order.
- Have the patient list part-time jobs, temporary jobs, second jobs, and summer jobs.
- Ask about military or wartime exposure (if applicable).
- Determine symptoms or illnesses related to work:
    "Describe the timing of symptoms in relation to work hours."
    "Has anyone else at work suffered the same or similar problems?"

Nonoccupational exposures could be related to illness or could be expected to produce problems. Ask about:

- Smoking
- Alcohol
- Geographic history: "Did you ever live near a facility that could have contaminated the surrounding area (e.g., mine, plant, smelter)?"

1 - Material safety data sheet: A written evaluation of a hazardous chemical, generally prepared by the substance manufacturer and given to the employer with the purchase of the substance. The Occupational Safety and Health Administration (OSHA) requires suppliers to include these data sheets with each shipment of industrial materials and requires employers to maintain them and make them available to physicians and workers.

- Family exposure: "Has anyone in the family worked with hazardous materials that they could have brought home?"
- Hobbies: "Are you exposed to any hazardous materials (e.g., ceramics, metals, glues)?" Remember that many products available over the counter are extremely hazardous to human health if not used safely.
- If retired, ask about previous occupations.

Many occupational diseases are not diagnosed because a work or exposure history was never taken. Two common conditions that should alert the provider include asthma and dermatitis *(Red Flag 1)*.

1 - As many as 1 in 10 cases of new-onset asthma or recrudescence of previously quiescent childhood-onset asthma have a potential link with occupation. Occupations at risk include hairdresser, baker, laboratory worker, and painter.

Occupational skin disease accounts for almost half of all occupational disease of American workers. Contact dermatitis accounts for 80–90% of occupational skin disease. It is one of the leading causes of days lost from the job due to work-related illnesses. Causal agents include poison oak, soaps and detergents, and latex.

Workers' Compensation and Reports

Workers' compensation is a legal system set up to guarantee an injured worker prompt but limited benefits and to give an employer sure and predictable liability. In exchange for prompt and complete medical care for a work-related injury, the injured worker gives up the right to sue the employer for negligence or for pain and suffering. The laws vary from state to state. Understanding the requirements of the state system and provision of necessary services to treat the condition will ensure the flow of benefits to the worker.

An important part of treatment for a work-related injury or illness is the report that goes back to the employer. This should address the following questions:

- Was the injury or illness work-related, in part or in full?
- Has the worker reached **maximum medical improvement (Definition 2)**?
- Is the worker capable of doing *any* work *(Brain 1)*?
- How long are the work restrictions to last?
- What treatment or tests were ordered?

2 - Maximum medical improvement: The date after which further recovery and restoration of function can no longer be anticipated, based on reasonable medical certainty.

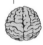

1 - Rather than state that the worker can or cannot work, it is better to state what activities the worker is capable of doing and let the employer decide whether the individual can work. Try to be as specific as possible. For example, do not order "light duty," but rather specify "no lifting more than 10 pounds with the left arm." Early return to work is associated with more rapid recovery and less disability from work-related injuries.

In most states, filing a workers' compensation claim has an implied consent for release of information for that claim. However, it is advisable to have the written consent of the employee before releasing information to the employer. In the report to the employer, he or she is entitled only to information regarding the work-related injury and nothing more. Releasing information to the employer regarding non–work-related medical conditions may expose the employer to liability under the **Americans with Disabilities Act (ADA) (Definition 3)**.

3 - Americans with Disabilities Act (ADA): Federal legislation forbidding discrimination by employers (with 15 or more employees) against individuals who currently have disabilities, are incorrectly perceived as being disabled, or have a record of disability.

Common Physical Examinations

Several specialty examinations are related to work. The most frequently requested are described here.

Preplacement

This evaluation is performed after the individual has been offered the job. The role of the provider is to determine if the individual is able to perform the essential job functions without injury to self or others *(Consultation and Referral 1)*. Essential job functions are determined

1 - It can be difficult during a clinical evaluation to determine work capacity, such as how many pounds and how often during a work shift an individual can safely lift. Referral to physical therapy can be very helpful for measurements of either one or two focused activities or for a broad spectrum of activities. When a full description of work capacity is needed, a **functional capacity evaluation (Definition 4)** can be useful. This is generally done with specialized equipment by a physical therapist with special training in this type of evaluation.

by the employer and provided to the physician. The report given to the employer should state only whether the individual can perform the job described or recommended restrictions. The restrictions should be described in detail. The employer then determines if there is availability of work.

Department of Transportation Physicals

The purpose of the evaluation is to certify drivers for the Federal Highway Administration. The patient will bring in a physical examination form and a certification card that must be signed by the examining physician. The certification remains valid for 2 years from the date of the examination. The examiner must determine if an individual has a medical condition that would render him or her unsafe to operate a vehicle on the highway. In this case, safety of the public, not the individual, is the issue. The criteria for certifying a driver as safe are outlined in the regulations. They can also be found on the World Wide Web at http://home.att.net/~NataH/. Certifying a driver who does not qualify under the regulations can place the examiner at risk of liability if the driver harms the public because of the disqualifying condition.

Independent Medical Examination / Disability Evaluations

An independent medical examination (IME) is usually requested by an insurance company, the Workers' Compensation Court, an attorney, or a case manager and is done to help settle a workers' compensation case. Questions the physician may be asked include:

- What is the diagnosis?
- What is the causation?
- Has the individual reached maximum medical improvement?
- Is there an **impairment**, and if so, what is the impairment rating? *(Defintion 5)* (Disability is decided by nonmedical people.)
- Are there any permanent restrictions?

Workers' compensation provides disability benefits. Other disability systems exist, such as Social Security, individual insurance policies, railroad, and various federal agencies. Each has specific requirements for qualification and the benefits available *(Consultation and Referral 2)*.

Fitness for Duty

This is an evaluation of an individual currently working, for ability to do the job without harm to self or others. This may be done on a regular periodic basis or an episodic basis when there is or appears to be a health problem that might interfere with attendance or performance. For example, an individual with diabetes mellitus working a night shift might have difficulty with control of blood sugars, causing frequent insulin reactions, and may require a restriction to work only during the day.

Putting It All Together

Many illnesses that arise from work or the environment present with symptoms similar to those of other common medical problems. Knowing how to take an occupational and environmental history will allow the physician to diagnose, treat, and prevent disease or injury.

4 - Functional capacity evaluation: A systematic method of measuring a patient's ability to perform meaningful tasks on a safe and dependable basis.

5 - Impairment: Anatomic or functional loss; such as amputation of a limb. In most states, the American Medical Association's *Guides to the Evaluation of Permanent Impairment, 4th edition* (or most recent), is used to determine the *impairment rating*. This is the impairment expressed as a percentage of the body as a whole or of an extremity.

2 - When a request is made for a disability evaluation, referral to a specialist in this area is recommended. It is best to contact the individual or agency the patient is seeking disability from to find out if there is a designated examiner. These examinations are costly and usually are not paid for by health insurance. Often the agency granting the disability will pay for the examination. Contact the Social Security Administration if the individual is applying for Social Security Disability, because designated examiners are retained for this purpose. If there is no designated examiner, contact the Workers' Compensation Court in your state, the American Board of Independent Medical Examiners, the American Academy of Disability Evaluating Physicians, or the American College of Occupational and Environmental Medicine to find an examiner in your area.

Many patients will need the services of a physician for workers' compensation claims and different specialty examinations. Knowledge of the laws and regulations that apply to the field of occupational medicine is essential to providing good care to the patient. A useful site on the World Wide Web for many aspects of occupational and environmental medicine is http://occ-env-med.mc.duke.edu/oem/index2.htm.

Selected Readings

1. Doege T: Guides to the Evaluation of Permanent Impairment, 4th ed. Chicago, American Medical Association, 1993.
2. Hartenbaum N: The DOT Medical Examination: A Guide to Commercial Drivers' Medical Certification. Beverly Farms, MA, OEM Press, 2000.
3. LaDou J: Occupational and Environmental Medicine, 2nd ed. Stamford, CT, Appleton & Lange, 1997.
4. Rom W: Environmental and Occupational Medicine, 2nd ed. Boston, Little, Brown, 1992.
5. Zenz C: Occupational Medicine, 3rd ed. St. Louis, Mosby, 1994.

The Business & Industry Health Group
6400 Prospect Suite 333
Kansas City, Missouri 64132
816/523-7770
FAX 816/523-5302

WORK ABILITY REPORT

Employee's Name__________ Chart Number__________

Employer__________

Date__________ Time In:__________ Time Out:__________

DIAGNOSIS __________

CARE PROVIDED ❒ Physician Exam ❒ X-Ray ❒ Physical Therapy ❒ Medication ❒ Other__________

WORK STATUS

❒ Return to regular work on__________

❒ Return to work on__________with the following restrictions:

❒ No exposure to cold, heat, water dampness, chemicals, paint, dust welding *(appropriate restrictions circled)*
❒ Keep affected area clean and dry
❒ No climbing of stairs or ladders
❒ No work around high speed or moving machinery
❒ No operating of mobile equipment
❒ Should be sitting ____% of time
❒ No work requiring repetitive bending of ________
❒ Other__________
❒ No repetitive shoveling
❒ No lifting over ____lbs.
❒ No push or pull over ____lbs. of force
❒ No reaching above shoulder level
❒ No kneeling or squatting
❒ Should be considered permanent
❒ No use of __________
❒ Limited use of __________

❒ Unable to work__________

FOLLOW-UP CARE

❒ Scheduled for physician appointment on **Date**__________ **Time**__________
❒ Scheduled for physical therapy on **Date**__________ **Time**__________
❒ Referral__________
❒ Released

____
Physician's Signature

If light duty is not available, then patient will be unable to work.

BIHG-031 (7/90)

Figure 1: Sample return-to-work sheet.
(From Zenz C: Occupational Medicine, 3rd ed. St. Louis, Mosby, 1994, with permission.)

46. Partner Abuse

Layne A. Prest, PhD, LMFT • W. David Robinson, PhD, LMFT

Synopsis

Partner abuse is one manifestation of the violence that takes place in a significant number of intimate relationships. Abuse is often a part of an intergenerational pattern of violence (against children, siblings, partners, or elders), taking place on emotional, psychological, physical, and sexual levels. Partner abuse is a leading cause and contributing factor to a variety of injuries, somatic complaints, and mental health conditions presented in the primary care clinical setting. The vast majority of the victims are female. An estimated 3–4 million women per year are abused, including 15–25% of patients who subsequently present to the primary care setting. Abuse is likely to take place in intimate relationships irrespective of socioeconomic, racial, ethnic, or religious background.

A careful, nonthreatening, and nonjudgmental interview is the basis for assessment and appropriate intervention. Assessing the victim's readiness for change and helping her develop a safety plan, including appropriate referrals, are crucial parts of the physician's management plan. Treatment of physical injuries, somatic complaints, and emotional symptoms requires a multidisciplinary approach. The most effective intervention often takes place in a continuity relationship and in concert with the legal and mental health systems in the community. Abused women are often so overwhelmed, hesitant, confused, embarrassed, or afraid that they may not reveal the abuse. Therefore, health care providers should maintain a high index of suspicion regarding these issues and routinely screen patients, especially those presenting with concerning physical or behavioral symptoms.

Differential Diagnosis

The "medical" differential will depend on the nature of the presenting signs and symptoms. Of course, physical injury should compel the provider to seriously consider abuse as a potential etiologic factor. However, most victims of domestic violence do not present physical symptoms of abuse in the primary care setting. From a biopsychosocial perspective, with a focus on the more psychosocially oriented diagnoses, the differential should include:

- Mood disorders
- Anxiety disorders
- Marital or family dysfunction not involving physical violence
- Substance abuse
- Other psychiatric disorders

History

When domestic violence is suspected, the health care provider should interview the patient alone in a private setting *(Red Flag 1)*. The interviewer should use a nonjudgmental manner and avoid blaming the patient for what is happening. The interview should include questions

 1 - This is especially true if the patient is accompanied by someone who may be the perpetrator of the abuse. A "red flag" should be raised if the person accompanying the patient is overly solicitous, controlling, attentive, or resistant or tries to influence the divulging of information.

about the current situation, past history of violence and abuse, the impact of the abuse on the patient (and others in the home, including children), and a discussion of the patient's short-term options and plans, including whether the patient can return home safely.

Opening Questions

Any number of the following or similar questions may be used to normalize the issues and create a less-threatening context.

- "Sometimes patients with these types of injuries (complaints) turn out to be in situations where they are being hurt by someone. Could it be that this is happening to you?"
- "It is pretty common for women to be hurt by their partners. Has anyone been hurting you by threatening, pushing, hitting, choking, restraining, or forcing you to do things sexually that you are uncomfortable with?"
- "We all argue or fight at home. What happens at your house when there are disagreements?"
- "Because so many women are involved with someone who hits them, threatens them, puts them down, and so on, I now ask all my patients about abuse. Is someone abusing you?"

Questions to Assess the Level of Violence in the Home

- "Do you ever feel afraid of, or threatened by, your partner?"
- "Do you feel safe at home?"
- "Has your partner ever destroyed things you care about?"
- "Has your partner ever threatened or abused your children?"
- "Has your partner ever threatened or abused your pets?"
- "Has your partner ever injured you? To what extent?"
- "Has your partner ever forced you to engage in sex that makes you feel uncomfortable?"

Questions to Assess the Control Tactics the Partner Is Using

- "Has your partner ever prevented you from leaving the house, seeing friends, getting a job, or continuing your education?"
- "Does your partner watch your every move? Call your workplace several times a day? Accuse you of having affairs with other people?"

Questions to Avoid

Avoid questions that imply blame or judgment or cause the patient to feel shame *(Brain 1)*.

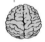

1 - The following questions should be **avoided:**
- What did you do to make him [her] hit you?
- What could you have done to diffuse the situation?
- Why don't you just leave?
- Do you get something out of the violence?

Questions to Assess Readiness for Change

Refer to the table on page 50 for the stages of readiness for change.

- "Have you ever thought that the way you are being treated by your partner was wrong?"
- "Have you ever thought that the way you are being treated by your partner was affecting your health?"
- "Have you ever thought that the way you are being treated by your partner was affecting your children?"
- "What have you thought you should do about this situation?"
- "Do you have a plan for what you will do when this happens again?"
- "Have you ever contacted (local support/social service agency specializing in abuse issues) for help?"

Questions to Assess Safety

- "Have you ever thought you were in danger? Are you in danger now?"
- "Have you ever thought about developing a plan for the safety of you and your children?"
- "When you leave here do you have a safe place to go?"
- "What signs are you able to see that s/he is getting angry or approaching a 'blow-up'?"
- "If you sense that s/he is building up to a point of hurting you again, where do you think you could go? Who could you call? What do you think would be safest for you to do?"
- "Would you be willing to talk with me or someone else about a plan to help keep you (and your children) safe?"
- "Do you need referrals to counseling or shelters?"

Thorough, well-documented medical records can provide important evidence should the legal system become involved. These records can actually benefit the patient by providing concrete, objective validation of the injuries or condition from which the patient suffers. It is best to use the patient's own words in recording the chief complaint and description of the abusive event.

The Appendix provides information on developing a safety plan.

Physical Examination

Perform physical exam as indicated by presenting complaints, signs, and symptoms, but pay particular attention to the following:

- Abdominal, back, and neck pain and headaches, etc.
- Central distribution of injury—face, neck, throat, chest, abdomen, genitals
- Bilateral distribution of injury to multiple areas
- History of repeated injuries or emergency room or clinic visits
- Contusions, lacerations, abrasions, human bites, or no physical evidence of trauma regardless of the patient's presenting problem
- Delay between onset of injury and presentation for treatment *(Red Flag 2)*
- Multiple injuries in various stages of healing
- Extent or type of injury inconsistent with patient's explanation
- Evidence of rape
- Chronic pain, psychogenic pain, pain due to diffuse trauma
- Pregnancy. Abused women are more likely to be beaten when pregnant. There is also an increased rate of miscarriage and self-induced, attempted, or successful abortions

2 - Information about a delay in seeking care helps explain the nature of the physical and emotional symptoms. The psychosocial concerns affect the timing in these situations. For example, situational factors (fear for safety, level of threat, financial constraints) may have prevented the patient from seeking care earlier or may be compelling the patient to seek care immediately.

In the medical record, record a complete description of the injuries, including type, number, size, location, resolution, possible causes, and explanations given *(Brain 2)*. Where applicable, the location and nature of the injuries should be recorded in a body chart or drawing (see figure on page 166) and be size proportionate. Many experts also recommend that health care providers take 35-mm or Polaroid-type pictures (with permission) of the injuries. It is helpful to provide an opinion on whether the explanation of injuries is believable. If the police are called, record

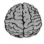

2 - Laws vary from state to state regarding mandatory reporting and other physician legal obligations. Check with your attorney or the state Domestic Violence and Sexual Assault Coalition for details.

the action taken as well as the name, badge number, and phone number of the investigating officer.

Testing

No testing is necessary unless indicated by physical examination or history.

Putting It All Together

More often than not in the primary care setting, the victim of partner abuse will present vague, somatic complaints rather than acute injuries. This presentation, in the context of other behavioral indicators (e.g., depressed or anxious affect, evasive demeanor, substance abuse, or history that doesn't explain the condition), should raise a red flag for the health care professional. Without change or intervention, partner abuse usually escalates in severity, starting with psychological violence (threats, intimidation, controlling money, and relationships) and proceeds to higher levels of physical and sexual violence (restraining, pushing, hitting, weapons, and forced sex). Abuse victims will often return to the abuser for a variety of reasons (fear, financial dependence, hope of change, shame, or keeping the family intact). It has been estimated that it may take victims an average of seven experiences or interventions in order to make the decision to leave the situation.

Management

Appropriate management begins with the initial interaction with the patient. Good interviewing may help the patient to begin thinking about his or her situation more clearly, giving thought to the emotional and physical consequences for him-herself, as well as any children that may be involved. In addition, the patient may be prompted to begin thinking about making changes and developing a concrete plan of action. The health care professional should pace her interventions according to the patient's readiness for change. Injuries and other somatic complaints should be treated appropriately. Medication (especially pain and psychopharmacologic agents) should be prescribed in conjunction with a plan to address the patient's emotional, social, and legal issues. Because of the associated acute and chronic stress, patients who are victims of partner abuse frequently experience comorbid conditions. Therefore the health care professional should be prepared to assess and treat anxiety, depression, post-traumatic stress disorder symptoms, and substance abuse, as well. Above all, it is important for the health care professional to attempt to provide nonjudgmental support and reassurance, resource and referral information, and reasonable follow up. A growing number of communities have agencies that provide shelter, legal, and medical advocacy, support services, and counseling for abuse victims. Remember to be familiar with the reporting statutes in your state. You may be required to report domestic violence to the local law enforcement officials. Anytime you learn about child abuse, you are required to report it. In preparation for your preceptorship experiences, find out what the reporting procedures are for the community. Know whom to contact and how *(Brain 3)*. Always report your suspicions confidentially to your preceptor before the patient leaves.

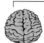

3 - Hotline numbers:
National Hotline: 1-800-799-SAFE
There's No Excuse for Domestic Violence (public education campaign): 1-800-777-1960
Family Violence Prevention Fund (resource information and training materials): 1-415-252-8900

Appendix

A safety plan developed by or with the patient is a helpful part of intervening in the cycle of violence. But it is most helpful if timed right (see stages of readiness for change). It is usually a mistake to jump into planning before the patient has signaled that she has thought about and become invested in changing her situation.

Some women may have to bolt from the home with no notice; others have some time to plan what they will need to take with them. The following items will be helpful to the woman after she leaves. Advise her to take them with her if she is able to do so or store them in a safe place that she can access if she does have to leave:

- As much cash as possible, a checkbook, an ATM card, and credit cards
- A small bag of extra clothing for the woman and her children
- Extra keys for the car and the house
- Important documents:
    Bank accounts and insurance policies
    Marriage license
    Abuser's date of birth
    Social security numbers (own, children's, abuser's)
    Birth certificates (own, children's)
    Prescription medication
    Special toy for each child

Selected Readings

1. Barnett OW, Miller-Perrin CL, Perrin R: Family Violence across the Lifespan. Thousand Oaks, CA, Sage Publications, 1996.
2. Grisso JA, Schwarz DF, Hirschinger N, et al: Violent injuries among women in an urban area. N Engl J Med 341:1899–1904, 1999.
3. Kyriacou DN, Anglin D, Taliaferro E, et al: Risk factors for injury to women from domestic violence. N Engl J Med 341:1892–1898, 1999.
4. Nebraska Medical Association: The Cure Can Begin with You: A Physician's Handbook on Domestic Violence. Lincoln, NE, Nebraska Medical Association, 1995.
5. Oriel KA, Fleming MF: Screening men for partner violence in a primary care setting: A new strategy for detecting domestic violence. J Fam Pract 46:493–498, 1998.
6. Rodriguez MA: Breaking the silence: Battered women's perspectives on medical care. Arch Fam Med 5:153–158, 1996.
7. Schornstein SL: Domestic Violence and Health Care: What Every Professional Needs to Know. Thousand Oaks, CA, Sage Publications, 1997.

47. Painful Joints and Arthritis

Gerald F. Moore, MD • Paul W. Esposito, MD

Synopsis

Soft tissue discomfort, painful joints, and **arthritis *(Definition 1)*** are very common problems. Most patients with musculoskeletal complaints will have self-limited soft tissue problems, **arthralgias**, and **myalgias *(Definitions 2)*** that will resolve within a few weeks. Various estimates suggest that up to 30% of the population have symptoms of arthritis at some time in their life. **Degenerative joint disease *(Definition 3)*** is the most common type of arthritis. Post-traumatic arthritis either resulting from injuries to articular joint cartilage or secondary to recurrent injuries caused by ligamentous instability of the joints is also frequent. Malalignment of joints following fractures also may cause painful joints by placing abnormal stresses on the joint.

Most diagnoses can be made with a careful and thorough history and physical examination. **Acute monarticular arthritis *(Red Flag 1)*** may be caused by trauma, fracture, or, in the absence of injury, acute septic arthritis or osteomyelitis. This complaint must be evaluated aggressively because a delay in appropriate therapy may result in destruction of the joint (e.g., untreated septic arthritis). Plain radiographs and laboratory analysis of joint fluid and peripheral blood usually can confirm clinical findings. Appropriate diagnosis and early treatment for more chronic forms of arthritis, such as **rheumatoid arthritis *(Definition 4)*** or degenerative arthritis, may result in significant improvement in the patient's well-being and activities of daily living. Inflammatory arthritis is initially treated with nonsteroidal anti-inflammatory drugs (NSAIDs), fractures are treated with immobilization or surgical stabilization, and infectious arthritis requires prompt, aggressive needle drainage coupled with appropriate IV antibiotics. Surgical debridement is occasionally warranted (always in hip infections).

Differential Diagnosis

Acute (< 3 Months)

- Soft tissue complaints (e.g., carpal tunnel)
- Trauma
- Septic joint
- **Gout *(Definition 5)***
- **Pseudogout *(Definition 6)***
- Tumor, leukemia

Chronic (> 3 Months)

- Soft tissue complaints (e.g., **fibromyalgia [*Definition 7*]**)
- Degenerative joint disease

1 - Arthritis: Inflammation of the joint.

2 - Arthralgia: Pain in the joint.
Myalgia: Pain in the muscles.

3 - Degenerative joint disease: Asymmetrical, large joint, activity-related complaints.

1 - Acute onset of a reddened, inflamed, monarticular process should prompt strong consideration for joint aspiration and antibiotic therapy if an infectious etiology is likely. An untreated septic joint may result in the development of bone destruction within a week.

4 - Rheumatoid arthritis: Bilateral, symmetrical, inflammatory arthritis of small joints.

5 - Gout: Acute inflammatory arthritis (typically of the great toe) associated with uric acid crystals found in the joint.

6 - Pseudogout: Acute inflammatory arthritis (typically of the knee) associated with calcium pyrophosphate crystals found in the joint.

7 - Fibromyalgia: Multiple soft tissue trigger points without arthritis.

- Rheumatoid arthritis
- **Connective tissue disease** *(Definition 8)*
- **Seronegative spondyloarthropathy** *(Definition 9)*

Inflammatory

- Rheumatoid arthritis
- **Systemic lupus erythematosus** *(Definition 10)*
- Gout or pseudogout

Noninflammatory

- Trauma
- Degenerative joint disease
- Fibromyalgia

Younger Age Group

- Trauma
- Infectious (septic joint)
- Rheumatoid arthritis
- Spondyloarthropathy

Older Age Group

- Degenerative joint disease
- Gout
- Pseudogout

Male

- Gout
- Spondyloarthropathy

Female

- Pseudogout
- Rheumatoid arthritis
- Connective tissue diseases
- Fibromyalgia

8 - Connective tissue disease: A group of disorders such as systemic lupus erythematosus that have multiorgan involvement.

9 - Seronegative spondyloarthropathy: Inflammatory disease of the spine with multiple etiologies.

10 - Systemic lupus erythematosus: Multiorgan, immune complex–mediated disease.

History

"Tell me about your joint complaints."

- "Was there an injury or activity that precipitated the pain? When did the pain start?"
- Preceding joint problems (Perthes disease or slipped capital femoral epiphysis as a child). Prior injury, change in activity level (sudden fitness rage in couch potato).
- "Was this precipitated by an accident or is it work related?" Make sure you check whether symptoms are related to repetitive tasks.
- "Do your joints swell or get red or hot?" (signs of inflammation).
- "Do you have stiffness in the joints?" (suggestive of synovial inflammation)
- "Do you have attacks or is the pain chronic?" Acute attacks suggest crystal-induced disease or septic arthritis.

- Fever or chills (suggestive of infection)
- Night pain (frequent in bony tumors)
- "Is one joint painful or are many painful?" Pattern can help diagnose type of arthritis.
- "Do your complaints always affect the same joints or do the symptoms migrate? Which joints are affected?" Rheumatoid arthritis usually involves the small joints of the hands and feet, and degenerative arthritis involves larger joints.
- "Are similar joints on both sides of the body affected?" Inflammatory arthritis is symmetrical, whereas gout and degenerative arthritis are typically asymmetrical. Most types of true arthritis will consistently affect the same joints.
- Systemic symptoms (e.g., fatigue in leukemia)
- Rash (seen in systemic juvenile rheumatoid arthritis or rheumatic fever)
- "What time of day do your joints bother you?" Morning suggests inflammatory disease; evening suggests more mechanical problem.
- "How long have you had joint problems?" Symptoms for less than 6 weeks suggest trauma or soft tissue disease. Symptoms lasting longer than six weeks would be consistent with rheumatoid arthritis or degenerative arthritis.
- "Do you have a history of arthritis in the family? Most types of arthritis are not familial, but occasionally some types of arthritis are found in multiple family members.
- "What have you taken for your complaints?" This may give you an idea of the severity of the problem.
- "Have you had any evaluation for this condition?" Obtain previous laboratory and radiographic studies for review.
- "Do you have any other symptoms?" Multisystem complaints may suggest an infectious or autoimmune etiology. Symptoms of systemic lupus erythematosus might include hair loss, recurrent nasal or oral ulcers, pleurisy, pericarditis, seizures, or psychosis.
- Travel history (e.g., Lyme disease in the Northeast, coccidiomycosis in San Joaquin Valley).
- Coexisting illness (e.g., sickle cell disease and *Salmonella* infections).

Physical Examination

- General observation. Note obvious discomfort or holding the joint still, refusing to bear weight.
- Vital signs for evidence of systemic involvement, fever
- Observe for signs of swelling, redness, or heat in the joints.
- Associated rashes (e.g., juvenile rheumatoid arthritis, viral-associated arthritis, or arthritis associated with psoriasis)
- Range of motion of the joints to document the extent of involvement
- Deformities such as osteophytes (spurs in degenerative joint disease), contractures with chronic pain, or instability (ligamentous injury)
- Palpation of the joints *(Brain 1)* for signs of synovial inflammation (**synovitis [*Definition 11*]**) such as swelling and warmth of the joint
- Check for tenderness *(Brain 2)* over soft tissue areas around the joint (e.g., bursa, tendons, ligaments).
- Systemic examination as appropriate for signs of systemic lupus, skin rashes such as psoriasis, and heart murmur.

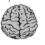
1 - Inflammation of a joint (synovitis) is graded from 0 to 4+.

11 - Synovitis: Inflammatory condition of the lining of joints.

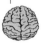
2 - Pain in a joint or soft tissue area is graded as follows:
1+ Patient complains of pain with palpation
2+ Patient visibly winces
3+ Patient withdraws from the discomfort

- Special tests as appropriate *(Table 1)*:
    Schober test for seronegative spondyloarthropathy
    Tinel's or Phalen's signs for carpal tunnel syndrome
    Yergason maneuver checking for bicipital tendinitis
    Test of the meniscus and collateral ligaments if instability of the
      knee is suspected
    Lachman, Apley, Drawer, McMurray tests

Table 1. Tests for Joint Pain Complaints

Test or Sign	What It Indicates
Schober test	Demonstration of decreased flexion of the lumbar spine
Tinel's sign	Physical finding in carpal tunnel syndrome (numbness and tingling in first $3^1/_2$ fingers after tapping median nerve at the wrist)
Phalen's sign	Physical finding in carpal tunnel syndrome (numbness and tingling in first $3^1/_2$ fingers after holding dorsum of hands together for up to 1 minute)
Yergason's maneuver	Pain at the bicipital groove of the humerus with supination of the forearm against resistance
Lachman's test	Checks for increased anterior–posterior movement of the tibia on the femur
Anterior drawer test	Checks for increased anterior–posterior movement of the tibia on the femur
Drawer test	Checks for instability of the collateral ligaments of the knee
Apley's test	Test for meniscal injury of the knee
McMurray's test	Test for meniscal injury of the knee

Testing

In general, no specific laboratory tests are diagnostic for arthritis. Soft tissue diseases have no systemic effects and will not have abnormal laboratory tests. Rheumatoid arthritis and degenerative joint disease can be diagnosed by doing a thorough history and physical examination. Radiographic findings may take years to develop and are therefore not helpful in making a diagnosis early in the disease process.

The erythrocyte sedimentation rate (ESR) and C-reactive protein tests are nonspecific indicators of inflammation. They are most useful in separating true inflammatory arthritis from soft tissue complaints when the history and physical examinations are not diagnostic. A complete blood cell count (CBC) may be helpful (e.g., elevated white blood cell [WBC] count with increased polymorphonuclear neutrophils [PMNs] may indicate infection or a low WBC count or anemia may indicate underlying neoplastic disease or systemic rheumatologic condition).

All patients with an acute inflammatory monarticular arthritis should have synovial fluid aspirated from the joint to check for an infectious or crystal etiology. Septic joints will have a high WBC count (usually > 50,000), but may have a negative Gram stain. The diagnoses of gout (caused by uric acid crystals) and pseudogout (calcium pyrophosphate crystals) can be made by finding birefringent crystals within the joint. Patients with gout may have an elevated serum uric acid level.

Rheumatoid factor *(Red Flag 2)* is an immunoglobulin M (IgM) antibody to IgG. It is neither sensitive nor specific for rheumatoid arthritis. The antinuclear antibody test *(Red Flag 3)* is sensitive for systemic lupus erythematosus (over 90% positive), but is also found in many other types of arthritis so it is not helpful as a screening test. Other antibody tests may be useful in confirming a diagnosis but are not useful as screening laboratory tests.

Radiographs of affected joints in two planes 90° apart (anteroposterior [AP] and lateral) may be helpful in disclosing trauma or long-term joint changes.

2 - A positive rheumatoid factor is not diagnostic of rheumatoid arthritis.

3 - The rheumatoid factor and antinuclear antibody tests are not useful as screening tests.

Putting It All Together

Most acute episodes of joint or muscle discomfort either will get better on their own (if local trauma) or will require prompt intervention for relief of pain. Prevention of destruction of the joint with a septic joint is dependent on rapid administration of antibiotics. In general, if trauma is not suspected, joint aspiration should be performed on all patients with an acute monarticular arthritis and appropriate treatment should be begun.

If the patient has had symptoms for more than a few months, the determination of the exact etiology of the problem may require a more thorough history and physical exam, laboratory testing, and radiographic evaluation. The presence of true joint involvement should be determined. Soft tissue complaints can be chronic in nature and may be treated by modification of activity, nonsteroidal medications, and corticosteroid injections when appropriate.

True joint disease can be either inflammatory or noninflammatory in character. If the symptoms are primarily mechanical (worse with activity and relieved by rest), degenerative joint disease, ligament or tendon damage, or other localized problems should be investigated. Inflammatory symptoms characterized by morning stiffness (> 30 minutes) or **gelling phenomenon *(Definition 12)*** are usually associated with rheumatoid arthritis, seronegative spondyloarthropathies, or connective tissue diseases. If an inflammatory condition is suspected, a thorough review of systems should be performed checking for symptoms of systemic autoimmune diseases such as systemic lupus erythematosus.

12 - Gelling phenomenon: Stiffness of a joint that occurs when the joint is inactive for some time.

Laboratory and radiographic testing are rarely helpful in the initial evaluation of the patient. Most serological studies are relatively nonspecific and therefore should be ordered primarily to confirm the diagnosis. The ESR is helpful if inflammatory conditions are thought to be present.

Management *(Consultation and Referral 1)*

Acute soft tissue and joint complaints often can be treated symptomatically with rest, heat, or ice (whichever gives the most relief) and appropriate physical therapy once the acute episode is over. NSAIDs, such

1 - Most routine problems can be treated by the generalist. Any questions about the correct diagnosis or the need for more aggressive therapy should be referred to either a rheumatologist or orthopedic surgeon.

as acetylsalicylic acid, naproxen, and ibuprofen, can provide pain relief as well as anti-inflammatory benefits (may take up to 3–4 weeks to achieve the anti-inflammatory effects). A septic joint usually requires up to a 6-week course of intravenous antibiotics. Acute crystal-induced disease usually will respond to anti-inflammatory medications or colchicine (decreases inflammatory cytokine release by inhibiting ingestion of crystals by WBCs).

The treatment of chronic joint disease should take into account any systemic manifestations. In general, the joint problems are initially treated with NSAIDs, modification of lifestyle, physical therapy, and adaptive devices. Inflammatory conditions such as rheumatoid arthritis may require disease-modifying drugs such as methotrexate, hydroxychloroquine, or sulfasalazine. Aggressive joint disease and systemic manifestations may require the use of corticosteroid preparations *(Treatment 1)*, which generally work well but have a high incidence of unacceptable side effects. Patients who fail to respond to more conventional therapy may require the use of combination drug therapy, cytotoxic agents, or surgical therapies. Newer treatments are being developed that utilize biologic agents *(Treatment 2)*. Even when treatment is not totally effective in relieving a patient's pain, patients are commonly grateful to know the cause and to be reassured and confident in the diagnosis.

1 - Corticosteroids provide excellent for control of acute symptoms but have many side effects when taken at high dosages or for a prolonged period of time.

2 - Etanercept, a tumor necrosis factor receptor binder, is one of a new group of biologic agents that is useful in the treatment of inflammatory conditions such as rheumatoid arthritis.

Selected Readings

1. American College of Rheumatology Ad Hoc Committee on Clinical Guidelines: Guidelines for the initial evaluation of the adult patient with acute musculoskeletal symptoms. Arthritis Rheum 39:1–8, 1996.
2. American College of Rheumatology Ad Hoc Committee on Systemic Lupus Erythematosus Guidelines: Guidelines for referral and management of systemic lupus erythematosus in adults. Arthritis Rheum 42:1785–1796, 1999.
3. Cash JM: Evaluation of the patient: A history and physical examination. In Klippel JH (ed): Primer on the Rheumatic Diseases, 11th ed. Atlanta, Arthritis Foundation, 1997.
4. Klippel JH: Appendix 1: Criteria for the classification of various types of arthritis. Primer on the Rheumatic Diseases, 11th ed. Atlanta, Arthritis Foundation, 1997.

Web Site

American College of Rheumatology: www.rheumatology.org. See fact sheets on common types of arthritis.

48. Peptic Ulcer Disease

Suzanne J. G. Cornwall, MD

Synopsis

Ulcers develop when the protective mucus lining cannot ward off the effects of the digestive acids and enzymes, causing a breakdown in the integrity of the wall of either the stomach (gastric ulcer) or the small intestine (duodenal ulcer). Peptic ulcer disease (PUD) includes both duodenal ulcers and gastric ulcers. Many factors have been found to cause ulcers. Nonsteroidal anti-inflammatory drugs (NSAIDs) are the most common external cause *(Brain 1)*, followed by alcohol and tobacco. *Helicobacter pylori* infection *(Definition 1)*, stress, excess gastric acid, excess pepsin secretion, and hyposecretion of protective mucus are also known precipitating factors. There appears to be an association between PUD and lower socioeconomic status and the elderly. PUD can occur at any age, but the incidence peaks in the fourth decade for duodenal ulcer disease and in the fifth decade for gastric ulcer disease. Duodenal ulcers are about three times more common than gastric ulcers.

The diagnosis of PUD may require only a trial of acid-blocking medications over a 4-week period. If symptoms persist, further testing is usually indicated, including simple blood, stool, or breath tests looking for *H. pylori*. The patient may need to undergo an **upper endoscopy** *(Definition 2)* so that the lining of the stomach can be visulized. A less invasive test would be the **upper gastrointestinal (GI) series** *(Definition 3)*.

Treatment may involve removing the offending agents (NSAIDs, alcohol, or caffeine), or the patient may be treated with various medications to suppress the acid. If the patient is infected with *H. pylori*, the bacterial infection is treated with antibiotics.

Differential Diagnosis

- Gastroesophageal reflux disease (GERD)
- Gastric carcinoma
- Crohn's disease
- Myocardial infarction (MI)
- Pancreatitis
- Cholelithiasis
- Abdominal aortic aneurysm (AAA)
- Zollinger-Ellison syndrome

History

"Tell me about your abdominal pain. What symptoms are you having?"

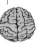
1 - Common NSAIDs include aspirin, ibuprofen (Motrin, Advil), naproxen sodium (Naprosyn, Aleve), indomethacin (indocin), ketoprofen (Orudis), celecoxib (Celebrex), and diclofenac sodium (Voltaren).

1 - *Helicobacter pylori (H. pylori)*: A corkscrew-shaped bacteria that attaches to the mucous membrane of the stomach. It can alter the immune system, allowing it to live with the host indefinitely. It thrives in a high-acid environment by making the enzyme urease. Urease generates ammonia, which neutralizes the acid and ensures *H. pylori's* survival. *H. pylori* also produces several toxins that cause inflammation and damage to the stomach's lining.

2 - Upper endoscopy: The patient is usually given intravenous sedation and a local anesthetic to the pharynx. A long, thin, flexible, fiber optic tube is passed through the pharynx, down the esophagus, through the stomach, and into the duodenum. The camera allows visualization of the anatomy, and a channel in the tube allows access for biopsies to be obtained.

3 - Upper GI series: The patient drinks a barium solution that outlines scarring, inflammation, ulcer craters, or deformities when x-rayed. The patient also may be asked to swallow crystals that cause gas to form in the stomach, allowing for expansion and aiding in the diagnosis of GERD.

Make sure that you elicit information specifically about:

- The presence of blood in the stools. "What color is your stool? Do you see blood in your stool?" *(Red Flag 1)*
- Vomiting up blood (coffee ground emesis) *(Red Flag 2)*
- Constitutional symptoms such as loss of appetite, weight loss, fever, chills, and night sweats *(Red Flag 3)*
- Radiation of pain. "Does the pain go into the chest, pelvis, back, or neck?" *(Red Flag 4)*

Other current history to obtain from the patient includes:

- "Have you experienced nausea or vomiting?"
- "Tell me about the quality of your pain. Is it burning or gnawing or does it give you the sensation of being overly hungry?"
- Intensity (scale of 1 through 10, 10 being most severe)
- Duration and timing. "When did it start? Is it constant? How long does it last?"
- "What kinds of things have you tried on your own to get relief? Has anything helped?"
- "Are there things that make it better or worse such as foods, medications, positions?"
- "Have you had similar symptoms in the past?"
- "Do you experience pain with swallowing (dysphagia)? Do liquids or solids get stuck (odynophagia) when you try to swallow?"

"Tell me about your past medical history."

- It is important to assess whether the patient has a prior history of cancer, coronary artery disease (CAD), heart attacks, or abdominal aortic aneurysm because these diseases may produce symptoms that mimic ulcer symptoms.

Other relevant factors of past medical history include:

- Current medications. NSAIDs, as well as other medications, can irritate the stomach and produce or exacerbate PUD.
- If female, last menstrual period and past pregnancies. Ectopic pregnancy or dysmenorrhea may produce symptoms similar to those of PUD.
- Surgeries or hospitalizations. Previous occurrence of PUD or past surgeries may have resulted in adhesions
- Other medical conditions (e.g., diabetes, high cholesterol, renal disease). Always be on the alert for other health risk factors.
- History of depression or anxiety, increased level of stress. Psychosocial stressors can exacerbate PUD or produce symptoms that are ulcer-like.
- Substance use (tobacco, alcohol, caffeine, past or present history of illicit drugs)
- Trauma. Recent truama can result in abdominal or gastric pain or discomfort.

"Does your abdominal pain affect you at home or work? Have you had to significantly alter your lifestyle or diet?"

"Do you have a family history of GI neoplasias or PUD?" PUD can have a genetic link.

1 - Bright red blood or melanotic (black, tarry) stools may indicate a perforation, hemorrhage, or underlying cancer.

2 - Vomiting up blood "coffee-ground emesis" may indicate a perforated ulcer.

3 - The presence of constitutional symptoms is more likely seen with infectious causes or neoplasia.

4 - Pain radiating into the chest, pelvis, back, or neck may indicate a perforation, AAA, pancreatitis, or MI (heart attack).

Physical Examination

- Note the patient's general appearance. Note grimacing, writhing around, or holding abdomen.
- Record vital signs, including temperature. Elevated temperature might indicate infection and possible perforation.
- Auscultate heart and lungs. Pneumonia can cause referred pain to the upper abdominal region. Congestive heart failure, acute MI, and pericarditis can mimic some signs and symptoms associated with PUD.
- If the patient has a positive family history for MIs or if the patient has risk factors for CAD, an electrocardiogram (EKG) is indicated.
- Look at the abdomen for color, scars, and symmetry.
- Listen to the abdomen. If bowel sounds are present, are they normal, high pitched, hyper- or hypoactive? Do you hear any aortic bruits?
- Percuss the abdomen. Is it dull, tympanic, or tender?
- Palpate the abdomen to check for guarding, rigidity, masses, rebound tenderness, and enlarged liver or spleen (hepatosplenomegaly).
- Check the femoral pulses.
- Perform a rectal exam and stool for blood.

With the exception of possible epigastric tenderness, the physical exam of a patient with uncomplicated PUD is generally normal. Lab tests will generally be unremarkable. Stool cards can be sent home with the patient to evaluate for any microscopic GI bleeding.

Diagnostic Testing

- Double-contrast upper GI with barium radiography. The ulcer will fill with barium and appears denser than the surrounding tissue. Inflammation or edema may produce a lucent band of tissue around the ulcer. Ulcers found in the duodenum are rarely malignant and should not require any further diagnostic studies. Gastric ulcers are associated with malignancy and will require endoscopic evaluation if they do not respond to treatment.
- Upper endoscopy is becoming the preferred diagnostic test. It is the most accurate and allows for biopsies to rule out a neoplasia, **Zollinger-Ellison syndrome** *(Brain 2)*, or Crohn's disease. It has a better success rate at locating duodenal ulcers. It also allows for testing of *H. pylori*.
- Serum or stool for *H. pylori* infection if not done with upper endoscopy.
- If the history and physical exam are not consistent with PUD, an abdominal ultrasound, amylase, lipase, hepatic function panel, hepatitis screening, and a complete blood cell count (CBC) may be needed to rule out other sources as mentioned in the differential diagnosis.

2 - The Zollinger-Ellison syndrome is caused by a non–beta islet cell tumor of the pancreas that secretes gastrin. Sixty percent of these tumors are malignant.

Putting It All Together

Most patients suffering from peptic ulcer disease will describe their pain as a gnawing, burning sensation localized to the mid-epigastric or left upper quadrant. The pain may radiate into the back. PUD will frequently wake the patient in the middle of the night. Patients may experience nausea, vomiting, bloating, or belching. It typically occurs 1–3 hours after eating. Partial relief may be achieved by drinking milk, eating, or taking over-the-counter H_2 blockers or antacids. Pain generally increases when the patient is supine. Alcohol, caffeine, citric acid, stress, NSAIDs, and smoking generally make PUD worse. *H. pylori* infection plays a major role in ulcer formation.

Patients presenting with the "typical" ulcer symptoms are usually younger than 45 years old, have no complications and no other significant medical history, and can be treated without the diagnostic work-up. Patients are usually treated for a period of 4 weeks. If no improvement occurs during this period and the patient adhered with medications and lifestyle modifications, treat him or her for an additional 4–8 weeks. Patients who fail to improve after 10 days of therapy or continue to have symptoms after 8–12 weeks need to undergo diagnostic testing to confirm that the diagnosis of PUD is correct.

Management

Symptom relief and prevention of complications are the main goal. Current therapies involve:

- Acid suppression with either H_2 blockers or proton pump inhibitors
- Protection of the mucosal lining from the acid or pepsin (misoprostol or sucralfate)
- Use of motility agents to speed up the passage of stomach contents into the intestine in order to decrease the exposure time to the various gastric acids
- Treatment of the *H. pylori* infection if present
- Discontinuing NSAIDs completely or switch to a cyclooxygenase-2 (COX-2) inhibitor agent
- Dietary modifications: avoid alcohol, citric-acid–containing foods and juices, and caffeinated and decaffeinated beverages. Decaffeinated beverages still contain tannic acid, which is irritating to the mucosal lining.
- Smoking cessation

Selected Readings

1. Friedman G: Peptic ulcer disease. Clin Symp 40:1–32, 1988.
2. Graber MA, Nugen A: Peptic ulcer disease: Presentation, treatment, and prevention. Emerg Med 31:66–78, 1999.
3. Ohning G, Soll A: Medical treatment of peptic ulcer disease. Am Fam Physician 39:257–270, 1989.
4. Robinson M: Acid-related diseases: A synopsis of pathogenesis, diagnosis, and treatment. Patient Care (winter):1–9, 1999.

49. Physical and Mental Disabilities

Cynthia R. Ellis, MD • Amy L. Ruane, EdS • Connie J. Schnoes, MA

Synopsis

The phrase "individuals with disabilities" covers a wide array of physical and mental difficulties in an estimated 43 million Americans. A *disability* results from a loss of physical ability (e.g., loss of sight, hearing, or mobility) or from a difficulty in learning or social adjustment that significantly interferes with an individual's normal growth, development, or functioning within the environment *(Table 1)*. A *handicap* is a limitation imposed on an individual by external or environmental demands that impairs the individual's ability to adapt or adjust to those demands. When an environment is not wheelchair accessible (e.g., a building without ramps, accessible only by stairs), a disability can become a handicap *(Brain 1)*.

Individuals with disabilities and their families interact with a variety of professionals with varied roles and responsibilities. This interdisciplinary team is responsible for the identification and diagnosis of the disability, explaining the results of the evaluation and testing, presenting treatment options, and facilitating intervention and advocacy. The ability to draw on the collective expertise and perspectives of the varied team members is a major advantage of an interdisciplinary team approach. This model is appropriate for treating patients with disabilities, because many patients have multiple problems and issues that go beyond the expertise of any single clinician or discipline. In addition to offering traditional health care services, physicians in an interdisciplinary team must be prepared to expand their usual role in the care of patients with disabilities.

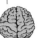
1 - Persons with disorders or disabilities should be described by using person-first terminology. That is, the individual comes before the disability. For instance, one should say "A child with mental retardation," not "A mentally retarded child."

The Physician's Role in the Interdisciplinary Team Approach

In addition to offering traditional health care services, the primary care physician must be prepared to collaborate effectively with professionals from several disciplines (for a description of the interdisciplinary roles and responsibilities of selected disciplines, see *Table 2*). In some cases, the physician will serve as the team leader or case manager because he or she traditionally has had the primary responsibility for diagnosis of the problem or disorder resulting in the disability or prescription of treatment. A second role the physician may play is that of a consultant on the interdisciplinary team.

Traditional Health Care Services

- Provide routine health care maintenance and general medical services with an understanding that patients with disabilities may require more than the usual preventive care and acute illness interventions.
- Conduct a comprehensive medical evaluation and diagnosis of dis-

Table I. Types and Examples of Disabling Conditions

Disability	Defintion
Developmental Disability	
Mental retardation	Significantly subaverage intellectual functioning (IQ < 70–75) existing concurrently with related limitations in two or more of the following adaptive skill areas: communication, self-care, home living, social skills, community use, self-direction, health and safety, functional academics, leisure and work, with onset before age 18
Learning disability	Average or near-average intelligence, yet achievement at unexpectedly low levels in one or more of seven areas: basic reading skills, reading comprehension, oral expression, listening comprehension, written expression, mathematical calculation, and mathematical reasoning
Pervasive developmental disorder	A spectrum of disorders (including autism) characterized by significant impairments in reciprocal social interaction, communication skills, and the presence of stereotyped behavior, interests, and activities. These disorders can range from mild to severe and are usually evident in the first 3 years of life.
Communication disorders	Impairment in understanding and/or transmitting information, including disturbances in speech production, comprehension, spoken and written language, or language-based learning
Physical Disability	
Myelomeningocele	A malformation of the spinal cord, skin, and vertebrae resulting in spinal cord or nerve root dysfunction
Cerebral palsy	A nonprogressive disorder of movement and posture, resulting from injury to the brain during early development
Muscular dystrophy	A group of genetically determined muscle disorders, many of which are progressive and disabling
Traumatic brain injury	Diffuse brain injury resulting from a traumatic event ranging in severity from mild or minor to severe with significant long-term sequelae
Spinal cord injury	Damage to the spinal cord with resulting functional impairment based on the level and completeness of the injury
Sensory Impairment	
Hearing loss	Reduction in the ear's responsiveness to loudness and pitch resulting in auditory impairment, which can range from mild to profound
Vision loss	Problems in any part of the visual apparatus, including the outer layers of the eye, the lens, the retina, the extraocular muscles, and the brain, that result in impairment ranging from mild to complete (blindness)
Mental Disability	
Psychiatric and behavioral disorders	A broad range of disorders that result in impairments in physical functioning, learning, and/or social functioning
Chronic Illness	
Acquired immunodeficiency syndrome (AIDS)	Infection with the human immunodeficiency virus (HIV) resulting in immunodeficiency and subsequent opportunistic infections
Epilepsy	A chronic condition with recurrent seizures that are not provoked by any known event, such as trauma or fever

abling conditions, including the identification of problems that require specific medical treatment or those that have implications for genetic counseling.

- Manage common medical complications associated with specific disabilities (e.g., cardiac, ophthalmologic, endocrine, orthopedic, and hematologic complications in Down syndrome).
- Recommend basic behavioral intervention strategies and psychopharmacotherapy in the treatment of problem behaviors associated with specific disabilities.

Collaboration with Other Disciplines *(Brain 2)*

- Determine the need for evaluations by professionals in other disciplines and make appropriate referrals.

Table 2. Interdisciplinary Roles and Responsibilities of Selected Disciplines

Discipline	Roles and Responsibilities
Audiology	Assess the severity and cause of hearing disorders Make recommendations about habilitative and rehabilitative procedures Determine appropriate amplification instruments
Genetic counseling	Assess genetic nature of disability Provide information regarding genetic disorders Assist with access to services and identification of additional resources Counseling regarding the risks of recurrence of genetic disorders, options for management of disorders, and reproductive alternatives
Medicine	Assess medical and developmental status and coordinate diagnostic work-up of suspected problems Provide primary medical care Recommend care of medical conditions related to diagnosis to prevent secondary disability Provision of a continuum of care involving the coordination of primary medical care and subspecialty services
Nursing	Provide and coordinate primary health services Case coordination Developmental screening Health education and anticipatory guidance Advocacy Counseling
Nutrition	Assess nutritional status Analyze nutritional and fluid adequacy of diet Recommend dietary and feeding interventions to support growth and development
Occupational therapy	Evaluate fine motor development, including manipulative and visuomotor skills Evaluate oromotor status related to feeding Address positioning, handling, adaptations, and compensatory strategies to decrease impact of disability and promote development Recommend and monitor fit and function of upper extremity orthoses
Physical therapy	Evaluate gross motor development Recommend positioning and handling to decrease impact of disability and promote development Prescribe manual techniques and physical agents (e.g., heat, cold, electrical stimulation, whirlpools) to relieve pain Recommend and monitor fit and function of adaptive equipment and lower extremity orthoses
Psychology	Conduct a cognitive evaluation Conduct a behavioral assessment Assess the psychologic and emotional factors involved in, and consequent to, physical disorders and disability Train parents and teachers in behavioral management Assist patients to develop personal or social skills, enhance their environmental coping skills, improve their adaptability to changing life demands, and develop problem-solving and decision-making capabilities Provide individual therapies for selective problems
Recreation therapy	Provide therapeutic recreation programs and services that assist patients in eliminating barriers to leisure, developing leisure skills and attitudes, and optimizing leisure involvement
Social work	Assess environmental variables impacting patient and patient–family resources Advocacy Provide family support and counseling Assist patients and families with resource identification and access
Speech-language pathology	Evaluate speech quality and oromotor status related to speech production Evaluate language development and communication intent Recommend, implement, and monitor interventions to improve overall communication strategies
Special education	Evaluate strengths and weaknesses Work with students, parents, and other professionals to develop the IEP and monitor its effectiveness Work with regular education teachers to integrate special education students in programs and activities with nondisabled students

- Understand and interpret the results of the evaluations by other professionals and effectively
incorporate these evaluations in the decision-making process. The contributions of the various
disciplines are not viewed in parallel; rather they are meshed into a shared vision of the whole.
- When indicated, serve as the team leader, which involves coordinating the duties of the different team members and acting as liasion with the patient, family, and other professionals.
- Maintain a central record and database containing all pertinent information about the patient.

2 - Each interdisciplinary team usually has a case manager that is responsible for coordinating services and ensuring communication among all team members. The physician should participate in, and consult with, team members throughout the evaluation and treatment planning process and offer continuing medical services that are included in the treatment plan.

Issues Facing Patients with Disabilities and Their Families throughout the Life Span

The primary care physician is in a unique position to assist and support patients with disabilities and their families as they deal with a broad range of issues across the life span *(Definition 1)*. It is important for the physician to maintain a free flow of information with the patient and family; facilitate communication between the patient, family, and all service providers; and assist in the development of policies and programs to meet the diverse needs of the patient and families. In addition, the physician must recognize and respect individual and family differences stemming from diverse racial, cultural, and economic backgrounds. In the context of providing comprehensive care to a patient and family over time, the primary care physician may be asked or find it relevant to address some of the following issues:

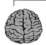

1 - Family-centered approach:
Physician–patient interaction in which the physician recognizes that the family is the only consistent part of the patient's team, whereas other service providers change. Family members act as partners with their health care providers.

- Acceptance of and adaptation to a disability
- Impact of a disability on family and friends
- Transition from childhood activities to adulthood
- Transition from educational programs (e.g., public school, vocational training) to work options (e.g., competitive employment, supported employment, volunteer work, day treatment programs, and sheltered workshops)
- Transition from pediatric to adult health care
- Home care versus community living (e.g., residential facilities, intermediate care facilities, community homes or alternate living units [ALUs], or independent living)
- Ethical issues (e.g., withholding treatment, organ donation, sexual and reproductive rights, and risks and benefits of genetic testing)
- Legal issues (e.g., competence in decision-making, wills, voting, criminal prosecution, and consent and legal guardianship)
- Funding for services and equipment
- Empowerment in care planning
- Identification of available and appropriate services and resources
- Access to recreation and leisure activities
- Sexuality and marriage
- Behavioral and emotional problems

Federal Mandates and Programs

The advocacy and protection of the needs and rights of patients with disabilities is an important function of health care providers. Primary care

Table 3. Landmark Legislation and Federal Assistance Programs for Individuals with Disabilities

Legislative Act or Federal Assistance Program	Provisions
Title V Social Security Act of 1935	Authorized federal funds to states to extend and improve maternal and child health services and services to "crippled children." Renamed the Children with Special Health Care Needs (CSHCN) Program in 1985.
Rehabilitation Act of 1973— PL 93-112	Mandated federal funds to provide a comprehensive plan for providing rehabilitation services to all individuals regardless of the severity of their disability. Section 504 of the Act prohibits discrimination on the basis of disability and implies that children with special needs are entitled to appropriate modifications within their regular or special educational program.
Education for All Handicapped Children Act—PL 94-142 (1975)	An "educational bill of rights" requiring that an evaluation, a free and appropriate public education in the least restrictive environment, a written individualized educational program (IEP)*, related services, parental participation, and due process be provided for all handicapped children, ages 5–18 years. The age range was extended to include children aged 3–21 years in 1977.
Education of Handicapped Children Act Amendments— PL 99-457 (1986)	Part H extends services to infants and toddlers with disabilities (birth through age 3 years) and their families through coordinated, interdisciplinary, interagency early intervention programs, including the development of an Individualized Family Service Plan (IFSP).†
Individuals with Disabilities Education Act (IDEA)— PL 101-476 (1990)	Reauthorization and expansion of the Education of Handicapped Children Act.
Americans with Disabilities Act (ADA)— PL 101-336 (1990)	Comprehensive civil rights legislation created to help integrate individuals with disabilities into every segment of society. It prohibits discrimination and requires accessibility and accommodation.
Supplemental Security Income (SSI)	Provides cash benefits to individuals who meet the Social Security Administration's (SSA) medical definition of disability and financial eligibility requirements. This program also provides a linkage to the Medicaid program for adults and children with disabilities.
Medicaid	Federally mandated public health program, including recipients of SSI, providing access to a range of medical services, ancillary therapies, home care, mental health services, case management, and transportation to medical services.

* An IEP is a written service plan for children aged 3 to 21 years providing information regarding the child's present level of performance, annual goals, short-term objectives, related services being provided, percentage of time the student spends in general education, and beginning and ending dates for special education services. The IEP must be updated on a yearly basis.
† The IFSP is similar to the IEP but for children aged birth through 2 years and focuses on the family. The IFSP is required to be developed by a interdisciplinary team that includes the child's parents.

providers should be familiar with landmark legislation defining services for individuals with disabilities as well as available federal assistance programs in order to assist their patients in advocating effectively for necessary medical, educational, and other services *(Table 3)*.

The Americans with Disabilities Act (ADA) outlines specific guidelines regarding the medical rights and protections for individuals with disabilities. An employer cannot require any medical tests, ask employees about medical or worker's compensation history, or ask general questions about an applicant's health until after the individual has been offered the job or promotion. Medical examinations after hiring are allowed only if they are required for all employees in comparable positions. The results of these medical tests cannot be used to retract an offer unless the employee is unqualified. In addition, individuals with disabilities must be offered medical insurance similar to that of other employees.

Selected Readings

1. Batshaw ML: Your Child Has a Disability. Baltimore, Paul H. Brookes, 1991.

2. Committee on Children with Disabilities: Pediatrician's role in the development and implementation of an Individual Education Plan (IEP) and/or an Individual Family Service Plan (IFSP). Pediatrics 80:340–342, 1992.
3. Rubin IL, Crocker AC: Developmental Disabilities: Delivery of Medical Care for Children and Adults. Philadelphia, Lea & Febiger, 1989.
4. Wallace HM, Biehl RF, MacQueen JC, Blackman JA: Mosby's Resource Guide to Chidlren with Disabilities and Chronic Illness. St. Louis, Mosby, 1997.

Web Sites

Advocates for Disabled Citizens (ADC): http://www.ald.net/adc/. Offers links to Web sites that address rights, needs, entertainment, recreation, and support for individuals with disabilities.

National Organization on Disability (NOD): http://www.nod.org/. Offers a wide array of topics and discussions related to individuals with disabilities.

50. The Prenatal Visit

Laeth Nasir, MBBS

Synopsis

Regularly scheduled visits focus on the progress of pregnancy, allow the physician to offer anticipatory guidance, monitor fetal growth, and detect abnormalities in a timely fashion. Regular prenatal visits also build rapport between the physician and the patient and allow the physician to detect and attempt to ameliorate adverse social or economic factors that might affect the pregnancy or postnatal course. Following an initial comprehensive visit, the patient with an otherwise uncomplicated pregnancy is seen monthly until the third **trimester** *(Definition 1)*, biweekly until 36 weeks, and weekly until delivery. Early in the pregnancy, the emphasis is on avoidance of toxins and teratogens as well as identifying risks for genetic abnormalities. Later, the physician's primary task is to monitor fetal growth and the early diagnosis of pathologic conditions specific to pregnancy.

1 - Trimester: Pregnancy is traditionally divided into these three parts, called trimesters. The first trimester is the period from the last menstrual period to 12 weeks of gestation, the second trimester runs from 13 to 28 weeks, and the third from 29 to 40 weeks.

Preconception or Periconceptual Care

Ideally, prenatal care begins before conception. Because most pregnancies are unplanned, the physician should discuss adequate and appropriate nutrition as well as avoidance of toxins and teratogens with all women of reproductive age. Particular demographic, social, and individual circumstances are risk factors for certain disorders and should be elicited by the physician in the preconceptual period in order to take full advantage of available primary prevention strategies. For the same reason, special attention should be given to ensuring updated vaccination status and elicitation of a family history of genetic disorders in this population of patients.

Initial Visit

History

- "When was your last menstrual period?" Obtaining accurate pregnancy dating is critical for later management decisions and timing of the delivery. The length of pregnancy is approximately 280 days from the first day of the last menstrual period in women who have a regular 28-day cycle.
- "Are you aware of any inheritable or genetic problems or illnesses that run in your family?" (e.g., Down syndrome, hemophilia, sickle cell disease, mental retardation). Patients may need to research the question with relatives.
- "Tell me about your overall health." *(Brain 1)*

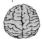

1 - Conditions such as diabetes, hypertension, and heart disease may significantly complicate the course of a pregnancy or require specialty referral for optimum management of the pregnancy. A history of surgery, particularly in the abdomen or pelvis, may have a bearing on the outcome of the pregnancy. A history of sexually transmitted disease or blood transfusions may put the patient at higher risk for infections such as hepatitis B or HIV.

- "Can you tell me about your previous pregnancies?" Ask about number, timing, type of delivery, difficulties or complications, miscarriages, and abortions.
- "What medicines do you take? Do you smoke or drink?" *(Red Flag 1)*
- "Where do you work? What jobs have you had in the past? Do you plan to change jobs in the future?" Certain occupations are associated with exposure to teratogens or increased risk of adverse outcomes such as preterm birth. Assess economic status and refer needy patients to federally sponsored nutrition and support programs such as WIC (Women, Infants, and Children).
- "Tell me about your diet." *(Brain 2)*
- "How is your husband [or partner] going to respond to the pregnancy?" Intimate partner abuse often begins during pregnancy. Identifying relationships at risk helps to ensure the safety of the patient and family (see Chapter 46).
- "Are you planning to breast-feed?" Educating women and their partners about the clear benefits of breast-feeding for the infant is important.
- "What else do I need to know about you or your pregnancy?"

Physical Examination

At the initial visit, current height and weight and an actual or estimated prepregnancy weight should be recorded. A complete physical examination and a pelvic examination should be performed. The pelvic examination should focus on the size of the uterus and abnormalities of the cervix or genitalia. **Clinical pelvimetry** *(Definition 2)* should be carried out.

Testing

Basic laboratory tests are performed routinely on the initial visit. These include:

- Hemoglobin and hematocrit. Screen for anemia and other hematologic conditions.
- Blood type, Rh factor and **irregular antibody** screening *(Definition 3)*
- Tests for hepatitis B, syphilis, and rubella. All can be transmitted to the fetus during pregnancy. Syphilis and rubella may result in fetal brain damage and congenital anomalies.
- HIV if the mother is in a high-risk category (see Chapter 40).
- Cervical cultures for gonorrhea and chlamydia, relatively common STDs that often result in inflammation of the genitourinary tract and can cause a number of complications, including preterm labor. Gonorrhea and chlamydia also can be transmitted to the neonate during delivery.
- Dipstick urinalysis for blood, protein, leukocytes, and glucose should be performed at the first visit and in all subsequent visits. Abnormalities may be the first or only manifestation of urinary tract infection, diabetes, or preeclampsia.
- Triple screen (serum alpha-fetoprotein, human chorionic gonadotrophin, and estriol) is offered to patients between the 15th and 20th weeks of gestation to screen for neural tube defects and Down syndrome.
- Other studies may be indicated depending on the past medical history or demographic factors.

1 - A complete medication history, including all prescribed and over-the-counter medication and herb and vitamin intake, should be elicited from all patients. The use of alcohol, tobacco, and illicit substances are the most important preventable causes of adverse pregnancy outcome in the United States. Intrauterine growth retardation, fetal alcohol syndrome, perinatal death, and a host of other adverse outcomes are associated with the use of these substances. The physician should actively and carefully screen all pregnant patients for the use of these substances, deliver an unequivocal message to quit to users, and help to provide the support necessary for women to stop the use of these substances.

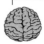

2 - Identifying patients with unusual or suboptimal diets is important to ensure good pregnancy outcomes. Multivitamin supplementation may be useful for all patients. It has been demonstrated that folic acid supplementation in the periconceptual period significantly reduces the incidence of neural tube defects. Therefore, in the United States, all potentially fertile women at average risk are recommended to take 0.4 mg of folate as a daily supplement. Because the average American diet is relatively poor in iron, it is recommended that pregnant women receive 30 mg of ferrous iron as a supplement daily.

2 - Clinical pelvimetry: A clinical estimate of the dimensions of the bony pelvis. Based on the findings, a judgment is made whether or not the pelvis is adequate to allow passage of the fetus during delivery.

3 - Irregular antibodies: Antibodies in maternal blood having the potential to cause fetal harm in a similar manner. A mismatch in blood types between mother and baby can cause the mother's immune system to attack the baby's blood, resulting in anemia or even death of the fetus.

Subsequent Visits

History

- "Have there been any problems since the last visit?" Be on the alert for symptoms suggesting underlying problems such as ectopic pregnancy, miscarriage, or preterm labor. These symptoms include:
    - Unusual back or abdominal pain, pelvic pressure
    - Intermittent abdominal cramping
    - Increase or change in vaginal discharge (may represent infection or leakage of amniotic fluid)
    - Vaginal bleeding. Early in pregnancy may may be due to miscarriage, ectopic pregnancy, or **hydatiform mole (Definition 4)**. Bleeding later in pregnancy may indicate placental abruption or placenta previa.
- "Have you had any headaches, excessive puffiness of the hands and face, visual changes, abdominal pain, or seizures?" **(Red Flag 2)**
- "Are you feeling the baby move?" **(Brain 3)**

Physical Examination

- Blood pressure and weight are important screens for preeclampsia and assessing nutritional status.
- Uterine size **(Brain 4)**
- Fetal heart rate. This is typically between 120 and 160 beats per minute and is an important sign of fetal well being.
- Leopold's maneuvers to determine the position of the baby and estimate fetal weight (done toward the end of pregnancy) **(Brain 5)**

Testing

- Dipstick urine for protein, leukocytes, bacteria, and glucose (see above)
- Ultrasonography to confirm gestational age, detect multiple pregnancy, and screen for structural abnormalities in the fetus
- Glucola test to assess pregnancy-induced gestational diabetes. Unrecognized diabetes can lead to significant problems including fetal macrosomia (abnormally large baby) and birth injuries.
- Group B *Streptococcus* (GBS) culture **(Brain 6)**

Counseling

Patients frequently have questions about certain routine activities and their effects on pregnancy.

- **Exercise:** Moderate levels of physical activity are generally well tolerated by pregnant women with low-risk pregnancies. It is recommended that pregnant women keep their heart rates below 140 beats per minute. Heavy lifting, prolonged standing, and work on industrial machines may be associated with poor pregnancy outcomes and should be avoided or modified.
- **Travel:** Pregnant women should avoid prolonged sitting because of the risk of venous thromboembolism. While traveling, women should ensure that they can increase the venous return in their legs by walking around for 10 minutes or so every 2 hours. In addition, preg-

4 - Hydatidiform mole: Proliferation of abnormal pregnancy-associated trophoblastic tissue. This frequently presents with abnormal vaginal bleeding and a uterus that is larger than expected at that stage of pregnancy. Most often this condition is cured by evacuation of the uterus through dilatation and curettage, but sometimes hysterectomy and chemotherapy are required.

2 - Preeclampsia, a pathologic condition specific to pregnancy, is typically asymptomatic in its early stages, but can present with excessive edema (particularly of the hands and face) headaches, visual changes, abdominal pain, and, in late stages, seizures. It manifests with hypertension, proteinuria, and edema. Early detection of this dangerous condition requires a high index of suspicion and appropriate testing because it is the #1 cause of peripartum and maternal mortality.

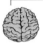

3 - Primiparous patients usually begin to feel fetal movement at about 18 weeks of gestation. Multiparous patients are usually able to appreciate movement about 2 weeks earlier. Patients should be counseled to obtain prompt medical advice if they stop feeling fetal movement or if there is a clear reduction in fetal movement from baseline levels.

4 - Monitoring the increase in uterine size is important to document adequate fetal growth. At about 12 weeks of gestation, the uterine fundus typically becomes palpable above the pelvic brim. At 16 weeks, the fundus is approximately halfway between the pelvic brim and the umbilicus, and at 20 weeks, it is at the level of the umbilicus. Between 20 and 30 weeks of gestation, the height of the uterine fundus, measured from the pelvic brim in centimeters, is approximately equal to the gestational age in weeks.

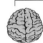

5 - This information allows the physician to make decisions on the route and timing of delivery. Leopold's maneuvers consist of 4 elements:
1. The uterine fundus is palpated to establish the presence of a fetal pole (head or breech). Absence of either suggests an oblique or transverse fetal lie.
2. The examiner palpates the sides of the uterus to determine the position of the fetal back.
3. The hands are placed just above the symphysis pubis and brought together to palpate the lower fetal pole.
4. The occipital protuberance is palpated to determine the position of the fetal head.

nant women who travel long distances should take a copy of their medical record in case of emergency.

- **Seat belt use:** Pregnant women should be advised to fasten their lap belts low across their pelvis rather than over their abdomen. This will reduce the amount of force transmitted to the fetus during an accident.
- **Sexual activity:** In women with an average-risk pregnancy, no restrictions are placed on sexual activity.
- **Weight gain:** Women with normal prepregnancy weight are expected to gain between 25 and 35 pounds during pregnancy. Underweight women may gain up to 40 pounds, and overweight women should limit weight gain to 15–25 pounds.

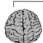

6 - GBS or *Streptococcus agalactiae* bacteria colonize the lower anogenital tract of many women. It is a leading cause of neonatal infections such as meningitis and septicemia. Neonates are exposed to the bacterium during the process of birth. Antepartum screening for carriage of this bacterium may be accomplished through vaginal and anorectal culture close to delivery. If the patient is found to be a carrier, intrapartum antibiotics may be administered to reduce the incidence of neonatal infection.

Selected Readings

1. Campos-Outcalt D: Twenty Common Problems in Preventive Health Care. New York, McGraw-Hill, 2000.
2. Fender G, Holland C: Key developments in women's health. Practitioner 245:258, 261–264, 2001.
3. Gabbe SG, Niebyl JR, Simpson JL: Obstetrics: Normal and Problem Pregnancies, 3rd ed. New York, Churchill Livingstone, 1996.
4. Nolan M: The influence of antenatal classes on pain relief in labour: A review of the literature. Pract Midwife 3:23–26, 2000.
5. Todd SJ, LaSala KB, Neil-Urban S: An integrated approach to prenatal smoking cessation interviews. Am J Matern Child Nurs 26:185–190, 2001.

51. Preoperative Evaluation

Paul M. Paulman, MD • Audrey Paulman, MD

Synopsis

The preoperative evaluation consists of a complete history, physical examination, and appropriate laboratory and x-ray evaluations to determine whether the patient can tolerate the planned anesthesia and operation. The other purposes of the preoperative evaluation are to detect medical conditions that may complicate the patient's operation and to determine if there are other problems that could be treated during the operation (e.g., a patient having a planned cesarean section could also undergo a tubal ligation).

Overview

If potential issues are detected during the operative evaluation, steps can be taken to correct or alter these problems for the benefit of the patient. The trend in pre- and postoperative care is toward shorter hospital stays and more care provided in the clinic and the patient's home. Therefore, it is important to include an assessment of your patient's home support system (family, friends, home medical services) during the preoperative evaluation.

If significant problems are detected, the planned anesthesia regimen or surgical procedure may be altered, delayed, or canceled. The degree of risk to the patient from anesthesia and the surgical procedure can be determined by using a variety of risk-stratification instruments. These instruments predict the risk of problems from anesthesia and surgery based on the patient's history, physical exam, laboratory findings, type of planned anesthesia, and planned operation. The basic types of anesthesia include blocking of nerve conduction (e.g., local blocks, field blocks, spinal and epidural blocks) and anesthetic techniques that produce altered states of consciousness (e.g., "general" anesthesia, "twilight sleep"). Each type of anesthesia has its own set of benefits and risks. The anesthesiologist will choose the anesthetic technique that best serves the patient's condition, planned operation, and the patient's need for pain control.

Table 1 shows one risk assessment instrument. As the class number increases, the patient's risk of anesthetic or operative complications increases.

As a student preceptee, you may be asked to assist with the preoperative evaluation for your preceptor's patients by performing the preoperative history and physical examination. Different clinical conditions demand different levels of preoperative evaluation and management, but regardless of the surgery scheduled, you should plan on completing a thorough history and physical examination.

Symptoms and physical findings may or may not be significant in the preoperative evaluation depending on the severity of the underlying condition, the temporal factors relating to the underlying condition, and the type of anesthesia and operation planned.

History

Here are some guidelines for your preoperative history. Other questions may need to be asked depending on the patient's clinical condition, operation, and the anesthesia planned.

Table I. American Society of Anesthesiologists Anesthetic Risk Classification	
Classification	**Description**
Class I	Patients younger than 80 years of age having no medical or psychiatric disturbance. The abnormal condition requiring surgery is limited, and there is no systemic disease. This patient reports no other illnesses or complaints and has been well (e.g., healthy young female for mole removal).
Class II	Mild to moderate illness caused by the surgical problem or another illness or abnormality (e.g., adults with asthma, patients under one year of age, and elderly patients)
Class III	Severe systemic disease related to the surgical condition or other illness causing disability (e.g., renal failure, stable coronary artery disease, history of myocardial infarction)
Class IV	Severe systemic problems that are life-threatening and not correctable by the surgery (e.g., end-stage renal disease, pulmonary failure, congestive heart failure)
Class V	Morbid patients with a poor chance of survival with or without surgery (e.g., severe head trauma, ruptured aneurysm)
Class VI	Any operation performed as an emergency in a patient who would be in class I–V (e.g., class I patient with incarcerated hernia).

Major Organ System Dysfunction

- "Do you have any nervous system problems (e.g., brain, spinal cord, or nerves)? Do you have seizures?"
- "Do you have any problems with blood clotting?"
- "Do you have easy bruising or bleed excessively when cut?"
- "Do you have any heart or blood vessel disorders?"
- "Do you have chest pain?"
- "Do you have a past history of stroke or high blood pressure?"
- "Have you had a myocardial infarction (heart attack)?"
- "Do you ever experience shortness of breath?"
- "Do you have asthma?"
- "Do you have diabetes?'

Adverse Reactions

- "Have you or anyone in your family ever had problems with anesthetic drugs or latex products, such as allergic reactions or hyperthermia?"
- "Have you or anyone in your family ever had a bad reaction to anesthetic medicines?"
- "Did you have any bad outcomes from previous operations?"
- "What are your allergies?"
- "Are you allergic to latex?" (Symptoms include rash, hives, and difficulty breathing.)

Conditions That May Cause Technical Problems for the Anesthesiologist

- "Have you ever had narrowing of the trachea?" (This could make it difficult for the anesthesiologist to maintain the airway.)
- "Have you ever had any neck surgery?"
- "Have you had any previous lower back surgery? (This could be problematic for delivery of spinal anesthesia.)

Other

- "What medicines do you take, including prescription, over-the-counter, and herbal medicines?" *(Brain 1)*

Condition ⇓	Hemoglobin	WBC	PT/PTT	Platelets	Electrolytes	BUN/Creatinine	Glucose	Liver Profile	Chest X-Ray	Electrocardiogram	Pregnancy Test	Type and Screen	Thyroid Function Tests	Drug Levels
Operation likely to cause bleeding	X											X		
Operation not likely to have bleeding														
Heavy smoker	X								X					
Infants	X													
Women of child bearing age	X													
Over age 50	X						X			X*				
Disease of heart or blood vessels						X			X	X				
Lung disease									X	X				
Liver disease		X	X					X						
Kidney disease	X				X	X								
Diabetes					X	X	X						X	
Thyroid disease													X	
History of Bleeding	X		X	X										
Possible pregnancy											X			
Undergoing cancer therapy	X	X							X	X				
Known cancer	X	X							X					
Seizure meds														X
Taking blood thinners	X		X											
Taking corticosteroids							X							
Taking water pills or diuretics					X	X								
Digoxin					X	X								

*Think about this in men over the age of 40, women over the age of 50.

Figure 1: Usual preoperative screening tests.
(From Paulman A, Paulman P: Perioperative Care. Leawood, KS, American Academy of Family Physicians, 2001, with permission.)

- "Do you have any anxieties or concerns about the planned anesthesia and operation?"
- "What kind of support system do you have following your surgery and during your recovery?" Plan for supportive care during recovery (e.g., post-hip replacement physical therapy).

Physical Examination

Here are some guidelines for your preoperative physical examination. Your history will guide your examination. Look for signs of major system dysfunction.

- **General.** Are the pulse, blood pressure, temperature, and respiration normal? Is the patient alert, oriented, and able to make an informed decision about the operation?
- **Skin.** Is there evidence of bruising, bleeding, or jaundice?
- **Nervous system.** Are there any major neurologic deficits, such as weakness, confusion, or loss of major sensory organ function?
- **Cardiovascular system.** Is there a heart murmur? Is there any evidence of leg and ankle swelling?
- **Respiratory system.** Is the patient short of breath? Are there abnormal lung sounds (e.g., wheezes, rhonchi, rales)?
- **Gastrointestinal system.** Are there any abdominal masses? Is the liver normal size? Is ascites present?

Neither the history nor examination list here should be considered complete or exhaustive for all conditions. The history, examination, and testing needs will vary depending on the clinical situation.

Testing

Your patient may require laboratory and radiographic evaluations depending on the planned anesthetic, operation, and the patient's medical condition *(Figure 1)*. Most preoperative evaluations will include one or more visits by your patient to the anesthesiologist and surgeon.

Another key area of the preoperative evaluation is patient counseling and education. If you know about an upcoming operation for one of your preceptor's patients, do some background reading about the medical condition, the planned anesthesia and operation, and the potential postoperative course and complications. Be sure to communicate with the patient's family and caregiver and defer any questions you can't answer to your preceptor *(Brain 2)*.

Selected Reading

Paulman A, Paulman P: Perioperative Care: Home Study Self-Assessment Program Monograph Edition 263. Leawood, KS, American Academy of Family Physicians, 2001.

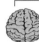

1 - Aspirin is found in numerous prescription and over-the-counter medications and can cause bleeding due to platelet dysfunction up to 10 days (sometimes longer) following ingestion. Be sure to ask your patient specifically about any aspirin-containing products, including pain relievers and cough and cold remedies. Aspirin and other nonsteroidal anti-inflammatory drugs (NSAIDs), including ibuprofen and naprosyn, can cause gastrointestinal bleeding in the postoperative period. Be sure to note the patient's use of any NSAIDs when you write your preoperative evaluation.

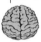

2 - Most surgeons are glad to have you observe or participate in your patient's operation and postoperative care. Contact the surgeon's office prior to the planned procedure and ask permission to participate in or observe your patient's operation. The surgeon's staff or the operating facility staff can help you with logistical questions (e.g., When is the operation? Where do I go? Where do I get surgical scrub clothes?).

52. Pressure Ulcers

Alexandra F. Suslow, MD • Jane F. Potter, MD

Synopsis

Pressure ulcers (PUs) are the result of pressure for a sufficient time to produce tissue injury. Unrelieved pressure for as little as 2 hours can damage skin because of inadequate perfusion. PUs are most often seen in immobilized, seriously ill, and disabled patients. They are not only a major source of morbidity for patients, but also are costly to the healthcare system and carry a high mortality rate.

Pressure ulcers often can be prevented. Although some of the factors associated with the development of PUs are preventable, suboptimal care is not always to blame every time a PU develops. The history and physical examination should focus not only on the presence of PUs, but also on general factors contributing to the problem, so that both a curative and a preventive plan of treatment can be developed. Therefore, a basic knowledge of the risk factors and the ability to correctly stage (classify) the depth of a PU are of the utmost importance for any clinician *(Table 1)*.

Careful documentation of the lesion(s) with serial measurements and, whenever possible, photographic records is extremely important. This documentation provides a basis for the development of an initial plan and serves as a point of reference for later management.

Differential Diagnosis

- True PUs
- **Venous stasis ulcers *(Definition 1)***
- **Ischemic foot ulcers *(Definition 2)***
- Infected traumatic skin lesions (e.g., skin tear)
- **Neuropathic ulcers *(Definition 3)***

History

Usually the best source of information will be the patient him- or herself. The history-taker is strongly encouraged to attempt to obtain the history from the patient whenever possible and obtain additional information from caregivers to fill in gaps. If a patient's condition is such that obtaining a direct history is not possible, the caregiver(s) may act as primary historian. Questions that can be helpful in obtaining a good history regarding PUs are:

"Tell me about your ability to move around." This information helps to identify those at high risk for developing pressure ulcers. Ask about:

1 - Venous stasis ulcers: Cutaneous ulcers in the area of drainage of a vein with sluggish blood flow. These ulcers are usually located on the medial aspect of the legs (very seldom on the foot) and tend to be accompanied by moderate-to-severe edema of the leg and pigmentation of the surrounding tissue. They tend to be small, superficial, with irregular margins and exudate covering the floor of the ulcer. They are easily movable with the skin and tend to be fairly tender.

2 - Ischemic foot ulcers: Cutaneous ulcers caused by minor trauma in patients in the advanced stages of peripheral arteriosclerosis. These ulcers tend to occur on areas most susceptible to trauma (e.g., the toes, heels, malleoli, and around the first and fifth metatarsals). Nondependent edema is usually minimal, pigmentation is absent, and the surrounding skin tends to be athrophic, fragile, shiny, and hairless. These ulcers tend to be deep, covered with necrotic tissue, and extremely painful.

3 - Neuropathic ulcers: Ulcers in diabetic patients who have developed neuropathy in their lower extremities. Because of reduced sensitivity to pain, minor skin irritations or minor trauma to the feet can develop into more serious wounds.

Table I. Classification of Pressure Ulcers

Stage	Description
Stage I	Erythema (blanchable or nonblanchable) of the intact skin
Stage II	Partial thickness or superficial skin loss involving epidermis or dermis. Ulcer presents as abrasion, blister, or shallow crater.
Stage III	Dermal involvement. Full-thickness skin loss with damage or necrosis to, but not through, underlying fascia.
Stage IV	Involvement of deep subcutaneous tissue. Full-thickness skin loss with extensive destruction, tissue necrosis, or damage to muscle, bone, or supporting structures. Undermining and sinus tracts may be present.

Adapted from Leigh IH, Bennett G. Pressure ulcers: prevalence, etiology, and treatment modalities, a review. Am J Surg 167:25S–30S, 1994.

- Ability to ambulate and transfer independently
- Ability to shift positions or maintain position
- Ability to sense when positional change is needed

" Do you have problems with loss of bladder or bowel function? Can you feel when you are soiled?"

- Incontinence
- Loss of sensation

Ask the collateral source or caregiver(s) " Does the patient have problems with memory?"

- Ability to communicate needs to caregiver
- Ability to cooperate with care
- Mental status changes
    Acute (medication, delirium)
    Chronic (stroke, Alzheimer's disease)

"Tell me about your past medical history."

- Medications currently used (neurologic agents, steroids and use of home remedies in the early stages of the lesion
- Exposure to known allergens or new chemical agents
- Falls, especially if the patient was lying down for a prolonged period of time
- Systemic diseases (diabetes, cancer, renal failure, autoimmune diseases)

" How did the sore (lesion) start? How long has it been there? Have you noticed any changes?"

- Traumatic injury
- Duration of the ulcer

"How are you doing overall?" *(Red Flag 1)*

- Weight loss
- Fevers or chills
- Pain in joints or around pressure points

"Have you noticed any changes on your skin?"

- Areas of discoloration
- Nonblanching areas of redness

1 - These questions are geared toward patients in whom a PU has been identified (regardless of stage) and are intended to elicit symptoms that point to more severe complications, such as sepsis or osteomyelitis.

- Dusky coloration to skin
- Any sores or blisters

Physical Examination

- General factors:
  Mental status
  Involuntary movements
  General health appearance
- Vital signs, including a recent weight (within 2 weeks)
- Visual inspection of the entire skin, with special emphasis on the bony prominences (sacrum, greater trochanters, heels, ischial tuberosities, lateral malleoli, and occipital area) *(Figure 1)*. Special attention should be paid to erythematous and dusky-colored areas of skin.
- Assessment of cardiovascular status emphasizing peripheral pulses, skin turgor, and capillary refill time in the extremities
- Complete neurologic exam, including mental status, pain perception, strength in the extremities, ability to independently reposition in bed and while sitting, and sensory integrity (light touch, pain, and vibration)
- If a PU is already present:
  1. Document locations, number of lesions, size and stage of each lesion and whether extension to deep underlying tissue can be seen (see Table 1).
  2. Notice the presence of blisters, **bullae,** or **eschars *(Definition 4)*.** An eschar may hide deep tissue injury.
  3. Look for the granulation of tissue (which is a sign of healthy healing tissue) and at the condition of surrounding skin.
  4. Examine for evidence of infection *(Red Flag 2)*.

Testing

- Complete blood count (CBC) and differential to assess for the presence of anemia and infection
- Complete metabolic profile including electrolytes, serum protein, albumin, and cholesterol levels to detect the presence of electrolyte imbalances and the presence of malnutrition
- If the patient has a cognitive status change and a history of previously intact mental status, neuroimaging may be indicated.
- Other imaging studies include a bone scan if there is suspicion of **osteomyelitis *(Definition 5)*.** If the bone scan is positive, a bone biopsy (the gold standard for the diagnosis of osteomyelitis) is highly recommended.
- Wound cultures are not recommended, because PUs are always colonized (often with multiple organisms) and the results of these tests will not contribute to the treatment of the lesion.

Putting It All Together

The history from the patient or someone who knows the patient and examination that shows the typical changes of skin injury over bony

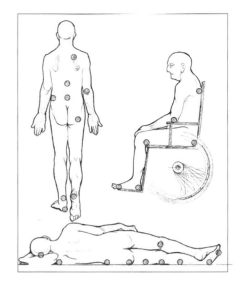

Figure 1: Common locations of pressure ulcers.
(From Williams ME: The American Geriatrics Society's Complete Guide to Aging and Health. New York, Harmon Books, 1995, with permission.)

4 - Bulla: Large vesicle appearing as a circumscribed area of separation of epidermis from subepidermal structures, caused by the presence of serum, sometimes mixed with blood.
Eschar: Thick, leathery, necrotic, devitalized tissue.

2 - Odor, purulent drainage, erythema of surrounding skin, fever, joint pain, or erythema in adjacent joints may point to sepsis or osteomyelitis.

5 - Osteomyelitis: Infection of bone marrow and adjacent bone often accompanied by severe destruction of the bone tissue. This condition carries a high rate of mortality, and treatment often involves surgical debridement of the area and prolonged antibiotic treatment.

prominences are sufficient to make the diagnosis of PU. This history and examination also will reveal the risk factors for the problem and suggest remedies.

The first order of management both for preventive and for curative therapies is to relieve the pressure without exerting pressure over other bony prominences. In both cases, it is also important to address the involved risk factors, including nutrition and the cause for decreased mobility. Management may be as diverse as treatment of arthritis with medications and physical therapy or treatment of Parkinson's disease.

Management

Management of PUs begins with prevention. Patients of any age who are immobilized are at high risk. Elderly persons tend to have higher incidence of incontinence (see Chapter 63), malnutrition, decreased mobility, and increased skin fragility. Be on the alert for early signs of problems, including:

- Areas of nonblanching erythema especially at pressure points (blanching may indicate a potential problem; nonblanching indicates a PU)
- Areas of dusky discoloration of the skin
- Soft boggy heels or elbows
- Urinary or fecal incontinence

The best way to prevent PUs involves:

- Pressure-relief measures (turning every 2 hours)
- Prevention of shearing (prevent sliding)
- Prevention of friction injuries (appropiate transfer techniques)
- Prevention of skin **maceration** *(Definition 6)*

6 - Maceration: Excessive softening of the skin caused by prolonged exposure to a humid, warm environment, such as occurs with urinary or fecal incontinence.

When PUs develop, curative management involves providing care to the wound as directed by the depth of the lesion. Be careful to detect and manage serious complications, including infections; dehydration, electrolyte imbalances, and anemia; and leg lesions hidden by eschar *(Consultation and Referral 1)*.

1 - It is appropriate to consult a skin care specialist such as an enterostomal nurse-specialist early in the management of the high-risk patient and in the management of ulcers that are refractory to conventional therapy.

Selected Readings

1. Evans JM, Andrews KL, Chutka DS, et al: Pressure ulcers: Prevention and management. Mayo Clinic Proc 70:789–799, 1995.
2. Leigh IH, Bennett G: Pressure ulcers: prevalence, etiology, and treatment modalities: A review. Am J Surg 167:25S–30S, 1994.
3. Orlando PL: Pressure ulcer management in the geriatric patient. Ann Pharmacother 32:1221–1227, 1998.
4. Patterson JA, Bennett RG: Prevention and treatment of pressure sores. J Am Geriatr Soc 43:919–927, 1995.
5. Vohra RK, McCollum CN: Pressure sores. Br J Med 309:853–857, 1994.
6. Williams ME: The American Geriatrics Society's Complete Guide to Aging and Health. New York, Harmony Books, 1995.

53. Rashes and Common Skin Problems

Richard P. Usatine, MD

Synopsis

A wide variety of rashes and common skin problems are seen on a daily basis in medical practice. These conditions are caused by infections, sun damage, trauma, inflammatory processes, immunologic disease, other systemic diseases, and diseases of the sebaceous follicle (acne). The recognition and treatment of these conditions can prevent disfigurement and death. Skin cancers are often curable when recognized early. Many skin diseases are predominantly cosmetic conditions, and improving the patient's appearance can have a significant impact on the patient's self-esteem and quality of life.

Differential Diagnosis

Pattern recognition is an essential technique in the diagnosis of skin conditions. The expert clinician is able to make rapid and accurate diagnoses through visual pattern recognition. However, even in dermatology, the history, physical examinations, and laboratory data enhance diagnostic accuracy. To develop your diagnostic skills, it helps to learn the basic patterns of the primary and secondary lesions listed in *Table 1*. This will give you the proper vocabulary and conceptual model to make keen observations and describe what you are seeing.

Although we are taught in medical school to perform the history before doing the physical exam, this is not the most efficient way to approach the diagnosis of a skin condition. When the patient has a skin complaint, look at the skin right away and ask your questions while you are doing so.

Physical Examination

- Look closely at the lesions to characterize the type of primary (basic or initial) lesions and secondary (or sequential) lesions present (see Table 1). A magnifying glass or loupe is helpful to distinguish the morphology of many skin conditions.
- Touch or palpate the lesions unless you believe the condition may be transmissible. If so, as in scabies, put on gloves before touching the skin.
- For some lesions, such as **actinic keratosis *(Definition 1)***, feeling the skin lightly helps you detect the scale. For deeper lesions, such as nodules and cysts, deep palpation is crucial.
- Look at the local distribution of the lesions to determine if the primary lesions are arranged in groups, rings, lines, or merely scattered over the skin. For example, the vesicles of herpes zoster (shingles) are usually grouped together because they follow a sensory nerve, whereas the vesicles of chicken pox are often scattered over the body.
- Determine which parts of the skin are affected and which are spared.

1 - Actinic keratosis: Premalignant superficial scaling skin lesions that have a small risk of becoming squamous cell carcinomas in untreated persons.

Table I. Primary and Secondary Skin Lesions

Type of Lesion	Description
Primary (basic)	
Macule	Circumscribed flat discoloration
Papule	Elevated solid lesion (up to 5 mm)
Plaque	Circumscribed, superficially elevated solid lesion (> 5 mm). Often a confluence of papules.
Nodule	Palpable, solid (round) lesion, deeper than a papule
Wheal (hive)	Pale-red edematous plaque; round or flat-topped and transient
Pustule	Elevated collection of purulence
Vesicle	Circumscribed elevated collection of fluid ($\leq$ 5 mm in diameter)
Bulla	Circumscribed elevated collection of fluid (> 5 mm in diameter)
Secondary (sequential)	
Scale (desquamation)	Excess dead epidermal cells
Crusts	A collection of dried serum, blood, or purulence
Erosion	Superficial loss of epidermis
Ulcer	Focal loss of epidermis and dermis
Fissure	Linear loss of epidermis and dermis
Atrophy	Depression in the skin from thinning of epidermis and/or dermis
Excoriation	Erosion caused by scratching
Lichenification	Thickened epidermis with prominent skin lines (induced by scratching)

- Look at the remainder of the skin, nails, hair, and mucous membranes for more clues. Think of yourself as a detective collecting clues. For example, look for nail pitting when considering a diagnosis of psoriasis.
- Don't be shy to ask patients to remove their shoes and clothing to show you areas of the body that are needed to make an accurate diagnosis.
- Complete skin exam for cancer detection:
  1. Look at the skin from head to toe. Skin cancer can occur at any site.
  2. Focus on the highest risk areas for skin cancer: the face, neck, back, and arms (areas that receive the most sun exposure).
  3. Patients at highest risk for skin cancer (fair skin, blond or red hair, blue eyes, or a family history of skin cancer) should get a complete skin exam regularly or yearly.
  4. Previous skin cancer or significant evidence of sun damage (erythema, mottled hyperpigmentation, wrinkling, scaling) increases the risk of skin cancer significantly.
  5. Use a systematic approach. Start with the head, looking at the face, ears, and scalp. To protect the patient's privacy and modesty, you may have the patient show you one segment of the body at a time with the gown on, rather than asking the patient to stand or sit stark naked in front of you. Don't forget to look in the axillae, under the breasts, between the buttocks, and on the soles of the feet. Even though these areas receive little sun, melanoma can occur in these regions. This is a good time to discuss sun exposure, protective clothing, and use of sunscreens.

History

Once you have started to look at the skin, your history will be become more focused. The following historical data can often help you make the diagnosis:

- Onset and duration of skin lesions: continuous or intermittent?
- Pattern of eruption: Where did it start? How has it changed?
- Any known precipitants: exposures to medications (prescription and over the counter), foods, plants, sun, topical agents, cosmetics, chemicals (occupation and hobbies)?
- Skin symptoms: itching, pain, paresthesia?
- Systemic symptoms: fever, chills, night sweats, fatigue, weakness, weight loss?
- Underlying illnesses: diabetes, HIV?
- Family history of acne, atopic dermatitis, psoriasis, skin cancers, dysplastic nevi (atypical moles that may indicate a higher risk for melanoma)?

Testing

Laboratory tests may be used to confirm or rule out a clinical diagnosis that was based on history and physical exam. The most important laboratory tests for the skin are:

- **Microscopy.** When considering a diagnosis of a fungal infection, it is helpful to scrape some of the scale onto a microscope slide. By adding 10% potassium hydroxide (KOH) with dimethyl sulfoxide (DMSO), you can look for the hyphae of dermatophytes *(Figure 1)* or the pseudohyphae and yeast forms of *Candida* or *Pityrosporum ovale*.
- **Cultures** may be useful to diagnose bacterial, viral, or fungal infections.
- **Blood tests** such as VDRL, ANA, and HIV titers *(Definition 2)* may be helpful to determine the etiology of unknown skin lesions.
- **Ultraviolet light** (black light) examination to look for fluorescence can be helpful in diagnosing tinea capitus (ringworm) and erythrasma (bacterial infection of the groin and axilla that fluoresces a coral red).
- **Surgical biopsy** can be used as a diagnostic and treatment tool. Having a reasonable differential diagnosis will help you choose the appropriate biopsy type.

Most Common Diagnoses

Dermatitis and Eczema (Rashes)

Dermatitis is a nonspecific term that means inflammation of the skin. Eczema is one type of dermatitis that demonstrates characteristic erythema, scale, or vesicles.

- **Eczema,** the most common type of skin inflammation, can occur in three stages: acute, subacute, and chronic. It is frequently seen on the hands or feet but can occur on any part of the body. Acute eczema may be vesicular and red, whereas subacute eczema lacks the vesicles and has more prominent scaling and cracking of the dry skin. In chronic eczema there is lichenification (thickened plaque with accentuation of the skin lines).
- **Atopic dermatitis** is a type of eczematous eruption that is itchy, recurrent, and symmetrical and often found on flexural surfaces *(Figure 2)*. These patients often have either a personal or family history of asthma, allergic rhinitis, or conjunctivitis. In infancy, atopic der-

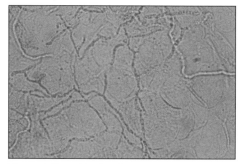

Figure 1: Fungal hyphae in a potassium hydroxide wet mount. The identifying characteristic is the branching, filamentous structure that is uniform in width.
(From Habif T: Clinical Dermatology: A Color Guide to Diagnosis and Therapy, 3rd ed. St. Louis, Mosby, 1996, with permission.)

2 - VDRL (Venereal Disease Research Laboratory): A blood test for syphilis.

ANA (antinuclear antibodies): A blood test for systemic lupus erythematosus and other autoimmune diseases.

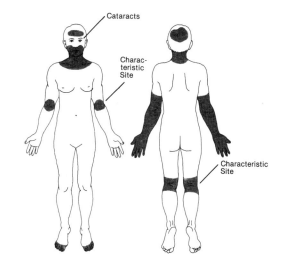

Figure 2: Atopic dermatitis.
(From Fitzpatrick TB, Polano MK, Surmand D: Color Atlas and Synopses of Clinical Dermatology. New York, McGraw-Hill, 1996, with permission.)

matitis often presents on the face. After infancy, the dry, scaling, and red lesions are found in flexural areas such as the antecubital or popliteal fossa.

- **Contact dermatitis** is an allergic response to an allergen such as the chemical found in the poison ivy or poison oak plant (*Rhus* dermatitis). These lesions are often linear and vesicular. Other contact allergens include nickel in jewelry and belt buckles and chemicals in deodorants.

Infestations

Scabies and lice are examples of infestations. Scabies is a rash caused by the *Sarcoptes scabiei* mite. It presents as a papulovesicular rash *(Figure 3)* with itching and it is typically seen on the hands and feet and around the waist, axilla, wrists, and groin. Acquisition of the mite requires skin-to-skin contact with someone previously infected. Typical symptoms include intense itching that is worse at night. The pathognomonic lesion of scabies is the burrow created by the mite crawling under the skin. The presence of a burrow is helpful in making the diagnosis, but its absence does not rule out scabies.

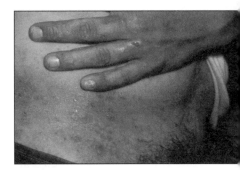

Figure 3: Scabies.
(Photo © Richard P. Usatine, MD.)

Seborrhea

Seborrhea, a superficial inflammatory dermatitis, is a common condition characterized by patches of erythema and scaling. The typical distribution of seborrhea includes the scalp (dandruff), eyebrows, eyelids, nasolabial creases, behind the ears, eyebrows, forehead, cheeks, around the nose, under the beard or mustache, over the sternum, axillae, submammary folds, umbilicus, groin, and the gluteal creases. These areas are regions with a greater number of pilosebaceous units producing **sebum** *(Definition 3)*.

 3 - Sebum: A complex lipid mixture that helps to maintain hydration of the skin.

The etiology of seborrhea is thought to be an inflammatory hypersensitivity to the yeast *Pityrosporum ovale* on the skin. Although this yeast can be a normal inhabitant of the skin, persons with seborrhea appear to respond to its presence with an inflammatory reaction *(Figure 4)*.

Seborrhea is characterized by remissions and exacerbations. The most common precipitating factors are stress, antibiotic use, and cold weather. The treatment of seborrhea should be directed at the inflammation and the *Pityrosporum*.

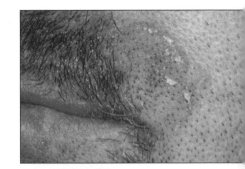

Figure 4: Seborrhea.
(Photo © Richard P. Usatine, MD.)

Psoriasis

Psoriasis is a chronic immunologic condition characterized by epidermal proliferation and inflammation. The lesions are well circumscribed, red, scaling patches, with white, thickened scale *(Figure 5)*. The distribution includes the scalp, nails, extensor surfaces of limbs, elbows, knees, sacral region, and genitalia. Psoriasis lesions may be called *guttate* when shaped like water drops, *inverse* when found in intertriginous areas such as the inguinal and intergluteal folds, or *volar* when found on the palms or soles. Psoriatic nail changes occur in 10–40% of persons with psoriasis. These nail changes include nail pitting, onycholysis (separation of the nail from the nail bed), and keratin debris under the nails.

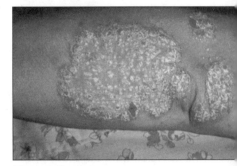

Figure 5: Psoriasis.
(Photo © Richard P. Usatine, MD.)

Bacterial Skin Infections

These are most often caused by *Streptococcus pyogenes* and *Staphylococcus aureus*.

- **Impetigo** is a superficial skin infection that is often characterized by translucent ("honey") crusts. It can be vesicular or bullous. Impetigo in children occurs often around the nose and mouth *(Figure 6)*.
- **Cellulitis** is an acute infection of the skin that involves the dermis and subcutaneous tissues. Cellulitis often begins with a break in the skin caused by trauma, a bite, or athlete's foot. It is most often seen on the legs and arms *(Figure 7)*.
- **Necrotizing fasciitis** ("flesh-eating bacteria") is a deep infection of the subcutaneous tissues and fascia. It often presents with diffuse swelling of the arm or leg, followed by bullae with clear fluid that may become violaceous in color. The patient has marked systemic symptoms *(Red Flag 1)*.
- An **abscess** is a localized collection of pus in a cavity and can occur in many areas of the skin and body. Abscesses that occur in or directly below the skin include furuncles, carbuncles, and the abscesses around fingernails (acute paronychias). A furuncle or boil is an abscess that starts in a hair follicle or sweat gland. A carbuncle occurs when the furuncle extends into the subcutaneous tissue. Incision and drainage is the treatment of choice for all types of abscesses.

Viral Infections

- **Warts** are caused by over 60 subtypes of human papilloma virus. Warts most commonly occur on the hands, feet, and genitals. The appearance of the wart is strongly related to its location. Warts on the hands (verruca vulgaris) are usually raised and hyperkeratotic. Warts on the soles of the feet (plantar warts) are flat, cause disrupted skin lines, and have dark dots visible in them. Flat warts (verruca plana) are usually seen in groups on the face and legs. Genital warts (condyloma acuminata) often have a cauliflower appearance and are transmitted sexually.
- **Herpes simplex virus** (HSV) types 1 and 2 produce vesicular eruptions on the skin with surrounding erythema. The lesions progress to crusts or ulcers before they re-epithelialize. However, the primary episode of HSV 1 can infect the entire mouth (gingivostomatitis) or be asymptomatic. Recurrent episodes of HSV 1 often occur on the lips and are commonly called *cold sores* or *fever blisters (Figure 8)*. Canker sores (aphthous ulcers) are not caused by HSV. HSV 2 is a sexually transmitted disease that can occur on the genitals, anus, buttocks, or in the mouth.

Fungal Infections

Fungal infections of the skin occur at many sites and are most often caused by dermatophytes, *Candida*, or *Pityrosporum* species. The dermatophytes cause tinea infections of the skin, which are commonly called ringworm, although there is no worm in ringworm. The typical dermatophyte infection of the body has an annular (ring-like) appearance with central clearing and redness and scale on the perimeter. Common dermatophyte infections are:

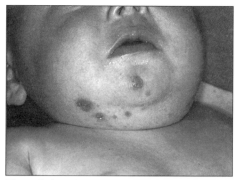
Figure 6: Impetigo.
(Photo © Richard P. Usatine, MD.)

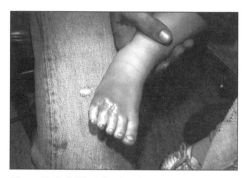
Figure 7: Cellulitis following foot trauma.
(Photo © Richard P. Usatine, MD.)

 1 - Necrotizing fasciitis can lead to cutaneous gangrene, myonecrosis, and shock. It is crucial to recognize necrotizing fasciitis because it is life- and limb-threatening and requires surgical treatment along with intravenous antibiotics. The major tip-off is that the patient looks and feels very sick.

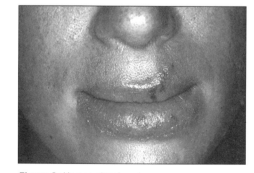
Figure 8: Herpes simplex virus.
(Photo © Richard P. Usatine, MD.)

- **Tinea capitis** (tinea of the head) causes patchy alopecia (hair loss) with broken hairs and some scaling *(Figure 9)*.
- **Tinea corporis** (tinea of the body) can occur on almost any part of the body. Small areas may respond well to topical antifungals *(Figure 10)*.
- **Tinea cruris** (tinea of the groin) may be red and scaling without the central clearing seen in tinea corporis.
- **Tinea pedis** (tinea of the feet) may be seen as macerated white areas between the toes or as dry red scaling on the soles or sides of the feet (moccasin distribution).
- **Onychomycosis** (tinea unguium) is a fungal infection of the nails.

Acne

Acne is a disease of the sebaceous follicle that occurs predominantly on the face, chest, and back. Acne typically begins during adolescence but can persist into adulthood. In some persons, significant acne may not begin until adulthood. Acne starts when the sebaceous follicle becomes blocked with sebum and desquamated cells. In inflammatory acne, there is also an overgrowth of *Propionibacterium acnes* within the follicle that leads to inflammation.

- **Comedonal acne** (obstructive, noninflammatory): The closed comedone ("whitehead") is a flesh-colored or whitish, slightly palpable lesion that is approximately 1–3 mm in diameter. The open comedone ("blackhead") is a flat or slightly raised, brownish or black lesion that measures up to 5 mm in diameter.
- **Inflammatory acne** (papulopustular, nodular, cystic, nodulocystic): Acne papules are pinkish or reddish inflammatory lesions that range from 2 to 5 mm in diameter. Pustules are superficial papules containing grossly purulent material. Acne nodules are solid, raised inflammatory lesions that exceed 5 mm in diameter and are situated deeper in the dermis than papules. The acne "cyst" is actually a large nodule that has suppurated and become fluctuant. Large deep inflammatory nodules are referred to as *cysts* because of the resemblance to inflamed epidermal cysts.

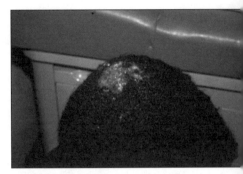

Figure 9: Tinea capitis.
(Photo © Richard P. Usatine, MD.)

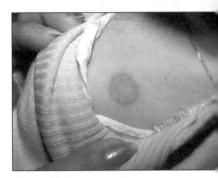

Figure 10: Tinea corporis.
(Photo © Richard P. Usatine, MD.)

Table 2. Acne Therapy by Severity

Type	Treatment
Obstructive or comedonal acne—mild	Benzoyl peroxide Tretinoin (Retin-A) or adapalene (Differin) Azelaic acid (Azelex) No place for oral antibiotics
Mild papulopustular	Topical antibiotics and benzoyl peroxide (Benzamycin) Consider oral antibiotics if topical agents are not working Tretinoin (Retin-a) or adapalene (Differin) Azelaic acid (Azelex)
Moderate papulopustular	May start with topical antibiotic, benzoyl peroxide, and oral antibiotic Oral antibiotics are often essential at this stage Tretinoin (Retin-A) or adapalene (Differin) Consider stopping oral antibiotics when topical agents are working well Consider birth control pills in females Consider isotretinoin (Accutane) if other therapies are not working in 6 months
Severe nodular or nodulocystic or scarring acne	May try all therapies listed above Isotretinoin (Accutane) is often needed

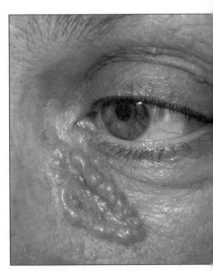

Figure 11: Basal cell carcinoma.
(Photo © Richard P. Usatine, MD.)

Acne Therapy by Severity

See **Table 2** for acne treatment.

Skin Cancers

The most common skin cancers are basal cell carcinoma (BCC), squamous cell carcinoma (SCC) and melanoma (approximately 80%, 16%, 4%, respectively). Sun exposure is the most important risk factor along with family history and skin type. BCCs are the most common skin cancer, and 85% of all BCCs appear on the head and neck region **(Figure 11)**. There are three major morphologic types: nodular, superficial, and sclerosing. The typical nodular BCC is pearly and raised with telangiectasias. The center may ulcerate and bleed, and become crusted. Sclerosing BCCs only account for 1% of BCCs and are flat and scarlike. Superficial BCCs look like SCC and are red or pink, flat, scaling plaques that may have erosions or crusts.

SCCs can look like a superficial BCC or can be more elevated and nodular **(Figure 12)**. SCCs frequently build up keratin and bleed easily. Recognizing and treating actinic keratoses is a method of skin cancer prevention. Because there is a spectrum from actinic keratosis to SCC in situ to full-blown SCC, it is sometimes necessary to biopsy a lesion that has features that appear more suspicious than your typical actinic keratosis **(Figure 13)**.

The incidence of melanoma has been on the rise in the U.S. in the last few decades. Early detection and treatment can prevent deaths and morbidity **(Brain 1)**.

Many benign growths can resemble melanoma, and a suspicious growth should receive a full-depth biopsy to make a definitive diagnosis **(Figure 14)**.

Basics of Dermatology Treatments

Major categories of treatment include medicine, surgery, and patient education. Many medicines for the skin are administered topically, including topical corticosteroids for inflammation and topical antibiotics for bacterial infections. Surgical biopsies and treatments include shave, punch and elliptical excisions. Patient education includes sun protection and safe sex practices. For the primary care physician, three situations should prompt consideration of a referral to a specialist for performing the biopsy:

1. Aggressive and recurrent skin cancer
2. The lesion is located in a sensitive area (cosmetic or functional)
3. Biopsy of a lesion is beyond the scope of one's skills

Putting It All Together

This chapter presents an overview of the diagnosis of common skin conditions. A great way to further your learning is to look at the many pictures of skin conditions found in published and on-line atlases and

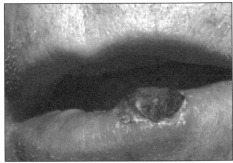

Figure 12: Squamous cell carcinoma.
(Courtesy of the Skin Cancer Foundation, New York)

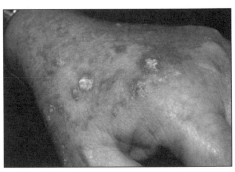

Figure 13: Actinic keratosis.
(Photo © Richard P. Usatine, MD.)

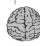

1 - ABCDE Guidelines for Diagnosis of Melanoma

A **A**symmetry. Most early melanomas are asymmetric (i.e., a line through the middle would not create matching halves). Common moles are round and symmetric.

B **B**order. The borders of early melanomas are often uneven and may have scalloped or notched edges. Common moles have smoother, more even borders.

C **C**olor variation. Common moles usually are a single shade of brown. Varied shades of brown, tan, or black are often the first sign of melanoma. As melanomas progress, the colors red, white, and blue may appear.

D **D**iameter. Early melanomas tend to grow larger than common moles— generally to at least the size of a pencil eraser (about 6 mm in diameter).

E **E**levation. Malignant melanoma is almost always elevated, at least in part, so that it is palpable.

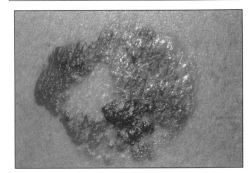

Figure 14: Melanoma.
(Courtesy of the Skin Cancer Foundation, New York.)

textbooks of dermatology. Many skin conditions (acne, seborrhea, psoriasis, eczema) are worsened by stress. Some skin conditions are the results of sexually transmitted infections or sun exposure. The physician should address lifestyle modifications that help the patient minimize exposures to risk factors for skin disease.

Optimal treatment and patient adherence depend on the patient having a good understanding of the diagnosis and treatment of the skin disease. Therefore, health education plays an important role in the treatment of skin conditions.

Selected Readings

1. Fitzpatrick TB, Polano MK, Surmand D: Color Atlas and Synopses of Clinical Dermatology. New York, McGraw-Hill, 1996.
2. Habif T: Clinical Dermatology: A Color Guide to Diagnosis and Therapy, 3rd ed. St. Louis, Mosby, 1996.
3. Usatine R: Skin problems. In Sloane P, Slatt L, Curtis P, Ebell M (eds): The Essentials of Family Medicine, 3rd ed. Baltimore, Williams & Wilkins, 1998.
4. Usatine R, Moy R, Tobinick E, Siegel D: Skin Surgery: A Practical Guide. St. Louis, Mosby, 1998.
5. Usatine RP, Quan MA: Pearls in the management of acne: An advanced approach. Prim Care 27:289–308, 2000.

54. The Red Eye

Joseph Kiesler, MD

Synopsis

The red eye is the most common ocular problem seen by primary care physicians. Although conjunctivitis accounts for the majority of these visits, orbital cellulitis, keratitis, iritis, acute primary angle-closure glaucoma, episcleritis, and scleritis are potential causes of vision loss that need to be excluded. A targeted history should ascertain the presence of pain or drainage, change in visual acuity, exposures, duration of onset, and chronicity of symptoms. The physical exam should focus on documenting current vision and inspecting the **conjunctiva (Definition 1)**, cornea, pupil, and surrounding soft tissues. Depending on the diagnosis, management may include warm compresses, topical antibiotics, eye patching, or a referral to an eye doctor for vision-threatening conditions.

1 - Conjunctiva: The palpebral tissue layer lining the inside of the eyelids and a bulbar layer covering the eye globe.

Differential Diagnosis

Non–Vision-Threatening

- Subconjunctival hemorrhage: bleeding beneath the conjunctiva
- Stye (external hordeolum): inflamed eyelash follicle
- Chalazion (internal hordeolum): inflamed meibomian cyst of the eyelid
- Blepharitis: inflammation of the eyelid
- Conjunctivitis: inflammation of the conjunctiva *(Brain 1)*
- Keratoconjunctivitis sicca: dry eyes
- Episcleritis: inflammation of a discrete area of the bulbar conjunctiva
- Superficial corneal abrasions
- Dacryocystitis: infected, blocked nasolacrimal duct typically occurring in infants

1 - Adenovirus is a common cause of epidemic, viral conjunctivitis ("pink eye"). *Staphylococcus, Haemophilus influenzae, Streptococcus pneumoniae,* and *Chlamydia* are the most common causes of bacterial conjunctivitis.

Vision-Threatening *(Red Flag 1)*

- Orbital cellulitis: infection of the orbital tissue
- Keratitis: inflammation of the cornea
- Iritis: inflammation of the iris and ciliary body
- Scleritis: inflammation of the sclera
- Acute angle closure glaucoma: closure of a preexisting, narrow anterior chamber angle obstructing aqueous drainage
- Hyperacute purulent conjunctivitis: associated with quick onset and copious amount of discharge, often *Neisseria* species

1 - These vision-threatening conditions should prompt an immediate consultation with an eye specialist.

History

"Tell me about how this began."

- Slow versus sudden onset *(Brain 2)*
- Time of day *(Brain 3)*

2 - Sudden onset is seen with trauma (foreign body or corneal abrasion), acute angle closure glaucoma, iritis, subconjunctival hemorrhage, and hyperacute purulent conjunctivitis.

- One versus both eyes: infectious conjunctivitis initially unilateral
- Preceding trauma: associated with possible foreign body or hemorrhage
- Worse upon awakening: suggests conjunctivitis

"What do you think might have caused your problem?"

- Work, home, or hobby exposures: explore allergic conjunctivitis, foreign body risks
- Recent infection in patient or close contact: possible viral conjunctivitis
- Use of contacts lenses: associated with conjunctivitis, corneal abrasion, foreign body

"Do you have any of the following symptoms?" *(Red Flag 2)*

- Decreased vision: rule out iritis, acute glaucoma
- Itching: associated with allergic conjunctivitis
- Scratchy sensation: suggests dry eyes, foreign body, blepharitis
- Burning: possible conjunctivitis
- Localized lump or tenderness: associated with hordeolum or chalazion
- Eye pain: rule out iritis, keratitis, acute glaucoma, scleritis, periorbital cellulitis, corneal abrasions
- Marked light sensitivity (photophobia): think iritis, keratitis, acute glaucoma, corneal abrasions, foreign body
- Mucus discharge: associated with allergic conjunctivitis, chlamydial infection
- Watery discharge: associated with viral conjunctivitis, chemical irritant
- Purulent discharge: associated with bacterial conjunctivitis, corneal ulcer, orbital cellulitis

"Tell me about your past medical history."

- History of allergies: possible allergic conjunctivitis
- History of collagen vascular diseases or on diuretics: may cause dry eyes
- Recurring eye problems: possible allergic conjunctivitis, corneal erosions, iritis
- Concurrent sexually transmitted disease (STD): may have related bacterial conjunctivitis
- Age > 50: acute angle glaucoma more likely

Physical Exam *(Figure 1)*

- General observation. Does the patient appear uncomfortable? Does the light in the room disturb the patient?
- Vitals
- Vision test. Record if it is with or without correction.
- Look for facial swelling or redness around the eye and eyelid which may be sign of cellulitis or **stye** *(Definition 2)*.
- Check the pupils for size, reactivity, accommodation, and irregularity. Iritis may have a constricted, irregular pupil
- Side-light the anterior chamber. Evaluate for acute angle closure glaucoma *(Brain 4)*.

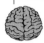

3 - Acute angle closure glaucoma may be triggered when the pupil dilates in a darkened environment.

2 - Decreased vision, marked photophobia, and eye pain are symptoms suggesting eye-threatening conditions

2 - Stye: An infection of the glands along the lash line. Localized swelling and tenderness of the eyelid occurs.

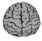

4 - Side-lighting: From the lateral side, shine the light source across the eye. If the anterior chamber is narrowed, the medial iris will not be illuminated.

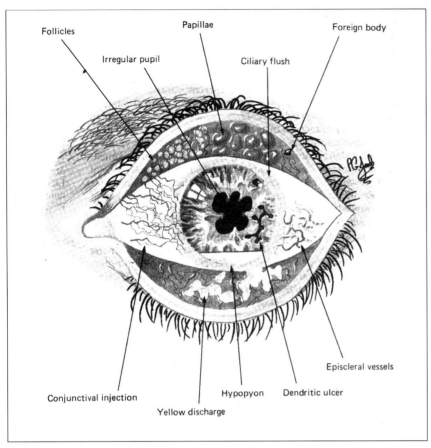

Figure 1: Physical signs of the eye.
(From Elkington AR, Khaw PT: The red eye. Br Med J 296:1720–1724, 1988, with permission.)

- Inspect palpebral (eyelid) conjunctiva. Redness with or without follicles and papules suggests conjunctivitis.
- Inspect bulbar (eyeball) conjunctiva
    Redness or ciliary flush surrounding the cornea suggest iritis.
    Focal inflammation with tenderness is associated with episcleritis or scleritis.
    Edema suggests allergic conjunctivitis.
- Look for presence and type of discharge.
- Extra-ocular movements—limited in orbital cellulitis.
- Evert the upper eyelid. Look for foreign body *(Brain 5)*
- Check for preauricular (in front of the ear) lymph nodes. These may indicate viral conjunctivitis.
- Look for haziness of cornea. Beware of acute glaucoma, iritis, and keratitis.

 5 - Everting eyelids:
1. Pull upper eyelid away from the globe.
2. Apply pressure on the outer surface of the eyelid with a swab while the patient looks down.
3. Evert the lid over the edge of the tarsus.

Testing

- Vision test using an eye chart
- Fluorescein exam *(Brain 6)*
    Branching (dendritic) ulcer pattern of the cornea is associated with herpes viruses.
    Any corneal defect will pick up the stain and may be due to abrasion, or ulcer.

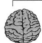 **6** - Fluorescein exam: Document the patient's vision before initiating this examination. Lightly wet the fluorescein strip with sterile water. Inform the patient that the dye will sting. With the patient looking up, touch the strip to the lower eyelid. Use a Wood's lamp to visualize defects.

- Cultures. If newborn or copious purulent discharge, rule out *Neisseria* species

Putting It All Together

Conjunctivitis will account for a majority of the "red eyes" presenting to the primary care doctor, but the most important item is to rule out vision-threatening conditions. The red flags for these include eye pain, history of trauma, sudden loss or change in vision, and marked sensitivity to light. An ophthalmologist should be consulted immediately whenever one of these conditions is suspected or the diagnosis is unclear. Patients may be fearful of losing their vision, and it is important to address this concern once a diagnosis has been made.

Management

Viral conjunctivitis is managed supportively with cold compresses and topical vasoconstrictors. Adenovirus is contagious for 7 days, so exposure to others should be restricted. If bacterial conjunctivitis is suspected or cannot be excluded, antibiotic eye drops or ointments should be used. Good hand-washing techniques need to be emphasized to decrease transmission to others. Primary treatment for allergic conjunctivitis involves elimination of the environmental irritant along with topical antihistamine or anti-inflammatory drops. For corneal abrasions, antibiotic eye ointment should be used, and the eye may be patched for symptomatic relief. Re-examination of the patched eye needs to occur each day until the abrasion is healed. Styes or chalazions often can be managed with antibiotic ointment and warm compresses. Vision-threatening conditions such as iritis, acute angle glaucoma, orbital cellulitis, or corneal ulcerations require immediate referral to an eye specialist **(Treatment 1)**.

1 - Topical steroids should only be used under the direct supervision of an ophthalmologist. It can make conditions such a herpetic infection significantly worse.

Selected Readings

1. Elkington AR, Khaw PT: The red eye. Br Med J 296:1720–1724, 1988.
2. Gaston H: Managing the red eye. Practitioner 233:1566–1572, 1989.
3. Hara JH: The red eye: Diagnosis and treatment. Am Fam Physician 54:2423–2430, 1996.
4. Leibowitz HM: Primary care: The red eye. N Engl J Med 343:345–351, 2000.
5. Morrow GL, Abbott RL: Conjunctivitis. Am Fam Physician 57:735–746, 1998.
6. Strong N: The acute red eye. Practitioner 232:116–120, 1988.

55. School Problems

Cynthia R. Ellis, MD • Amy L. Ruane, EdS

Synopsis

The majority of school problems are minor in nature and require minimal intervention to correct. However, more severe academic and behavioral problems can interfere significantly with a child's progress in school and require more intensive intervention. Significant academic and behavioral problems affect approximately 10% of the school age population in the United States; of these, learning disabilities affect approximately 5%, attention deficit–hyperactivity disorder (ADHD) affects approximately 3–5%, and mental retardation affects approximately 1%. The differential diagnosis of "school problems" is extensive, and a comprehensive, interdisciplinary evaluation may be needed to clarify the underlying reasons for school dysfunction. Furthermore, it is not uncommon for children with significant problems to fall into more than one category of disability or impairment. In addition, there may be an interaction of multiple variables underlying their dysfunction.

This chapter does not cover all of the many different school problems that impact children. Instead, this chapter lists some of the most prevalent categories and provides information about each. Most school problems are nonspecific and related to situational factors. However, the history, nature, and severity of each child's complaints need to be evaluated to determine the complexity of the problem and guide further evaluation. The history, physical examination, and testing completed during the initial visit are important to rule out the presence of a medical disorder, determine the family history of specific disorders, identify environmental stressors and supports, and lead to the most probable broad diagnostic categories. This can then serve as a guide for determining whether additional assessment is necessary and facilitate the development of a treatment plan.

Differential Diagnosis

Developmental Disability

- **Mental retardation (MR):** MR is characterized by significantly subaverage intellectual functioning (IQ < 70–75), existing concurrently with related limitations in two or more of the following adaptive skill areas: communication, self-care, home living, social skills, community use, self-direction, health and safety, functional academics, leisure, and work. MR manifests itself before age 18.
- **Learning disability (LD):** People with LDs usually have average or near-average intelligence, yet achieve at unexpectedly low levels in one or more of seven areas: basic reading skills, reading comprehension, oral expression, listening comprehension, written expression, mathematical calculation, and mathematical reasoning. Learning disabilities represent a heterogeneous group of conditions that can range from mild to severe.
- **Pervasive developmental disorders (PDD):** PDD represents a spectrum of disorders (including autism) characterized by significant impairments in reciprocal social interaction and communication skills and the presence of stereotyped behavior, interests, and activities. These disorders can range from mild to severe and are usually evident in the first 3 years of life.
- **Communication disorders:** Impairment in understanding and/or transmitting information, including disturbances in speech production, comprehension, spoken and written language, and language-based learning.

Sensory Impairment

- Hearing loss
- Vision loss

Psychiatric and Emotional Disorders

- **Attention deficit–hyperactivity disorder (ADHD):** ADHD is a neu-robehavioral disorder characterized by inattention, impulsivity, and hyperactivity of greater than 6 months' duration that causes functional impairment in two or more settings. Although it may not be diagnosed until school age, the onset of symptoms must be before age 7 years.
- **Oppositional defiant disorder (ODD):** ODD represents a recurrent pattern behavior of greater than 6 months' duration that is excessive-ly negativistic, defiant, and disobedient toward parents, teachers, or other authority figures. This hostile behavior leads to impairment in social and academic functioning.

Psychosocial Issues

- Poor motivation
- Social skills deficit
- Family dysfunction
- Ineffective schooling

Chronic Illness

History

The following questions should be addressed to the parent or caregiver.

"Let's talk about how school is going. What are your current concerns?" *(Red Flag 1)*

- Any subjects particularly difficult for the child
- Failing grades
- Excessive tardiness, or absences
- Difficulty following directions or paying attention
- Consistently incomplete or inaccurate assignments
- Poor peer relations; few or no friends
- Doesn't respect authority, violates school rules
- Disruptive during class, fighting

"What are his [her] teachers reporting?"

- Academic performance relative to grade level
- Behavioral concerns in the classroom
- Problems with peer interactions
- Concerns about motivation

"How long have these problems been going on?"

- Age of onset of first concerns
- Previous academic or behavioral problems

"Has any testing or intervention been recommended in the past?"

1 - These academic and behavioral concerns are red flags for further evaluation and may be indicative of a more serious underlying dis-ability or disorder. It is imperative for the clini-cian to identify these issues early so that appropriate intervention can begin as soon as possible.

- Referrals for evaluations by the school or other agencies
- Special education services received by the child in the past or currently

"Are there any significant health or emotional concerns that you feel may be related to the current school problems?" *(Brain 1)*

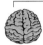

1 - Historical information regarding past medical history, developmental milestones, family history, and social history may provide important clues to current problems.

- Significant change in overall health status
- Concerns for vision or hearing
- Multiple somatic complaints
- Sleep problems
- Lack of age-appropriate activities and interests
- Changes in mood
- Self-esteem

"Were there any concerns regarding his [her] behavior or development prior to entering school?"

- Attainment of developmental milestones
- Temperament concerns

"Have any other family members experienced similar difficulties?"

- Family history of significant behavioral or academic problems
- Family members diagnosed with any developmental disorders

"What is the home learning environment like?"

- Recent environmental changes (e.g., move, divorce)
- Lack of homework supervision
- Resistance to homework
- Argumentative
- Mood changes

Physical Examination *(Red Flag 2)*

General observations (including dysmorphic features, tics, activity level)

2 - Although the physical examination is generally normal, any abnormalities detected should be pursued with a further medical work-up specific to the exam findings. Chronic illnesses and other medical conditions can be related to school difficulties.

- Routine vital signs
- Growth measurements, including head circumference
- General screening exam
- Complete neurologic examination

Testing

Vision and hearing screening are indicated to rule out sensory impairments. A mental status exam (includes an evaluation of the child's physical appearance, orientation, cooperation, activity level, use of speech and language, mood and affect, content of thought, flow of thoughts, cognition, memory, insight, judgment, and presence of suicidal or homicidal ideation) will help identify psychiatric and emotional disorders. Question the child to get an idea of their current emotional status. Look for signs of depression, anxiety, and low self-esteem. Does the child feel he or she has any control over what happens to him or her or hope for change in the current situation?

Parent ratings scales (e.g., Connors Parent Rating Scale–Revised) are available with standardized norms to assess a child's functioning for a number of clinical conditions. The selection of a rating scale is indicated by the clinician's initial diagnostic impression.

Self-report measures on a variety of conditions (e.g., depression, anxiety, ADHD) can be completed by most children over 8 years of age. The selection of a rating scale is indicated by the clinician's initial diagnostic impression.

Developmental screening or neurodevelopmental testing should be considered to obtain an indication of the child's cognitive abilities, language skills, and adaptive behavior *(Brain 2)*.

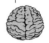

2 - An assessment of a child's cognitive functioning may assist the clinician in determining if a referral for additional psychoeducational testing is indicated.

Laboratory testing is based on indications from the history or physical examination, such as obtaining a lead level with a history of developmental delay or pica, or ordering a chromosome analysis if dysmorphic features are found on physical examination.

Putting It All Together

The conclusion of the initial visit may lead the clinician to the most probable broad diagnostic category. In many cases, there will be multiple diagnostic categories to consider. The clinician must assess the nature, complexity, and intensity of the problems. If the problem revealed is simple in nature and easily identifiable, such as a vision problem or slight distractibility, the clinician can suggest an appropriate intervention (e.g., further vision testing and correction or development of a behavioral plan for distractibility). Understanding more complex or severe problems will require additional information from multiple sources, particularly the school and teacher, and intervention generally requires an interdisciplinary approach. The more serious school problems usually are not due to a single factor but result from the interaction of multiple school, child, and family variables. The primary care provider should use the first and subsequent visits to clarify the reasons for the school dysfunction and facilitate appropriate evaluation and intervention.

Management

The selection of a specific management strategy is based on the nature and severity of the underlying problems causing the school dysfunction. Therefore, it is imperative to gather the appropriate additional information needed to identify the cause(s) of the school problems. The physician should obtain a release of information from the parents to contact the school and obtain educational records. All records should be reviewed, and, if needed, additional information can be obtained from the teacher using direct contact or through checklists and rating scales. Relevant records should also be obtained from any other care providers (e.g., daycare providers, mental health providers, and medical subspecialists). A follow-up appointment should be scheduled to review the additional information obtained and determine the need for further evaluation or develop an initial treatment plan.

Psychoeducational testing is indicated when mental retardation or a learning disability is suspected. The patient should be referred back to his or her local school system or to a qualified psychologist for a comprehensive evaluation. Psychiatric consultation may be indicated if there is evidence of a significant psychiatric or emotional disorder.

Underlying medical conditions that are identified, such as a seizure disorder or sleep disorder, can be treated. Pharmacologic and behavioral interventions should be initiated when indicated for specific diagnoses, such as ADHD *(Treatment 1)*. The physician's role in counseling the parents of a child with school problems may include delineation of expectations based on the student's abilities, assistance in understanding the legal rights of students and families, guidance regarding common school difficulties, and advice regarding the development of specific behavioral interventions.

Educational intervention is very important for any child with school dysfunction. Thus, coordination and collaboration between the physician and school personnel are essential to optimize the child's functioning in that environment *(Consultation and Referral 1)*.

Follow-up, either by phone or office visits, should occur on a regular basis, depending on the severity of the problems and the efficacy of the interventions utilized, until the problems have resolved or the underlying disorder has stabilized.

1 - There is often overlap between ADHD, LD, and other disorders. If an initial treatment strategy is unsuccessful, additional evaluation should be undertaken to confirm the initial diagnosis or look for comorbid diagnoses.

1 - Local school systems are experts in providing regular and special education services to children from birth to age 21 years and are an important resource for physicians managing children with school problems.

Selected Readings

1. American Association on Mental Retardation: Mental Retardation: Definition, Classification, and Systems of Support. Washington, DC, AAMR, 1992.
2. American Psychiatric Association: Diagnostic and Statistical Manual of Mental Disorders, 4th ed. Washington, DC, APA,1994.
3. Dworkin PH: School failure. Pediatr Rev 10:301–312, 1989.
4. Fox AM, Mahoney WJ (eds): Children with School Problems: A Physician's Manual. Ottowa, Canadian Pediatric Society, 1998.
5. Kazdin AE: Conduct Disorder in Childhood and Adolescence. Thousand Oaks, CA, Sage Publications, 1995.
6. Lerner JW: Learning Disabilities: Theories, Diagnosis, and Teaching Strategies. Boston, Houghton-Mifflin, 1997.

56. Sexually Transmitted Diseases

William Henry Hay, MD

Synopsis

The term *sexually transmitted disease* (STD) refers to a variety of conditions transmitted primarily via genital contact. As a group, these diseases are extremely common and result in a large burden of morbidity and mortality *(Brain 1)*. It is important to keep in mind that many STDs are frequently asymptomatic, so the physician must maintain a high index of suspicion, and testing should be done on anyone who is found to be at risk after taking a sexual history. If a patient has or is at risk for any particular STD, he or she is at risk for all the others, and the appropriate screening tests should be done. Appropriate treatment should be followed up by testing for cure and counseling to prevent future infections. If a patient is found to have an STD, it is imperative that his or her partners be informed and treated appropriately.

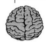

1 - An estimated 15 million Americans contract an STD each year, and half of all Americans will contract one by age 35.

Differential Diagnosis

- **Urethritis *(Definition 1)***: *Chlamydia*, gonorrhea, *Trichomonas*
- Vaginitis: *Trichomonas*
- Cervicitis: *Chlamydia*, gonorrhea, *Trichomonas*
- **Pelvic inflammatory disease (PID) *(Definition 2)***: *Chlamydia*, gonorrhea
- Genital ulcer: herpes, syphilis (also chancroid, but rare in U.S.)
- Genital growth: genital warts (condyloma)
- Systemic infection: human immunodeficiency virus (HIV), hepatitis B and C, secondary and late syphilis, primary herpes, PID

1 - Urethritis: Inflammation of the urethra often presenting with frequency, urgency, or painful urination or discharge.

2 - Pelvic inflammatory disease (PID): Infection of the uterus and adnexa characterized by tenderness in these areas, often accompanied by fever, discharge, and abnormal uterine bleeding. The patient may be quite ill, and long-term consequences include chronic pain and infertility.

History

When is it appropriate to take a sexual history? It is obviously necessary if the patient's stated concern is an STD, but populations at higher risk, such as those between 15 and 24 years of age, should be screened routinely. As a rule, some level of sexual history is appropriate on almost any adult or adolescent patient, at least as part of a general physical examination.

How the physician approaches this sensitive subject is very important. It is helpful to be cognizant of one's own feelings about asking these questions. If the physician appears nervous, anxious, or judgmental, the patient's comfort with giving complete and truthful answers will be affected. Avoid closed-ended questions. Patients tend to give the minimum information necessary to answer the question and may understand terms, such as *protection* and *sexually active*, differently from the questioner. It is also important to avoid assumptions about the patient's sexual behavior and orientation.

If the patient has not presented specifically about an STD or other sexual health concern, the physician should explain the rationale for these questions: "Because sexual health is an important issue, I am going to ask you a few questions about your sexual history. Sometimes these types of questions can be uncomfortable, but I think that they are important so that I can get a full picture of your health. Of course you don't have to answer all my questions." For many patients, the first two or three questions in the following list are all you need to ask to assess risk. More thorough questioning can be reserved for those found to be at risk or for those who have specific questions or concerns about their sexual health.

- "Are you sexually active?" If the patient says no, ask: "When were you last sexually active?" *(Brain 2)*
- "How many sex partners do you currently have? If one, when did you last have another partner?"
- "How many partners have you had in the last year? How many since you became sexually active?"
- "Are your partners men, women, or both?"
- "Do any of your sex partners have sex with any other partners?"
- "What sorts of sexual activity do you engage in?" (Possible follow-up: "Do you engage in vaginal, oral, or anal sex?") *(Brain 3)*
- "What forms of protection do you and your partner use during sexual activity? How consistently do you use them?"
- "Have you or any of your sex partners used needles to take recreational or street drugs?"
- "Have you or any of your partners ever had a sexually transmitted disease?"
- "Have you or any partner ever traded sex for food, money, drugs, or a place to sleep?"
- "Have you ever been forced into sexual activity?"
- For female patients: "Are you using any birth control? Have you missed any periods? Could you be pregnant?"
- "Do you have any of the following symptoms?" *(Brain 4)*
  - Fever or chills
  - Painful or frequent urination
  - Urethral or vaginal discharge
  - Genital sores or growths
  - Abdominal, genital, testicular, or rectal pain
  - Recent changes in menstruation
  - Rashes
- "What concerns do you have about this problem?" *(Brain 5)*

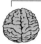

2 - It is important to follow up on negative responses. Research suggests that many teens who engage in oral sex do not consider themselves sexually active.

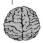

3 - Information about types of sexual practices should be elicited so the clinician will know where to obtain cultures and be better able to provide appropriate counseling about safer sex.

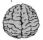

4 - These symptoms and signs are targeted at acute infections. More generalized questioning and examination are required for systemic diseases such as HIV and later stage syphilis.

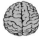

5 - Patients' concerns may be very different from the physician's. They may think that their symptoms imply other conditions. They may be concerned with the impact this will have on their relationships and their future fertility.

Physical Examination

- Vital signs including temperature
- Oral exam if symptomatic or a history of oral sex obtained
- Genital and possibly rectal exam (e.g., sores, discharge, tenderness)
- Inguinal lymph nodes (frequently enlarged or tender with STDs)
- General skin exam for rashes (e.g., a sign of syphilis)

Testing

- Chlamydia: antigen or DNA detection tests on swab of urethra or cervix. Cultures, although more difficult and expensive, may be needed if pharyngeal or rectum specimens must be obtained.
- Condyloma: Visual inspection may be enhanced by application of 4–10% acetic acid (vinegar) to area for 5 minutes.
- Gonorrhea: similar to chlamydia
- Hepatitis B: serum hepatitis B surface antigen
- Hepatitis C (HCV): serum anti-HCV antibody
- Herpes: viral culture of ulcers or serum herpes simplex IgM antibody
- HIV (see Chapter 40)
- Syphilis:
    - For primary syphilis (ulcer present) use dark-field microscopic exam or direct fluorescent antibody test of swab of an ulcer.
    - Later stages: serum RPR (rapid plasma reagin)
- *Trichomonas*: saline exam of urethral or cervical/vaginal swab
- Pregnancy screen
- Pap smear

Putting It All Together

STDs are extremely common and often asymptomatic. The physician should routinely inquire about sexual history, especially with high-risk groups such as adolescents. If the patient has or is at risk for one STD, he or she is at risk for and should be tested for other STDs. Proper follow-up including partner notification is essential.

Management

Follow-up should include retesting for cure and treatment of any additional STDs identified. Appropriate immunizations, currently limited to hepatitis B virus, should be started.

Counseling should include a discussion of safer sex practices to avoid future infections. The patient should be instructed in the use of barrier methods, which include condoms, the female condom, and latex dental dams (flat pieces of latex placed over the vagina or anus). The patient should be instructed that such methods are to be used during all sexual contacts. Safer sex also includes limiting the number of sexual partners and the careful selection of sexual partners.

When any STD is diagnosed, it is vitally important that the patient's sexual partners are contacted and advised to be seen by a physician for testing or treatment. This is important not just for the partner's health, but to prevent reinfection of the patient. How far back to trace partners will depend on which infection is being treated. The physician may need to help the patient notify his or her partners (e.g., having the patient bring the partner in during the follow-up visit). Local health departments also can be a resource in partner notification.

Selected Readings

1. 1998 Guidelines for the Treatment of Sexually Transmitted Diseases: Proceedings of a meeting. Clin Infect Dis 28 (Suppl 1):S1–S90, 1999.
2. Centers for Disease Control and Prevention: 1998 Guidelines for treatment of sexually transmitted diseases. Morb Mortal Wkly Rep 47(RR-1):1–111, 1998. Available at http://www.cdc.gov/mmwr/preview/mmwrhtml/00050909.htm. Accessed April 7, 2002.
3. Gevelber MA, Biro FM: Adolescents and sexually transmitted diseases. Pediatr Clin North Am 46:747–766, 1999.
4. Schaffner W, Sondheimer S, Trotto N: STDs: Are you up-to-date? Patient Care 33(10):74–103, 1999.

Web Site

National Center for HIV, STD and TB Prevention, Division of Sexually Transmitted Diseases: http://www.cdc.gov/nchstp/dstd/disease_info.htm. Accessed April 7, 2002.

57. Sleep Disorders

Jeffrey L. Susman, MD

Synopsis

Difficulties with sleep are very common but often go undiagnosed. The initial evaluation should concentrate on separating acute from chronic sleep problems and ascertaining whether the problem is with falling asleep, maintaining sleep, or abnormal daytime drowsiness. Sleep habits (commonly termed sleep hygiene) should be explored. Underlying causes of sleep problems include medical, psychiatric, and environmental issues. The impact on daily function is important to assess. When a **primary sleep problem** *(Definition 1)* is suspected, further evaluation, including a formal sleep study **(polysomnogram)** *(Definition 2)*, is often required. Treatment should be directed toward precipitating factors, improving sleep hygiene, and the specific sleep disorder.

1 - Primary sleep problem: Disorders primarily attributable to changes in sleep. May include dyssomnias (problems with the amount or timing of sleep such as sleep apnea syndrome) and parasomnias (disturbances that occur during sleep such as sleepwalking).

2 - Polysomnogram (sleep study): Measurement of brain waves, eye movements, muscle activity, breathing, heart rate, and other physiologic measurements during sleep. Provides diagnosis of sleep apnea syndrome, restless legs syndrome, and many other sleep problems.

Differential Diagnosis

Medical Problems

- Gastroesophageal reflux disease (GERD)—may mimic **sleep apnea syndrome** *(Definition 3)*
- Benign prostatic hypertrophy (BPH)—patient's sleep may be disrupted by need to go to bathroom
- Congestive heart failure (CHF)—nocturnal breathing problems
- Neuropathy—pain may disrupt sleep
- Diabetes mellitus (hypoglycemia)
- Arthritis—pain
- Lung disease

3 - Sleep apnea syndrome: Cessation (apneas) or reductions (hypopneas) of airflow during sleep caused either by obstruction of naso-oral airflow or a cessation of the central drive to breathe. Presenting symptoms include daytime sleepiness, snoring, and nocturnal breathing cessation.

Psychiatric Disorders

- Depression—may cause early morning awakening
- Anxiety including situational anxiety
- Obsessive-compulsive disorder
- Dementia—fragmented sleep, naps, day–night reversal

Drugs

- Alcohol—can cause disrupted sleep, especially dream (rapid eye movement [REM]) sleep
- Nicotine
- Caffeine—some patients are very sensitive to any form of methylxanthine (coffee, tea, cola drinks, chocolate) and should avoid it entirely
- Beta blockers
- Corticosteroids

- Bronchodilators
- Diuretics
- Antidepressants, particularly selective serotonin reuptake inhibitors (SSRIs)
- Thyroid hormone

Sleep Hygiene Problems

Some sleep problems are caused by poor sleep habits *(Table 1)*.

Table 1. Good Sleep Hygiene or Habits

- Awake at the same time each day.
- Go to bed when sleepy, and decrease time spent in bed.
- Don't take naps unless part of an established sleep schedule.
- Use the bed only for sleeping.
- Avoid stimulants (e.g., caffeine), alcohol, and smoking.
- Don't become a "clock watcher."
- Exercise ≥ 6 hours prior to bed.
- Try a glass of warm milk prior to bedtime.
- Make sure the bedroom environment is comfortable.
- Schedule "worry time" prior to bedtime.

4 - Sleep cycle disorders: Sleep problems caused by a mismatch between the physiologic tendency for sleep and wake and the desired sleep-wake cycle.

5 - Restless legs syndrome and periodic leg movements in sleep: Disorders characterized by limb movements that disrupt normal sleep. The restless legs syndrome occurs prior to sleep onset and is associated with an irresistible urge to move one's legs. Periodic limb movements in sleep are leg twitches that occur when individuals are in non-dream sleep.

Sleep Disorders

- Sleep apnea syndrome
- **Sleep cycle disorders *(Definition 4)***
- **Restless legs syndrome and periodic leg movements in sleep *(Definition 5)***
- Many other rare sleep problems

History

- "Tell me about your sleep problem. How long has it been going on? What other medical problems do you have? What medicines, including supplements and over-the-counter remedies, do you take?" The initial history should focus on uncovering the time course and nature of the sleep problem and potential precipitating causes. The first step is to evaluate whether the problem is acute or chronic (going on for shorter or longer than a month) *(Figure 1)*. Standardized sleep history forms or sleep logs or diaries can be helpful.
- "How has your sleep problem affected your life? Your job? Your relationships? Have you had any accidents or near accidents related to sleepiness? Do you tend to fall asleep doing repetitive or boring activities such as driving, reading or working? How are things going at home? On the job? Are there any changes in your life? Tell me about your sleep habits and your sleep patterns." Acute problems suggest transient psychophysiologic causes of insomnia, a change in environment, or poor sleep habits. More chronic problems, especially those characterized by daytime functional impairment *(Red Flag 1)*, warrant further evaluation (see Figure 1). A history of shift work should be ascertained. Poor sleep habits may impair sleep—encourage good sleep hygiene (see Table 1).

1 - Functional impairment, including problems with falling asleep unintentionally or sleepiness that results in accidents (especially motor vehicle accidents), suggests a more serious cause of the sleep problem, and a diagnosis should be aggressively pursued.

- "Tell me more about your sleep problem. Is it primarily a difficulty falling asleep, staying asleep, or being sleepy during the day? Do you or your bed partner notice any abnormal movements, snoring, or

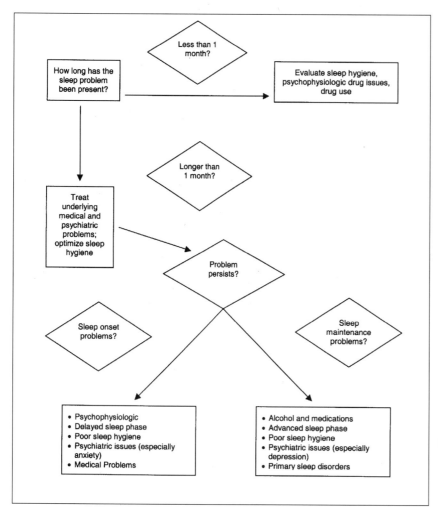

Figure 1: Evaluation of sleep disorders.

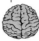

1 - Sleep Changes with Aging:
- Tend to go to bed earlier and get up earlier
- Less deep sleep and dream sleep
- More awakenings during the night
- More time in bed, but less time asleep (sleep less efficient, but total sleep requirement about the same)

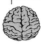

2 - The prevalence of snoring increases with age. The majority of middle-aged Americans snore, men slightly more than women. Weight loss, avoidance of sedatives, and sleeping in a side position may be helpful. A careful evaluation for sleep apnea is important.

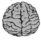

3 - Sleep phase or cycle changes commonly occur in normal adolescents—who tend to go to bed later and get up later—and normal elders—who tend to go to bed earlier and get up earlier. Sleep changes associated with jet lag and shift work are other common examples of a mismatch between the physiologic and desired sleep-wake cycle.

2 - Many patients will self-medicate with alcohol and other substances, over-the-counter and prescription sleeping pills, and other potentially harmful or ineffective interventions. Although appropriate self-care is important, many individuals will unwittingly exacerbate a problem such as sleep apnea or unknowingly forego effective treatment for a condition such as depression.

other unusual things that happen during sleep?" If the problem is more chronic, it is helpful to ascertain whether it is a difficulty with falling asleep, staying asleep, or daytime sleepiness (see Figure 1). The age of the patient is important, as predictable changes in sleep occur with aging **(Brain 1)**. Restless legs syndrome and periodic limb movements in sleep will often disrupt sleep and may result in daytime sleepiness. Sleep apnea syndrome will be suggested by snoring **(Table 2)**, although most snorers do not have sleep apnea **(Brain 2)**. Sleep cycle or phase disorders are characterized by shifts in the normal temporal occurrence of sleep **(Brain 3)**.

- "What treatments have you tried?" Note especially over-the-counter remedies, "natural" or "alternative" therapies, prescription sleeping pills, alcohol, and other drugs. In addition, a wide variety of nonpharmacologic devices, ranging from nasal strips to special pillows, are used by many patients **(Red Flag 2)**.

- "What do you think is causing your sleep problem?" Solicit the patient's concerns, theories about his or her problem, and any other pertinent history.

Table 2. Signs and Symptoms Suggestive of Obstructive Sleep Apnea Syndrome

- Snoring
- Daytime somnolence
- Complaints of poor sleep and awakening from sleep unrefreshed
- Nocturnal breathing cessation (as reported by bed partner)
- Enlarged tongue, tonsils, uvula, and other ear, nose, and throat (ENT) abnormalities promoting nasal-oral airway obstruction
- Morning headache
- High blood pressure
- Decreased libido
- Obesity
- Unusual body movements at night (as reported by bed partner)
- Cor pulmonale

Physical Examination

- Vital signs. Pay particular attention to hypertension.
- Oropharynx. Evaluate the tongue, epiglottis, neck, and oropharynx for enlargement.
- Thyroid. Note enlargement, asymmetry, or nodularity.
- Lungs. Look for evidence of chronic obstructive pulmonary disease (see Chapter 21).
- Heart. Check for **cor pulmonale *(Definition 6)*, pulmonary hypertension *(Definition 7)***, and CHF.
- Periphery. Check for edema.
- Mental status examination. Note signs of substance abuse, depression, anxiety, or other psychiatric disorders.

6 - Cor pulmonale: Hypertrophy of the right ventricle resulting from lung disease.

7 - Pulmonary hypertension: Hypertension in the pulmonary system; it may be due to cardiac or pulmonary disease.

Testing

No testing is indicated unless an underlying primary sleep disorder is suspected. If so, a sleep study or polysomnogram in an accredited sleep laboratory may be indicated. Home polysomnograms are of unproven diagnostic accuracy. The evaluation of thyroid function is often important, especially in the differential diagnosis of sleep apnea syndrome. Other tests will be dictated by the careful history and physical examination.

Putting It All Together

The history and physical examination are key to accurate diagnosis. A sleep log or more complete history from a bed partner may be gathered over several visits. When the problem is acute, the evaluation should focus on uncovering transient psychophysiologic issues, especially stress and anxiety. When the sleep problem is chronic, evaluation for underlying medical, psychiatric, and primary sleep problems should occur. The evaluation should uncover if the problem is related to sleep onset, sleep maintenance, or daytime sleepiness, which will help direct the work-up. Patients with more chronic problems or a suspicion of disorders such as sleep apnea or restless legs syndrome will often warrant a sleep study.

Management

Initial efforts are directed to most effectively treating precipitating causes of the sleep difficulty. Underlying disorders should be treated and appropriate sleep habits encouraged. Many nonpharmacologic approaches, including behavioral therapies (e.g., sleep restriction and cognitive behavioral therapy), are effective. If the problem is unresponsive to such therapy, or an underlying primary sleep problem such as sleep apnea syndrome or restless legs syndrome is suspected, a sleep study (polysomnogram) may be essential. *(Consultation and Referral)*. Specific treatments are available for the primary sleep disorders including more unusual problems that may be uncovered by a polysomnogram. Sedative-hypnotic medications should be used cautiously, with clear goals in mind, in the context of a total plan for improving sleep. Sedative-hypnotic medications are associated with serious side effects (e.g., falls), particularly in elders, and can cause withdrawal when used on a chronic basis *(Red Flag 3)*.

Treatment is directed to underlying causes of the sleep disorder, especially medical and psychiatric conditions, establishing better sleep habits, and specific therapies for primary sleep disorders. Short-term or intermittent sedative-hypnotic use may be helpful for transient psychophysiologic sleep disorders, but it is important to educate the patient and establish clear goals of care. The sleep apnea syndrome is usually treated with nasal continuous positive airway pressure (CPAP; a mask-like device that delivers oxygen under pressure and acts as a splint to keep the airway open) or surgery. Restless legs syndrome responds best to dopaminergic medications such as levodopa–carbidopa.

1 - Consultation with a sleep specialist should be considered when an underlying primary sleep problem is suspected. Recalcitrant problems of the sleep cycle, sleep apnea, or unresponsive sleep difficulties often warrant further expert evaluation. An otolaryngologist assessment may be helpful in patients with sleep apnea.

3 - Sedative-hypnotics may impair daytime functioning, cause falls, and be associated with withdrawal. Their use should be monitored closely. Sedative hypnotics should be used regularly for sleep problems for no more than 1 month.

Selected Readings

1. Mahowald MW: What is causing excessive daytime sleepiness? Postgrad Med 107:108–123, 2000.
2. National Heart, Lung, Blood Institute Working Group on Insomnia: Insomnia: assessment and management in primary care. Am Fam Phys 59:3029–3038, 1999.
3. National Sleep Foundation: Doctor, I Can't Sleep. Palo Alto, CA, National Sleep Foundation, 1993.
4. Venugopal M, Susman JL: Insomnia in the elderly: Toward a good night's sleep. Consultant 40:1234–1247, 2000.

58. Sore Throat

Mark H. Ebell, MD, MS • Jose Romero, MD

Synopsis

Sore throat is a frequent cause for a trip to the doctor's office, and the cause is usually a self-limited viral infection. However, about one-third of children and 10% of adults have an infection caused by group A beta-hemolytic streptococcal (GABHS) bacteria. Antibiotic treatment may benefit such patients. The absence of cough, and with the presence of tonsillar exudates, swollen lymph glands (cervical adenopathy), and fever increase the likelihood of GABHS infection. Rapid antigen tests can be helpful in patients who have an intermediate likelihood of GABHS pharyngitis. Those with a very low probability of GABHS pharyngitis can be treated symptomatically, and those with a very high probability should be considered for empiric antibiotic therapy. Infectious mononucleosis is a relatively common cause of sore throat in teenagers and older children, although testing is often inconclusive until later in the course of the illness. In patients with a high likelihood of infectious mononucleosis, an enlarged spleen is a frequent complication. Ascertaining the spleen size is an important part of the examination in any patient with a sore throat. Patients who have an enlarged spleen should not engage in activities that might lead to blunt abdominal trauma.

Differential Diagnosis

- **Viral pharyngitis.** Approximately 70% of infectious sore throats in children and 90% in adults are caused by viral infection. Epstein-Barr virus infection (infectious mononucleosis) can cause a prolonged infection and is most common in children and teenagers, where it causes approximately 5% of sore throats. Other viral pathogens that cause sore throat are enterovirus, adenovirus, and herpes simplex virus.
- **Bacterial pharyngitis.** GABHS bacteria causes about 10% of sore throats in adults and about 30% in children. *Chlamydia pneumoniae* and *Mycoplasma pneumoniae* bacteria have also been implicated as causes of sore throat.
- **Nonpharyngitis causes** of sore throat. This includes gastroesophogeal reflux disease (GERD), postnasal drip, allergy, upper respiratory infection, irritation from chronic or persistent cough, and thyroiditis.

History

One of the purposes of history-taking is to differentiate viral from bacterial causes of pharyngitis.

"Tell me about your sore throat."

- Onset of sore throat pain (gradual onset more common in viral disease, whereas sudden onset more indicative of GABHS)
- Duration of pain (> 1–2 weeks suggests noninfectious cause or infectious mononucleosis)
- Pattern of "double-sickening" *(Brain 1)*

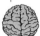
1 - "Double-sickening" refers to a pattern where a patient initially has symptoms of a cold or viral upper respiratory infection. Initially, the symptoms begin to resolve, but the patient then develops new, more severe symptoms. This pattern is often seen with sinus infection, otitis media, or other secondary bacterial infection.

"What other symptoms do you have, in addition to sore throat?"
(Red Flag 1)

- Fever or chills (presence increases risk of GABHS)
- Swollen glands (presence increases risk of GABHS)
- Sores inside the mouth (frequently seen in herpetic gingivostomatitis)
- Red eyes (frequently seen in adenovirus infection)
- Cough (absence increases risk of GABHS)
- Fatigue (especially prominent in infectious mononucleosis)
- Allergic symptoms (sensitivity to specific exposures such as animals, dust, mold or plants, sneezing, itchy eyes)
- Headache or facial pain (more frequent in sinus infection)
- Nasal discharge (frequent in viral upper respiratory infection or sinus infection)
- Difficulty swallowing or excessive drooling (frequently seen in younger children with herpetic gingivostomatitis)
- Skin rash (seen in both infectious mononucleosis and GABHS)

"Does anyone at home, daycare, school, or work have similar symptoms?"

1 - Red flags for serious disease include a muffled or "hot-potato voice," toxic appearance, or altered mental status seen in peritonsillar abscess, enlargement of the spleen (infectious mononucleosis), and signs of airway obstruction due to extremely enlarged tonsils.

Physical Examination

- General appearance. If patient appears very ill and uncomfortable, consider peritonsillar abscess, severe GABHS infection, or airway obstruction.
- Briefly examine the skin of the chest and back for a rash. A fine, follicular rash that has the tactile feel of fine sandpaper and has faint red tint ("scarlatinaform rash") is rare but strongly associated with GABHS pharyngitis.
- Inspect oropharynx and tonsils, if present, looking for pharyngeal exudates, tonsillar exudates, and tonsillar enlargement (all make GABHS more likely). Petechial rash on the palate is rare but is strongly associated with GABHS pharyngitis. Also, inspect both the anterior and the posterior pharynx for ulcers (make herpes and enterovirus more likely, respectively). Herpes virus will cause the gums to be swollen and bleed easily.
- Palpate anterior and posterior cervical triangles, periauricular region, and occipital nodes (latter associated with infectious mononucleosis).
- Inspect nasal passages.
- If sinus infection is suspected based on history, percuss sinuses, and transilluminate. Both of these maneuvers are difficult to do with small children.
- Auscultate lungs if patient has cough or tachypnea.
- Examine the skin of the abdomen for a scarlatinaform rash and palpate the abdomen for any enlargement of the liver or spleen. Splenomegaly is frequently seen in infectious mononucleosis. The liver is also frequently involved, but may not be palpably enlarged or tender.

Testing

Two types of tests are available for the diagnosis of GABHS pharyngitis: rapid antigen tests and throat cultures. The latter are positive in 90% of cases of GABHS pharyngitis and are very specific. However, they take 2 days to perform, so a decision must be made on treatment before the results are available. Rapid antigen tests are increasingly accurate and, when used with information from the history and physical examination, can be used to guide management. A rapid antigen test should be considered when the patient has an intermediate probability of GABHS pharyngitis.

In young patients with signs and symptoms of possible infectious mononucleosis (fatigue, splenomegaly, posterior cervical, periauricular and occipital adenopathy), confirmatory testing should be considered. Note that during the first week, 1 out of 5 patients with infectious mononucleosis will have a negative test result. This decreases to 1 in 7 during the second week of symptoms, and 1 in 30 during the third week of symptoms. In addition to serologic testing, a complete blood count (CBC) will be normal to slightly elevated. The differential frequently will show the presence of more than 40% atypical lymphocytes or the combination of > 50% lymphocytes and > 10% atypical lymphocytes. Both results are strong evidence for the presence of infectious mononucleosis.

Putting It All Together

Most cases of sore throat are self-limited and are usually caused by viral infections that require only symptomatic treatment. Even in patients with GABHS pharyngitis, treatment with an antibiotic reduces the duration of symptoms by 12–24 hours. On the other hand, antibiotics may reduce the risk of rheumatic fever (a rare, but serious complication of GABHS infection).

Management

Rational management of sore throat begins with a careful history and physical examination. Special attention should be paid to the four cardinal symptoms of GABHS pharyngitis:

- Absence of cough
- Fever by history or measured in the office
- Tonsillar exudate
- Cervical adenopathy

Using the clinical rule described in *Table 1*, patients can be divided into three groups according to their risk of GABHS pharyngitis. Those with a very low probability of GABHS pharyngitis (< 3%) can usually be reassured and receive symptomatic treatment. They require neither testing nor treatment. Those with a very high probability of GABHS pharyngitis should be considered for empiric antibiotic therapy. Patients with an intermediate probability of GABHS pharyngitis should have their therapy guided by the results of a rapid antigen test. Patients who have a negative rapid antigen screen and a low-to-moderate risk of GABHS pharyngitis based on their history and physical examination do not require a throat culture to confirm the absence of GABHS.

Patients with suspected viral pharyngitis should be encouraged to drink plenty of fluids, take an antipyretic if they have fever, and consider the use of 2% lidocaine gargle, throat lozenges, or nonsteroidal anti-inflammatories (ibuprofen) to reduce the pain of sore throat *(Brain 2)*.

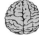
2 - Patients may often expect or even request antibiotics for what is apparently a viral condition. Studies have shown, however, that patient satisfaction is determined by the amount of time spent explaining the condition and the quality of that explanation and is not related to whether or not the patient actually received a prescription for antibiotics.

Table I. McIsaac's Modification of Centor's Strep Score

1. Add up the points for your patient:		2. Find the risk of strep.		
Symptom or sign	Points	Total Points	Likelihood Ratio	Percentage with Strep (Patients with Strep/Total)
History of fever or measured temperature > 38°C	1	-1 or 0	0.05	1% (2/179)
Absence of cough	1	1	0.52	10% (13/134)
Tender anterior cervical adenopathy	1	2	0.95	17% (18/109)
Tonsillar swelling or exudates	1	3	2.5	35% (28/81)
Age < 15 years	1	4 or 5	4.9	51% (39/77)
Age ≥ 45 years	-1			
Total:		Note: Baseline risk of strep is 17% in this population		

Data from a group of 167 children over the age of 3 and 453 adults in Ontario, Canada. (Adapted from McIsaac WJ, Goel V, To T, Low DE: The validity of a sore throat score in family practice. CMAJ 163:811–815, 2000.)

Children and teenagers with suspected infectious mononucleosis require close follow-up and should be warned against participating in contact sports. It is not unusual to see a coexisting GABHS pharyngitis infection in these patients as well as airway obstruction due to massive tonsillar enlargement. Such patients may require hospitalization, intravenous steroids, and close monitoring.

Selected Readings

1. DeMeyere M, Mervielde Y, Verschraegen G, Bogaert M: Effect of penicillin on the clinical course of streptococcal pharyngitis in general practice. Eur J Clin Pharmacol 43:581–585, 1992.
2. Gerber MA: Diagnosis and treatment of group A streptococcal pharyngitis. Semin Pediatr Infect Dis 9:42–49, 1998.
3. Green M: Non-streptococcal pharyngitis. Semin Pediatr Infect Dis 9:56–59, 1998.
4. Hamm RM, Hicks RJ, Bemben DA: Antibiotics and respiratory infections: Are patients more satisfied when expectations are met? J Fam Pract 43:56–62, 1996.
5. Hoffman S: An algorithm for a selective use of throat swabs in the diagnosis of group A streptococcal pharyngo-tonsillitis in general practice. Scand J Prim Health Care 10:295–300, 1992.
6. Komaroff A, Aronson MD, Pass TM, et al: Serologic evidence of chlamydial and mycoplasmal pharyngitis in adults. Science 222:927–928, 1983.
7. Poses RM, Cebul RD, Collins M, Fager SS: The importance of disease prevalence in transporting clinical prediction rules. Ann Intern Med 105:586–591, 1986.
8. Sloane P, Slatt L, Curtis P, Ebell MH: Essentials of Family Medicine, 3rd ed. Baltimore, Williams & Wilkins; 1998.

59. Substance Abuse

W. David Robinson, PhD, LMFT • Layne A. Prest, PhD, LMFT

Synopsis

Problematic substance use takes on many forms, including misuse, abuse, dependence, and addiction *(Definition 1)*. Alcohol, prescription drugs, illegal drugs, and other substances (e.g., glue, gasoline, propellants) can be used for their intoxicating effects. The highest rates of illicit drug use are found in the 16–20 age group. Alcohol abuse is a leading cause of preventable mortality and morbidity. The 18–29 age group has the highest prevalence of problem drinkers.

Substance abuse can be found in families of all socioeconomic, racial, and ethnic groups. Substance abuse can negatively affect the lives of family members at many levels because of associated relational, social, and legal difficulties. Paradoxically, substance abusers are often enabled by family members who may rationalize or cover for their addictive behavior patterns.

The impact of the substance on the individual and the family depends on the type of drug, length of use, amount being used, and any comorbid conditions. Physicians need to regularly include substance abuse screening in their encounters with patients. Denial is often a complicating factor when working with these individuals and families. For this reason, physicians must provide a safe, nonjudgmental environment so patients can share their struggles. Successful intervention with these patients is based on (1) the individual's desire to stop *(Brain 1)*, (2) effective detoxification, (3) treatment of dual diagnoses, (4) in- or outpatient treatment, and (5) relapse prevention (e.g., individual and/or family treatment or Alcoholics Anonymous).

1 - Abuse: The use of a substance to intoxication or excess.

Addiction: A person's emotional and behavioral response to the physiologic and psychological need for a substance whererin the person seeks out, uses, or consumes the substance despite adverse physical, emotional, spiritual, vocational, or relational consequences.

Dependence: The physiologic need to have a substance in order to avoid withdrawal.

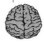

1 - It is important to intervene at the appropriate level in a patient's readiness for change (see table on page 50). The goal should be to help the patient progress to the next level. Progress toward abstinence is still progress. In this slow process, trying to push a patient too fast may result in not having any influence at all.

Differential Diagnosis

With substance abuse, a variety of possible comorbid conditions may either contribute to or result from the substance abuse:

- Mood disorders
- Anxiety disorders
- Other psychiatric disorders (e.g., schizophrenia, bipolar disorder)
- Marital or family dysfunction
- Partner or child abuse
- Physical injury to self or engaging in dangerous behaviors (driving while intoxicated; falls, especially in the elderly)
- Overdosing

Alcohol abuse may present with the following symptoms:

- Gastrointestinal tract disorders (chronic inflammation, malignancies, Mallory-Weiss tears, esophageal varices, peptic ulcer disease)

- Malnutrition
- "Fatty liver"
- Alcoholic hepatitis
- Cirrhosis
- Pancreatitis
- Nervous system disorders (numbness, weakness, fatigue)
- Cardiovascular system disorders (fatigue, hypertension, palpitations, shortness of breath, arrhythmia)
- Withdrawal

History

Many substance-abusing patients deny they have a problem. For this reason, they usually will not present with substance abuse as the initial focus. Therefore, looking for simple clues such as work absenteeism, marital discord, and vehicular and everyday accidents can help uncover substance abuse. It is important to conduct the interview in a matter-of-fact, nonjudgmental way. Effective interviewing and assessment often includes brief screening methods such as the CAGE questionnaire *(Table 1)*.

Table 1. The CAGE Method*

C	Have you ever felt that you ought to **c**ut down on your substance usage?
A	Have you ever been **a**nnoyed by people criticizing your substance use?
G	Have you ever felt **g**uilty or bad about your substance use?
E	Have you ever had to use the substance first thing in the morning to get your day going, steady your nerves, or to treat a hangover (**e**ye-opener)?

*One positive response indicates high risk for abuse.
Adapted from Ewing JA. Detecting alcoholism: The CAGE questionnaire. JAMA 252:1905–1907, 1984.

Initial screening:

- "What brings you in today? What symptoms are you experiencing?" See associated chapters for specific problems (i.e., abdominal pain, gastritis).
- Determine the extent of patients' use of drugs and alcohol by asking in a matter-of-fact way if they drink or use drugs *(Table 2)*. Normalize the questions about substance use (history portion of the interview) by stating that these questions are asked of all your patients. Insert these questions with other screening questions (e.g., safe sex, smoking).

If substance abuse is suspected, probe for more information:

- "Sometimes symptoms like these are related to a person's lifestyle; for example, diet, exercise, stress level, family strife, or substance use."

Once that problem is understood and alcohol or substance use surfaces, address the following issues as appropriate:

- "How long have you used this substance?" *(Red Flag 1)*
- "When was the last time you used it?"
- "Do your physical symptoms worsen after use?"
- "Do you use the substance to alleviate the symptoms or cope with problems?"

1 - The patient is at high risk for abuse if the patient was 14 years or younger when he or she began using alcohol, drugs, or both.

Table 2. Differentiation of Substance Abuse

Use Pattern	Description
Substance misuse	Occasional use of a legal or illegal substance to excess
Substance abuse	A maladaptive pattern of substance use occurring within a 12-month period that causes impairment in social or occupational functioning (job, legal, and interpersonal problems)
Substance dependence	A maladaptive pattern of substance use occurring within a 12-month period, leading to significant impairment or distress, and characterized by either tolerance or withdrawal (even if withdrawal does not happen because the patient uses a substance to relieve or avoid withdrawal symptoms)

- "What is the quantity you are using?" Try to exaggerate the option. For example: "Did you drink 12 to 15 beers last time you drank?" This allows patients to state that they drank less.
- "Are you using any other substances?" Use of multiple substances is common.
- If alcohol, "What are you drinking? Beer? Wine? Hard liquor?"
- "When do you start using the substance during the day?"
- "Do you find that you need more and more of the substance to get the desired effect?" Patient may have developed *tolerance* to the substance *(Definition 2)*.
- "Have you been in any trouble with the law?"
- "Are you having any trouble with family members because of your substance use?"
- "Are you having any work or occupational problems?"
- If family members are present, the physician may ask about their concern about the patient's substance abuse. This may need to be in a private setting, and physical abuse should be assessed (see Chapter 46).

2 - Tolerance: The process of the body adapting to the presence of a substance to the extent that it takes more of a substance to achieve the desired level of intoxication.

Physical Examination

Conduct a routine physical exam looking for physical findings associated with the substance being used:

- Vital signs, especially tachycardia (e.g., signs of withdrawal, agitation)
- General appearance (e.g., is the patient oriented, well-groomed?)
- Skin (e.g., track marks, extremity edema)
- HEENT (e.g., nasal atrophy, perforation associated with inhaled substances)
- Pulmonary (breathing problems can be caused by a variety of substances)
- Abdominal exam (e.g., liver enlargement, tenderness)
- Central nervous system (CNS) (e.g., tremor, neuropathy, confusion, delirium)

Testing

2 - Make sure you get informed consent from the patient. If testing is employer-mandated, inform the patient about his or her rights and possible problems that can occur if the drug test turns up positive.

Drug testing may be required as part of a pre-employment physical exam *(Red Flag 2)* and may include:

- Drug screen (urine or blood)
- Liver function test
- Basic metabolic panel
- Complete blood cell count (CBC)
- HIV and hepatitis A, B, and C

Putting It All Together

Substance abuse is a very broad topic. It can present in a variety of ways, and its manifestations are often subtle. The patient and, many times, the family will deny that substance use is an issue for them. The primary care physician should be proactive in addressing substance use. It is also important to assess the patient's stage of readiness so as to intervene at the appropriate level. In working with substance abuse, a biopsychosocial perspective is the most influential because of the effects on individuals and families at multiple levels.

Management

Management of substance abuse is a difficult process because of the abuser's denial *(Brain 2)* and family members' enabling behaviors *(Brain 3)*. Management also can be frustrating because relapse is common. However, the benefits of helping patients recover from substance abuse can be rewarding. Substance abuse recovery directly influences the health of the individual, thus reducing health care costs. Recovery also reduces stress on the family, increases the likelihood that the individual can be a productive member of society, and decreases the occurrence of criminal behaviors.

The first step in working with substance-abusing patients is to help them understand that their behaviors are negatively affecting their own health and the welfare of their families. A family meeting can be an initial step in starting the treatment process. Once the individual is willing to seek treatment, options need to be explored. The choices are often determined by the individual's insurance. For individuals who are physically addicted to the drug, in-patient detoxification is often necessary. Once the long-term substance abuser has gone through physical withdrawal, in-patient, long-term treatment may be necessary. This option, however, is often not reimbursed by third-party payors. Other options include intensive outpatient treatment, outpatient psychotherapy (individual, marital, and family), group therapy, and support groups (see Appendix).

All can be helpful in the recovery process. However, because these options are often short-term, physician follow-up for physical problems and recovery maintenance is very important.

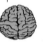

2 - Challenge the patient to a week of sobriety if he or she claims it isn't a problem and have the patient follow up. If this fails, help the patient readdress the extent of the abuse; depending on the patient's response:
- Encourage another trial week using the new insight
- Encourage patient to attend Alcoholics Anonymous
- Encourage patient to attend individual psychotherapy
- Negotiate treatment plan including appropriate follow-up (two weeks or less)

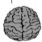

3 - When seeing a patient who has a family member with a substance abuse problem:
- Ask how patient is dealing with the substance abuse and its effects on him/her and the family.
- Find out if the patient also has a substance abuse problem
- Validate the patient's frustrations with the substance abuse
- Help the patient understand enabling behaviors and encourage her or him to develop some healthy boundaries.
- Offer the patient help through Al-Anon or individual psychotherapy.

Selected Readings

1. Ewing JA: Detecting alcoholism: The CAGE questionnaire. JAMA 252:1905–1907, 1984.
2. Prochaska J, DiClemente C: Toward a comprehensive model of change. In Miller W, Heather N (eds): Addictive Behaviors: Processes of Change. New York, Plenum Press, 1986, pp 3–27.

Appendix: Referral and Information Organizations

Al-Anon Family Group
National Referral Hotline
800-344-2666

Alcoholics Anonymous (AA)-Worldwide
475 Riverside Drive
New York, NY 10115
212-870-3400
www.alcoholics-anonymous.org

American Society of Addiction Medicine
4601 North Park Avenue
Suite 101, Upper Arcade
Chevy Chase, MD 20815
301-656-3920
E-mail: asamoffice@aol.com

Drug Abuse Information and Treatment Referral Line
800-662-HELP; Spanish 800-66-AYUDA

Narcotics Anonymous and Nar-Anon Family Group
Nationwide referral line: 202-399-5316

National Alcohol Screening Day
(Project Headquarters)
781-239-0071

National Clearinghouse for Alcohol and Drug Information
P.O. Box 2345
Rockville, MD 20847-2345
800-729-6686
www.help.org

National Council on Alcoholism and Drug Dependence
12 West 21st Street
New York, NY 10010
800-622-2255 or 800-475-4673
www.ncadd.org

National Institute on Drug Abuse
5600 Fishers Lane, Room 10-05
Rockville, MD 20857

Nationwide helpline: 800-662-HELP
www.nida.nih.gov

60. Thermal Injuries

Jeffrey D. Harrison, MD

Synopsis

Thermal injury refers to topical injury of the skin from temperature extremes as well as elevated or decreased body temperature. The morbidity from these injuries involves pain, disfigurement, and dysfunction, whereas the major mortality involves inhalation injury and carbon monoxide poisoning. Electrical injury is a specialized type of burn that often requires burn center treatment because of the large area of injury that occurs below the skin. Hyperthermia can lead to disordered thermoregulation and death if untreated. Frostbite injuries from cold can cause as much morbidity to the patient as any burn injury and may take weeks or months to reveal their full damage. Hypothermia is a lowered body temperature and can be a comorbidity in many injuries and trauma.

Injuries Due to Heat

Differential Diagnosis

Burns can be classified in the following way *(Table 1)*:

- Superficial burn or first-degree
- Partial-thickness burns or second-degree
- Full-thickness burns or third-degree

Three specialized types of burns exist that need consideration:

- Chemical burns
- Electrical burns
- Inhalation injuries, including upper airway burns and carbon monoxide poisoning

Hyperthermia or elevated body temperature could indicate:

- Heat exhaustion: body temperature > 37.8°C with weakness, fatigue, and moist skin
- Heat stroke: body temperature > 41°C with loss of thermoregulatory mechanism (no sweating)

History

In assessing topical burns, pertinent historical information includes:

- What is the duration of the exposure?
- What body parts were exposed? (face, digits, and genitalia are more serious)
- What agent caused the burn (e.g., water, grease, etc)?
- What time did the burn occur? *(Brain 1)*
- What was the environment in which the burn occurred? *(Brain 2)*

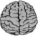

1 - The time of the burn is important for determining the volume and rate of fluid replacement in extensive full- and partial-thickness burns.

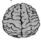

2 - The burn environment is important because other nonburn injuries may exist, such as smoke inhalation in an enclosed space and internal injuries from explosions.

308

Table 1. Burn Classification

Classification	Description
Superficial or first-degree (e.g., sunburn)	Erythematous and painful Involve only the epidermis Do not blister
Partial-thickness or second-degree	Painful and erythematous Often blister Extend to the dermal-epidermal junction May appear mottled with local swelling May have wet or weeping surface
Full-thickness or third-degree	Painless (due to destruction of the nerve endings) Dry surface May appear pale, white, and leathery or have a red, mottled appearance Can initially appear as partial thickness, but will lack sensation

Chemical exposures history:

- What agent is involved?
- What is the concentration of the agent?
- What was the duration of contact?
- What was the amount of agent involved?

Electrical injury history:

- What are the entry and exit sites?
- What was the source of the electricity (lightning, power line)?

Hyperthermia:

- What was the patient doing?
- Where was the patient?
- Prior problems with heat?
- Sweating or not? *(Red Flag 1)*

1 - Patients with heat stroke have lost their thermoregulatory ability and will not sweat. This is a life-threatening condition.

Pertinent past history for all thermal and cold injuries:

- Diabetes (delayed tissue healing)
- Cardiovascular disease
- Pulmonary disease
- Allergies and sensitivities
- Tetanus status *(Brain 3)*
- Smoking history (increased carbon monoxide levels)

3 - A fully immunized patient (3 doses) should have a booster if > 5 years have passed since the last booster.

Physical Examination

All thermal injury victims should first have the ABCs of life support addressed *(Brain 4)* along with an initial set of vital signs, including weight. For topical burn victims, the initial evaluation should focus on the depth of the burn (see Table 1) and the percent of body surface area (BSA) involved. Initially, it may be difficult to determine if a burn is superficial or partial thickness.

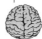

4 - Airway, breathing, and circulation: This would include the presence of a patent airway, adequate ventilation and breathing, and a perfusing circulatory system.

Estimate the BSA involved. The BSA can broken down into multiples of 9% ("the rule of nines") *(Brain 5)*.

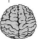

5 - This has importance in determining the need for a burn center transfer as well as the volume of IV fluid the patient would need.

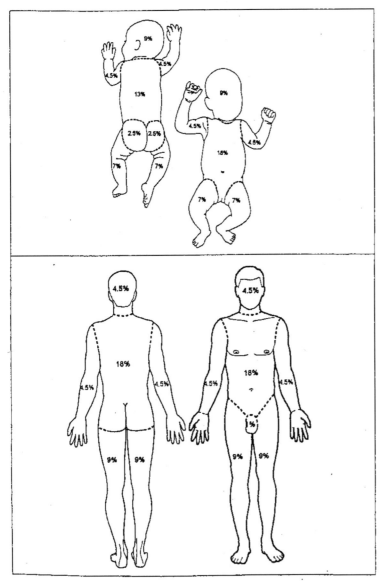

Figure 1: Rule of nines.
(From American College of Surgeons Committee on Trauma (ed): Advanced Trauma Life Support for Doctors. 6th ed. Chicago, IL, American College of Surgeons, 1997, with permission.)

- Head and each upper extremity compose about 9% (greater in infants)
- Each lower extremity comprises 18% (less in infants)
- Front and back of the torso=18%
- The palms, excluding the fingers, comprise about 1% of the BSA in most individuals *(Figure 1)*

Assess for associated injuries to the airway *(Red Flag 2)*:

- Facial burns
- Singed eyebrows and nasal hair
- Carbonaceous sputum
- Inflammatory changes in the oropharynx

 2 - The greatest cause of morbidity and mortality involve airway problems. Hot air and gases can cause upper airway burns, which lead to swelling and obstruction just above the vocal cords.

Assess for hyperthermia

- Elevated core body temperature (rectal > 41°C)
- Altered mental status
- Anhydrosis: indicates heat stroke (loss of thermoregulatory mechanisms)
- Moist skin: indicates heat exhaustion

Testing

Superficial burns and limited partial thickness:

- No specific lab or x-ray testing is needed

Patients with possible inhalation injuries:

- Carbon monoxide level **(Red Flag 3)**
- Chest x-ray

Patients who have sustained electrical shock injuries:

- Urine myoglobin **(Brain 6)**
- Electrocardiogram (EKG)
- Continuous EKG monitoring

Heat exhaustion and heat stroke:

- Electrolytes
- Urinalysis

Putting It All Together

The majority of patients who present to the clinic with burns will have superficial or partial-thickness injuries involving limited body surface area. Their greatest concern will be pain relief and the risk of possible scarring. The practitioner should perform a brief history and exam to determine the need for more advanced levels of care. Specifically, the search for full-thickness burns and concomitant injury (e.g., inhalation, falls) should be done. If no serious problem is found, the focus should move to controlling pain pharmacologically and covering the injured areas to prevent irritation of the injured nerve endings. The integrity of burned skin is lost; therefore, protection from infection is paramount in treating burn injuries.

In those cases where inhalation injury is suspected based on a history of an enclosed setting or evidence of upper airway burn (facial burn, nasal singeing, carbonaceous sputum), the possibility of carbon monoxide poisoning and upper airway obstruction also should be considered. These patients are best managed in a burn center or appropriate hospital setting.

Electrical injuries can appear far less serious than they actually are. The history and exam should focus on the source of electricity as well as the entry and exit sites. These patients can have injury to the cardiac conduction system and to large volumes of muscle tissue.

Heat exhaustion is characterized by elevated temperature, moist skin, and tachycardia. It occurs in hot environments where the patient has both water and sodium depletion. The patient is usually thirsty, weak, and anxious. Treatment is focused on rehydration and lowering the

3 - Carbon monoxide has 240 times the affinity for hemoglobin as oxygen does; this prevents the hemoglobin from carrying oxygen to the tissues. The half-life of carbon monoxide is 4 hours when the patient is breathing room air; it is decreased to 40 minutes when breathing 100% oxygen. Those with levels below 20% usually have no symptoms; from 20–40% there is nausea, headache, and confusion; coma will develop above 40%; and death occurs at 60%.

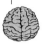

6 - Urine myoglobin is a breakdown product from muscle injury; high levels can cause renal failure.

body temperature. If left untreated, heat exhaustion can lead to heat stroke.

Heat stroke is a life-threatening condition resulting from the failure of the body's thermoregulatory mechanism. The classic findings include elevated body temperature (> 41°C), impaired level of conscious, and absence of sweating. This condition requires immediate reduction of the core body temperature to at least 39°C. Evaporative methods are the treatment of choice using cool water and fans; immersion in ice baths is contraindicated. Fluid replacement through an IV is indicated as is close observation of electrolyte levels.

Management

Management of topical burns begins with stopping the burning process by removing any offending substance, be it chemical residue or charred clothing. *Table 2* outlines treatment for cutaneous burns.

Inhalation injury treatment:

- 100% oxygen
- Endotracheal intubation
- Carboxyhemoglobin level
- Burn center transfer

Electrical injury treatment:

- Cardiac monitoring
- Maintain urine output at 100 ml/hour
- Consider burn center
- Sterile dressing for entry and exit injury

Chemical injury treatment:

- Brush away dry powders
- Copious irrigation for at least 20–30 minutes
- Longer irrigation for alkali

Heat exhaustion treatment:

- Place in cool, shaded environment
- Oral or intravenous isotonic saline hydration (1–2 L)
- 24 hours of rest

Table 2. Cutaneous Injury Treatment

Depth of Burn	Treatment
Superficial	Clean dressing Topical antibacterial, such as silver sulfadiazine (Silvadene) Non-narcotic pain medication
Partial-thickness	Cover with sterile dressing Silvadene if not transferring Leave intact blisters Debride broken blisters Pain control—consider narcotics Update tetanus 24-hours follow-up
Full-thickness (most will need burn center transfer) *(Brain 7)*	Cover with sterile dressing Avoid ointments Determine fluid needs *(Brain 8)*

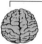

7 - Patients should be taken to a burn center if they exhibit any of the following:
- Partial- or full-thickness burns > 20% BSA
- Partial- or full-thickness burns on hands, feet, face, genitals, or major joints
- Full-thickness > 5% BSA
- Significant electrical burns
- Inhalation injury

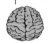

8 - The formula for fluid replacement in burn victims is 2–4 ml/kg/%BSA burned. This should be administered in the first 24 hours after injury where half the volume is given in the first 8 hours. Normal saline or lactated Ringer's is the solution of choice.

Heat stroke treatment:

- Rapid reduction of core temperature (< 39°C)
- Remove clothing
- Cool water (15°C) or mist
- Fan or air current across patient
- IV fluid replacement (normal saline)
- Monitor electrolytes and urine
- Avoid re-exposure

Injuries Due to Cold

Differential Diagnosis

- Frostbite: freezing injury to the skin
- Hypothermia (body temperature < 35°C)

History

- What was the temperature of the exposure?
- What was the duration of the exposure?
- What was the environment in which the injury occurred? *(Brain 9)*

Physical Examination

In patients with frostbite and cold exposure, it may be difficult to determine the extent of the injury until weeks or months after demarcation of nonviable tissue has occurred.

Superficial frostbite:

- Pale gray skin that is pliable
- May develop blisters within 24–48 hours

Deep frostbite:

- Skin will feel woody
- Develop dark (hemorrhagic) blisters after several weeks
- Will appear cool and mottled even after rewarming
- Can be edematous for up to 1 month

Hypothermia is characterized by a low body temperature; findings include:

- Depressed level of consciousness
- Cold to the touch
- Gray and cyanotic skin
- Depressed vital signs *(Brain 10)*

Testing

No lab or x-rays are usually indicated for frostbite. For those with hypothermia, lab testing includes:

- Complete blood count (CBC)
- Electrolytes and glucose
- Alcohol (frequently a compounding morbidity) and toxin screen
- Electrocardiographic monitoring (increased risk of ventricular fibrillation)

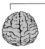

9 - Immobilization, concomitant trauma, prolonged time, and moisture all increase the severity of cold injury.

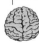

10 - Favorable findings on initial exam include pinprick sensitivity, normal color, warmth, large clear blisters, and edema. Unfavorable findings on initial exam include cold cyanotic distal tissues, small dark blisters, and absence of edema. Those body areas most frequently involved are the nose, ears, fingertips, and toes.

Putting It All Together

Patients who have sustained freezing skin injury need rapid rewarming of the affected skin while at the same time avoiding aggressive manipulation of the injured area. The history should focus on the duration and severity of the exposure. A history of prior freezing injury is a risk factor for a poor outcome. As with burn injury, the risk of infection is increased for these patients.

Hypothermia is a lowered body temperature often characterized by a decreased level of consciousness, depressed vital signs, and cold skin. The history should focus on the duration of exposure and other comorbidities (alcohol is frequently involved). Rapid rewarming is the key to treating these patients. Cardiac monitoring is indicated during the rewarming process.

Management

Frostbite:

- Rapid rewarming with circulating water that is 104–110°F for 20–30 minutes or until skin flushed
- Keep injured tissues elevated
- Avoid trauma
- Leave blisters intact
- IV pain medications if painful injury
- Update tetanus

Hypothermia (patient temperature 30–35°C):

- Passive rewarming
- Warm blankets and clothes
- Warmed IV fluids

Hypothermia (< 30°C):

- Active rewarming
- Peritoneal lavage
- Hemodialysis
- Cardiopulmonary bypass
- Cardiac monitoring

Selected Reading

American College of Surgeons Committee on Trauma (ed): Advanced Trauma Life Support for Doctors, 6th ed. Chicago, IL, American College of Surgeons, 1997.

61. Trauma

Jeffrey D. Harrison, MD

Synopsis

Students primarily will be observers in the care of the trauma patient. However, an understanding of the basic principles of trauma care will help the student become an informed spectator and ready to assume increased responsibility with added experience. Trauma-related deaths have a trimodal distribution. The first peak of death occurs within seconds to minutes of the injury and generally is caused by lacerations of the aorta, spinal cord, brain stem, and other large vessels. Very few of these injuries are treatable, and prevention is the only way to decrease the number of deaths from these conditions.

The second peak occurs minutes to hours after the injury. Patients within this group may survive with rapid assessment and resuscitation, the basic principle of advanced trauma care. The cause of death in this group includes subdural hematoma, epidural hematoma, tension pneumothorax, splenic lacerations, and pelvic fractures.

The third peak of death occurs days to weeks after the injury and is due to sepsis and multiorgan failure. Early care has a direct effect on the outcome in this group.

Three underlying concepts to early trauma care are essential:

- Treat the greatest threat to life first.
- The lack of a definitive diagnosis should not delay appropriate interventions.
- A detailed history is not required to begin the evaluation of an injured patient.

All trauma patients should be evaluated by the ABCDE approach *(Brain 1)*.

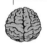

1 - ABCDE approach to trauma:
A Airway
B Breathing
C Circulation
D Disability
E Exposure

Differential Diagnosis

The goal of the primary evaluation in the trauma patient is to identify those conditions that are immediately life-threatening and correctable.

Absence of a patent airway is the greatest risk to the patient. Possible causes include:

- Altered mental status, decreased level of conscious
- Mid-face trauma

Inadequate ventilation (breathing) is the next greatest risk:

- Tension pneumothorax: increased intrapleural pressures due to a valve-like mechanism that allows air to enter the pleural space from the lung but not to escape

- Pulmonary contusion: trauma to the lung parenchyma resulting in fluid and blood in the alveoli, interstitial spaces, and bronchi
- Flail chest: fracture of four or more ribs resulting in paradoxical respiratory motion leading to hypoventilaton
- Open pneumothorax: a defect in the chest wall allowing communication of the pleural space with the environment
- Hemothorax: an accumulation of blood in the pleural space resulting from injury to the lung, chest wall, mediastinum, or diaphragm

Inadequate perfusion (circulation) is the next condition that must be identified:

- Hypovolemia (most common cause)
- Internal bleeding (spleen, liver, great vessels)
- Fractures of the pelvis or long bones
- External bleeding from lacerations and amputations

Neurologic injury (disability) is the next area to be identified:

- Subdural hematoma: bridging vein injury resulting in blood collection in the plane between the dura and arachnoid
- Epidural hematoma: dural artery injury resulting in a blood collection between the skull and dura
- Diffuse axonal injury: prolonged post-traumatic coma that is not due to a mass lesion or ischemic insult

History

A complete history is not essential in the evaluation and treatment of the trauma patient. Instead use the mnemonic AMPLE to guide the history *(Brain 2)*. The most essential piece of information that must be obtained is the mechanism of the injury. If the patient cannot provide this information, it should be obtained from prehospital personnel (EMTs), family members, or other observers.

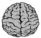

2 - AMPLE mnemonic:
A Allergies
M Medications
P Past illness
L Last meal
E Events involving the injury

Key questions to consider when evaluating motor vehicle accident victims include:

- Seat belt usage (tenfold reduction in serious injury)
- Ejection from the vehicle (300% increase in serious injury)
- Vehicular damage
- Other passenger deaths
- Steering wheel or windshield damage

In gunshot wounds, the key questions include:

- The caliber of the gun
- Location of entry and exit wounds
- Distance from the gun to the victim

In falls, key questions include:

- The distance of the fall
- Body area affected by initial impact
- Type of surface struck

Other pertinent factors include:

- Prehospital interventions by rescue personnel

- Vital signs (particularly trends in pulse, respiratory rate, and blood pressure)
- Tetanus status *(Brain 3)*

Remember, when dealing with major trauma, a detailed history is not required to begin treating serious injuries.

 3 - If a patient has had three primary immunizations, a booster should be given if more than 5 years have lapsed. For patients who have not received three primary immunizations, tetanus immune globulin and a booster dose should be given.

Physical Examination

The goal of the examination is to identify the most rapid causes of death. The ABCDE approach is followed.

Airway patency is the first priority, and the provider examines the patient for objective signs of airway obstruction by *(Red Flag 1)*:

- Looking for agitation, obtundation, cyanosis, or retractions
- Listening for abnormal sounds such as gurgling, snoring or **stridor** *(Definition 1)*
- Feeling the trachea to assure a midline position

 1 - Any patient with an altered level of conscious is at increased risk for airway obstruction. All trauma patients should be given supplemental oxygen and should be assumed to have a cervical-spine injury until proven otherwise.

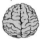 **1** - **Stridor:** High-pitched sounds made during inspiration, indicating upper airway obstruction.

Breathing or adequate ventilation is the next priority. This is evaluated by:

- Looking for a symmetrical chest rise with inhalation
- Listening with the stethoscope on both sides of the chest for equal breath sounds
- Percussing the chest wall for hyperresonance *(Brain 4)*

 4 - An asymmetric chest rise indicates a flail chest or malpositioned endotracheal tube (if the patient was previously intubated). Unequal breath sounds or hyperresonance can indicate a pneumothorax, flail chest, or hemothorax.

Circulation or recognition of the shock state is the next priority in the exam *(Definition 2)*. Exam priorities are:

- Checking pulses for tachycardia and a narrowed pulse pressure (the difference between the systolic and diastolic blood pressure)
- Looking for external hemorrhage (bleeding is the most common cause of shock in the trauma patient)
- Checking skin color
- Determining level of conscious (inadequate perfusion of the brain can cause confusion or agitation)
- Looking at the neck veins for distention (tension pneumothorax or pericardial tamponade)

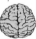 **2** - **Shock:** A clinical state characterized by inadequate organ perfusion and tissue oxygenation. It is not defined by the blood pressure.

Disability refers to doing a brief neurologic exam. This is important to have as a baseline because any future neurologic examination will be compared to this evaluation. Key components include:

- The patient's level of conscious *(Brain 5)*
- Pupillary size and response *(Red Flag 2)*

 5 - The AVPU mnemonic is a helpful way to describe the patient's level of consciousness when the patient is alert, responds to voice, and responds to pain, or is unresponsive to all stimuli.

Exposure is the final part of the initial exam.

- Completely undress the patient
- Maintain body temperature and avoid hypothermia

2 - The patient's pupillary size and response to light also should be documented because unequal size can indicate increased intracranial pressure from bleeding or swelling, a situation that mandates immediate neurosurgical consultation.

Once the initial examination is completed and the patient is stabilized, a head-to-toe exam should be performed. This includes:

- Gathering a complete history
- Performing a detailed physical examination on all body parts (including the back)

Table 1. Glasgow Coma Scale

Variable	Patient Response	Score
Eye opening	Spontaneous	4
	To speech	3
	To pain	2
	None	1
Best motor response	Obeys	6
	Localizes	5
	Withdraws	4
	Abnormal flexion	3
	Extension response	2
	None	1
Verbal response	Oriented	5
	Confused conversation	4
	Inappropriate words	2
	Incomprehensible	2
	None	1

- Reassessing all vital signs and previously performed exams
- Performing a detailed neurologic exam, including the Glasgow Coma Scale. The Glasgow Coma Scale is a more detailed neurologic evaluation and should be performed once the patient has been stabilized **(Table 1)**.

Testing

In the trauma patient, several basic tests need to be run; however, none of them should delay the resuscitation of the patient.

Three portable x-rays should be considered in all trauma victims:

- Lateral cervical spine film **(Brain 6)**
- Anteroposterior (AP) chest film (may reveal life-threatening injuries such as pneumothorax or aortic tear in the form of wide mediastinum)
- AP pelvis (fractures may indicate large volumes of blood loss, raising suspicion for shock and need for blood transfusion)

Other imaging should be ordered based on clinical findings but not until the patient has been stabilized.

Trauma patients should have:

- Continuous EKG monitoring to look for arrhythmia
- Continuous pulse oximetry to assess oxygenation **(Brain 7)**
- Colorimetric carbon dioxide detector attached to an endotracheal tube or arterial blood gas (ABG) analysis to follow ventilation **(Brain 8)**

Initial blood testing in trauma patients should include:

- Complete blood cell count (CBC)
- Chemical analysis
- Pregnancy testing **(Red Flag 3)**
- Type and cross match **(Brain 9)**

6 - Cervical spine film should be done in those with trauma above the clavicles or mental status changes. This film can prove a cervical spinal (c-spine) injury is present, but a normal film does not exclude a c-spine injury. An adequate c-spine film must show all 7 cervical vertebrae including the C7–T1 interspace. If this cannot be obtained either a specialized view (swimmer's view) or a computed tomography (CT) scan of the cervical spine must be performed.

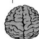

7 - The oxygen saturation (SaO_2) should be kept at > 95%. Although this is a useful noninvasive adjunct to follow oxygenation, it does not provide meaningful information regarding ventilation.

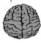

8 - A low pH (< 7.35) and a high pCO_2 (> 40) suggest inadequate ventilation (respiratory acidosis).

3 - A positive pregnancy test should not delay or cause the omission of any essential intervention or diagnostic test in the mother. The best chance for fetal survival rests with rapid resuscitation and stabilization of the mother.

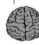

9 - Complete cross match usually will take about an hour, and this blood is the ideal replacement. Type- and Rh-specific blood will take about 10 minutes to be available in most labs; this is the next preferable choice, although minor incompatibilities may exist. Type O-negative blood is indicated when type-specific blood is unavailable.

Putting It All Together

The manner in which trauma patients present can be overwhelming, and it is imperative to follow a rapid and thorough system to ascertain life-threatening injuries. In the typical office encounter, a thorough history, exam, and assessment can be performed. In trauma patients, a rapid assessment with a highly focused history and physical is performed followed by near-simultaneous treatment.

During the initial encounter with a trauma patient, the ABCDE system should be followed, with diagnosis and treatment of problems addressed as they are found. Establishment of a patent airway is the first priority along with the addition of supplemental oxygen while maintaining cervical spine protection. Assurance that adequate ventilation is occurring should be performed next by observation of chest rise and auscultation of breath sounds. If endotracheal intubation or chest tube insertion is indicated, it should be performed here. Evaluation of the circulatory system is the next step, which includes recording the blood pressure, palpation of the peripheral pulses (for presence, quality, and heart rate), and control of external hemorrhage (by direct pressure). Two large-bore peripheral IVs (≥ 16-gauge) should be started at this time. A baseline neurologic exam including pupillary light response and level of conscious is performed next. A Glasgow Coma Scale scoring can be performed here or during the complete exam once the patient is stabilized. Finally, all trauma patients should be completely undressed, but care should be taken to maintain body temperature.

Once these initial steps are completed and the patient is stabilized, the process should start over with reassessment of previously made diagnosis and interventions followed by a thorough head-to-toe exam. As problems are discovered, they should be treated. The three basic imaging studies (c-spine, chest x-ray, and AP pelvis) are accomplished along with indicated blood work. Also at this time, consideration should be given to the need for early surgical consultation and possible transfer to a trauma center.

Management

The overall theory in managing trauma patients is to expeditiously recognize and treat those conditions that are most immediately life-threatening.

Airway loss is the earliest cause of death, so control becomes paramount. Keep airways open by:

- Performing chin lift or jaw thrust maneuver
- Ensuring an oropharyngeal airway or nasopharyngeal airway patency
- Endotracheal intubation *(Red Flag 4)*

Ventilation and breathing are the next earliest causes of death. The following help maintain ventilation:

- Bag-valve mask or endotracheal intubation with ventilatory assist (1 breath every 5 seconds).
- Ensure proper tube position (equal breath sounds).
- Cover open chest wounds.
- Splint unstable chest wall sections.

4 - To prevent iatrogenic spinal cord injuries, care must be taken to ensure midline cervical spine immobilization with any airway maneuver.

- Place chest tube for pneumothorax or hemothorax.

Circulatory collapse is the next cause of death. To prevent this:

- External bleeding should be controlled with direct pressure.
- Two large-bore IVs should be should be placed peripherally (≥ 16-gauge).
- A 2-L bolus of lactated Ringer's solution (warmed) should be given to adults.
- A 20-ml/kg bolus of lactated Ringer's should be administered to children.
- Repeat boluses as needed *(Red Flag 5)*.

5 - Lack of response to the bolus is an indication for surgical consultation and possible blood transfusion.

Neurologic injury is the next priority:

- If Glasgow Coma Scale < 13, obtain neurosurgical consultation.
- Ensure adequate oxygenation.
- Promote mild hyperventilation via endotracheal intubation.
- Maintain euvolemic state (avoidance of overhydration or hypovolemia).
- Avoid dextrose-containing or hypotonic solutions.

Selected Reading

American College of Surgeons Committee on Trauma: Advanced Trauma Life Support for Doctors, 6th ed. Chicago, American College of Surgeons, 1997.

62. Urinary and Vaginal Symptoms in Adults

Maria M. Sandvig, MD

Synopsis

Vaginitis means inflammation of the vagina and is characterized by a vaginal discharge with an irritated vagina or cervix and increased vaginal mucus. When accompanied by vulvar inflammation, it is referred to as *vulvovaginitis*. Vaginitis is the most common gynecologic problem encountered by physicians providing primary care to women, and *Chlamydia* is the most commonly reported STD in the US. Young, sexually active patients often present with vaginal discharge, but women of all ages may be affected by vaginitis. Vaginal symptoms may be caused by bacterial, fungal, or protozoan infections, chemical irritation, or atrophy of vaginal tissues. A new pathogen or imbalance in the "vaginal ecosystem" leads to vaginitis. The vaginal equilibrium can be altered by sexually transmitted diseases (STDs), antibiotics, douching, oral contraceptive pills (OCPs), other hormones, sexual intercourse, intravaginal medications, stress, endocrine disorders, and a change in sexual partners.

Urinary symptoms may be related to a vaginal infection or a separate urinary tract infection, often called a *bladder infection* or *cystitis*. Women often know by their symptoms of dysuria, frequency, and urgency that they have a bladder or urinary tract infection (UTI). See **Table 1** for definitions of terms relevant to urinary and vaginal problems.

Differential Diagnosis

- Sexually transmitted infection
- Chemical irritation
- Yeast vaginitis
- Bladder infection
- Prostatitis (inflammation of the prostate)
- **Pelvic inflammatory disease** *(Definition 1)*
- Pregnancy (increased vaginal mucus production)
- Foreign body in vagina (old tampon or used condom)

 1 - Pelvic inflammatory disease: An ascending infection from the vagina or cervix that can lead to tubo-ovarian abscess, infertility due to scarred fallopian tubes, and increased risk for ectopic pregnancy. Signs include pelvic pain, abdominal pain, fever, cervical motion tenderness, and mucopurulent cervical discharge.

History

Common presenting complaints include: "I have a discharge," "My boyfriend has a discharge," "It hurts to pee," "I itch down there," " My stomach hurts a lot," and "I've got this terrible smell when I have sex," and "I want a Pap smear" *(Brain 1)*.

 1 - Many patients mistakenly think Pap smear means gynecologic exam to rule out infection.

Patients are often very concerned about being labeled as having an "STD." Thus, learning to obtain the history in a respectful, nonjudgmental manner can be key to building a relationship that will allow for the most accurate diagnosis, the most cost-effective and expedient therapy, and the greatest likelihood for future prevention. Work toward taking the history with the same attitude and facial expression you would have if you were asking questions about a sinus or upper respiratory infection.

Table 1. Common Terminology

Term	Definition
Atrophic vaginitis	A vaginal irritation seen when the estrogen levels decrease in peri- or post-menopausal women due to thinning and drying of the mucous membranes
Bacterial vaginosis	An overgrowth of bacterial species (*Gardnerella* and anaerobic bacteria), which leads to a malodorous discharge
Candidal vaginitis	A yeast infection that leads to a thick white discharge with intense pruritsus
Cervicitis	Inflammation of the cervix, often caused by an STD (e.g., chlamydia or gonorrhea) or a chemical exposure (e.g., spermicide) that appears red and may bleed easily if touched with a cotton swab, cytobrush, or spatula
Chemical irritation	A reaction to a foreign substance such as soap, perfumes, douching, minipads, latex condoms, or spermicide
Cystitis	Inflammation of the urinary bladder, also known as bladder infection or urinary tract infection (UTI)
Discharge	Mucus in the vagina that can originate from the vaginal walls or the cervical os
Dysuria	Pain with urination
Ectopic pregnancy	Pregnancy located outside of uterus, often in fallopian tube
Ectropion	Columnar epithelium on the ectocervix. It appears red as opposed to the pink squamous epithelium, and extends from the cervical os. It may bleed easily
Friable	Refers to mucosa that bleeds easily when touched with speculum or cotton swab
Frequency	Urinating more times than usual
Lesion	Excoriations, ulcers, blisters, or papillary structures seen on vulva, vagina, or cervix
Trichomonas vaginalis	A protozoal infection that can lead to a thin white or yellow, frothy discharge, vaginal itching, and pelvic discomfort or pain
Urethritis	Inflammation of the urethra that, when present in women, is often associated with vaginal gonorrhea, chlamydia, *Trichomonas,* or atrophic changes
Wet mount	Mucus mixed with a drop of saline examined under microscope
Yeast vaginitis	See candidal vaginitis

Here are some examples of history questions (after first *listening* to complaints):

- "Tell me about your symptoms."
- "How much discharge? What color is it?" *(Table 2) (Brain 2) (Red Flag 1)*
- "How many days have you noticed it?"
- "How many partners have you had intercourse with in the past 6 months? How long have you been with your present partner(s)?" Risk of STDs increases with number of sexual partners (see Chapter 56).
- "Do you use condoms? All the time or most of the time?"
- "Have you recently been on antibiotics?" Antibiotic use increases the risk of developing yeast vaginitis.
- "Do you douche? If so, how often and with what agent?"
- "Could you be pregnant?"
- "Is the discomfort at the opening of the vagina or inside?"
- "Do you practice oral or rectal sex?"
- "Do you have burning with urination? Fever? Abdominal pain?" *(Red Flag 2)*
- "Are you urinating more frequently than usual? Do you have a sense of urgency? Or inadequate emptying (or that you cannot get all the urine out)?"

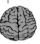

2 - Some girls may experience a scant, white, creamy discharge prior to and during puberty due to the change in hormone levels. When any vaginal discharge touches underwear, it may turn yellow from oxidation.

1 - Vaginal bleeding in postmenopausal women is cancer until proven otherwise.

2 - Severe abdominal pain with fever and vaginal discharge may be a sign of pelvic inflammatory disease. Severe abdominal pain with pregnancy and spotting or bleeding may be due to ectopic pregnancy.

Table 2. Vaginal Discharge Etiologies

Etiology	Chief Complaint	History	Physical Findings	Special Notations	Wet Mount
Normal	White discharge	N/A	Changes throughout the month with cyclical hormone changes Discharge is clear to white and is watery to mucoid pH < 4.5	Educate about normal cycles Discharge on clothing can turn yellow from oxygen	Normal squamous cells and few WBCs
Atrophic vaginitis	Burning Vaginal dryness	Peri- or post-menopausal	Vaginal mucosa is pale, dry, and sometimes red with irritation		Increased WBCs
Chlamydia/gonorrhea	Yellowish discharge Pelvic discomfort or pain	New or non-monogamous sexual No condoms	Thin yellow or green discharge Pelvic pain ranging from mild discomfort to severe Purulent cervical discharge	Check for other STDs; treat for both	Increased WBCs
Bacterial vaginosis	White or yellowish Homogenous discharge Fishy odor	Douches more than once a month	Thin, malodorous white to gray discharge, pH > 4.5		Clue cells—squamous cells with tattered edges and stippled cytoplasm
Chemical irritation	Itching Burning Profuse discharge	Douches Spermacides New lotions or soaps	Clear to white discharge Reddish vaginal mucosa	This can change the pH, making conditions more favorable for other infections	Increased WBCs
Trichomonas	Itching Burning Dysuria Profuse yellow-to-green discharge Pelvic discomfort or pain	Unprotected intercourse	Frothy light yellow or white discharge, pH > 4.5 Mobile, flagellated protozoa on wet mount	May be asymptomatic (unknown if weeks or months)	Flagellated protozoa, larger than WBC, smaller than squamous cell
Yeast	Itching Burning Thick white discharge	Diabetic Recent antibiotics BCPs	Thick white discharge that is adherent to vaginal wall	May be a normal finding if asymptomatic	Budding yeast and pseudohyphae seen on wet mount or on prep with KOH
Birth control pills	Profuse white discharge without pain or itching	On BCPs	Same as "Normal" except discharge is often much thicker and more profuse	Educate patient when BCPs begin	N/A

WBCs = white blood cells; KOH = potassium hydroxide; BCPs = birth control pills

Physical Examination

- **Vital signs.** Check for fever, and check pulse for tachycardia (could indicate dehydration or severe pain).
- **Abdominal.** Suprapubic pain is often seen with UTI. Palpate for masses or enlarged uterus (pregnancy).
- **Lymph.** Tender inguinal lymph nodes are found with vulvar lesions and cervicitis.
- **Back.** Check for tenderness in the costovertebral angle (over the kidney) for pyelonephritis.
- **Pelvic.** Perform external exam to look at the labia majora and minora for excoriations, papules, pustules, vesicles, ulcerations, and erythema. Check the pubic hair for evidence of pubic lice. Labial vesicles and ulcers suggest herpes. Syphilis is the "universal masquerader" and can look like anything! (e.g., red rash, nonpainful ulcer)!
- **Internal inspection.** Insert speculum carefully. Evaluate mucus in vagina for color, consistency, amount (scant, moderate, copious), and location (cervical os, vaginal walls). Check condition of vaginal mucosa (dry, erythematous, pink and moist). See Table 2 for characteristic mucus for each condition.
- **Cervix.** Women who have a large ectropion (glandular mucosa on the ectocervix) may notice a heavier amount of vaginal mucus.
- **Bimanual exam.** Pain with movement of the cervix indicates pelvic inflammation. Adnexal mass could be tubo-ovarian abscess or ectopic pregnancy.
- **Musculoskeletal.** Nonradicular low back pain or ache may indicate pelvic infection.

Testing

To diagnose a UTI, a urinalysis and spun microscopic exam of the urine are performed. Positive urinalysis findings may include presence of nitrites, leukocyte esterase, and blood. Many white blood cells (WBCs) in spun urine in the absence of many squamous cells is indicative of UTI *(Brain 3)*. Often, a urine culture is done to identify the bacteria causing infection.

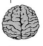

3 - A urinalysis with many red blood cells associated with back pain or flank pain may indicate a renal or ureteral stone and should be evaluated with further imaging studies and treated appropriately.

To diagnose vaginitis and cervicitis, a wet mount of vaginal mucus often helps to identify the cause of the symptoms. See Table 2 for specific wet mount findings. A DNA probe for gonorrhea and chlamydia is routinely obtained if an STD is suspected. New diagnostic modalities are becoming available, including urine tests, that employ DNA amplification to identify the organism causing infection.

Putting It All Together

Although vaginal and urinary complaints are often similar, a diagnosis of cystitis or vaginitis can be made by a careful history, physical exam, wet mount, and urinalysis. Cystitis or a bladder infection will present with symptoms of dysuria, but no vaginal discharge. Other common symptoms include increased urinary frequency, hesitancy, suprapubic discomfort, and a sense of inadequate emptying *(Red Flag 3)*. Vaginitis and cervicitis present with complaints of increased discharge, odor, and

3 - A urinary tract infection associated with fever, nausea, vomiting, and back pain may indicate pyelonephritis (kidney infection) and should be treated with parenteral antibiotics or oral antibiotics with close follow-up.

itching with a mucus discharge. Seeing characteristic changes on the physical exam and wet mount nails down the diagnosis. Infection, chemical irritation, or atrophy (aging) often causes an abnormal vaginal discharge. If there is infection, it is either sexually transmitted (gonorrhea, chlamydia, and/or *Trichomonas*) or not (yeast and bacterial vaginosis). However, at times, an infection usually considered to be sexually transmitted may not be such, as when *Trichomonas* has been contracted by shared towels or vibrators. Properly used condoms with spermicide can help prevent many STDs.

Atrophic vaginitis can be seen when the skin inside a woman's vagina becomes thinner near or after menopause due to lower estrogen levels. This mucosa is more susceptible to inflammation and infection.

Bacterial vaginosis is caused by an overgrowth of anaerobic bacteria in the vagina. This can occur when there is a change in the ecosystem of the vagina from semen, douching, or medications.

Chemical irritation can cause vaginal discharge and discomfort and is often caused by perfumed lotions, deodorant soaps, and spermicides.

Gonorrhea and chlamydia may cause symptoms of dysuria or a yellow-green discharge but also may be asymptomatic. It takes about 4 days to show symptoms after being exposed to gonorrhea and about 1 week to ≥ 1 month to have symptoms after exposure to chlamydia. Either of these infections can cause serious medical problems, including pelvic inflammatory disease, pelvic organ scarring, infertility, and an increased risk of ectopic pregnancy.

Trichomonas is asymptomatic in 20–50% of women, meaning a person might carry it for weeks, months, or even years without knowing it. A yellow-green or white frothy discharge and itching are generally the main complaints *(Red Flag 4)*.

4 - Treatment of *Trichomonas* with metronidazole is contraindicated during the first trimester of pregnancy.

Yeast likes to grow in a dark, moist environment. As such, it is important to educate patients about keeping the genitalia dry (change clothes after a workout, remove wet bathing suit). Other risk factors for yeast infection includes recent antibiotic use, uncontrolled diabetes, and HIV infection.

Management

Treatment is based on the cause of the vaginal symptom, as deduced by the history, physical examination, and complementary testing *(Consultation and Referral 1)* (see Table 2).

1 - Indications for referral:
- Recalcitrant vaginal discharge that does not respond to conventional therapy may be a sign of malignancy and should be referred to a gynecologist.
- Any STD in a child must be referred to a trained professional who can evaluate for sexual abuse.
- Other reasons for referral include suspicion of ectopic pregnancy and tubo-ovarian abscess.

Selected Readings

1. Centers for Disease Control and Prevention: 1998 Guidelines for prevention of sexually transmitted diseases. MMWR 47:1–111, 1998.
2. Faro S: Vulvovaginits: In Rakel R (ed): Conn's Current Therapy. Philadelphia, W.B. Saunders, 1999, pp 1088–1093.
3. Haefner H: Current evaluation and management of vulvovaginitis. Clin Obstet Gynecol 42:184–195, 1999.
4. Majeroni B: Bacterial vaginosis: An update. Am Fam Physician 57:1285–1289, 1998.
5. Nyirjesy P: Vaginitis in the adolescent patient. Pediatr Clin North Am 46:733–745, 1999.

6. Sobel JD: Vulvovaginitis in healthy women. Comprehens Ther 25:335–346, 1999.
7. Woodward C: Drug treatment of common STDs. Part I: Herpes, syphilis, urethritis, chlamydia and gonorrhea. Am Fam Physician 60:1387–1394, 1999.

63. Urinary Incontinence

Saira Asadullah, MD • Wendy L. Adams, MD, MPH

Synopsis

Urinary incontinence (UI) is the involuntary loss of urine in a quantity or frequency sufficient to cause a medical, social, or hygienic problem. It may be an acute or chronic condition. It is twice as common in women as in men and increases with age. Most of these patients are undiagnosed and remain untreated. Patients are often hesitant to discuss symptoms with their physician because of embarrassment or because they consider urinary incontinence a normal part of aging. Although UI is common among elderly people, it is not a normal part of aging. A complex integration of muscular, neurologic, and psychologic functions is required to properly store urine and to empty the bladder appropriately. In elderly people, a combination of factors often contributes to incontinence. Treatment can usually improve symptoms and sometimes cure the condition altogether.

For most patients, a history and physical examination will give you the diagnosis. History should be taken in a relaxed, unhurried fashion, with strong emphasis on preserving the patient's dignity. Ask about the length of time the patient has had incontinence and the mode of onset. There may be an association with an event such as prescription of a drug, surgery, or acute illness.

Differential Diagnosis

- **Acute urinary incontinence** is often reversible. It may occur with the onset of an acute illness or a new medication and resolve with treatment of the underlying problem. The most common causes are urinary tract infection and medications *(Brain 1)*.
- **Chronic urinary incontinence** may be reversible but generally requires more detailed investigation. Most often, chronic urinary incontinence in elderly people is a multifactorial problem, so the approach to diagnosis and treatment should target all potentially treatable contributors *(Table 1)*.

History

"What happens when you lose your urine and get wet?" The following features may give you a clue to the cause:

- Volume of urine lost. Large volume suggests urge incontinence, smaller volume suggests stress or overflow.
- Sudden urge to urinate (urge incontinence). Often this will be precipitated by running water, hand washing, cold temperatures, or the sight of one's garage or front door.

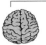
1 - The mnemonic DIAPPERS can help determine causes of acute urinary incontinence[4]:

D **D**elirium or confusional state may cause somnolence or inability to organize the activities needed for normal toilet use.

I **I**nfection of the urinary tract may cause incontinence, which is sometimes the only presenting symptom of urinary tract infection in elderly women.

A **A**trophic vaginitis and urethritis often contribute to incontinence.

P **P**harmaceuticals such as diuretics, anticholinergics, cholinergic agonists, psychotropics, narcotic analgesics, alpha-adrenergic blockers, calcium channel blockers and alcoholic or caffeinated beverages

P **P**sychological disorders, such as severe depression or psychoses

E **E**xcessive urine output from congestive heart failure, medications, hyperglycemia, hypercalcemia

R **R**estricted mobility or dexterity may prevent efficient use of the toilet.

S **S**tool impaction can precipitate incontinence, especially in persons who are disabled or on anticholinergic medications. These patients often have concurrent fecal incontinence.

When Foley catheters are removed, patients may experience acute transient incontinence due to urinary tract infection or because of the disruption of normal bladder function.

Table 1. Types of Chronic Urinary Incontinence

Type of Incontinence	Symptoms	Causes
Urge incontinence (the most common and most disabling type of incontinence in elderly women and men)	Sudden strong desire to urinate coupled with involuntary urine loss	1. Involuntary contraction of the bladder (detrusor) 2. Rapid bladder filling from diuretics or metabolic disorders 3. Local irritants, such as bladder stones or tumors
Stress incontinence (this type is uncommon in men unless there has been neuromuscular damage from urologic surgery)	Occurs with increased intra-abdominal pressure such as coughing and laughing	1. Changes in the pelvic floor support tissues and lower urinary tract ("urethral hypermobility") 2. Incompetent sphincter
Overflow incontinence	Dribbling, sensation of incomplete emptying, difficulty starting stream	1. Impaired detrusor contractility, 2. Bladder outlet obstruction that may be caused by enlarged prostate, urethral stricture, or large cystocele
Functional incontinence (may be the sole cause of incontinence but also often complicates other types of incontinence)	Varies—often resembles urge incontinence	Physical, cognitive, or psychiatric disability that interferes with normal toilet use
Mixed incontinence	More than one type of symptom, most often stress and urge incontinence	Usually more than one cause
Detrusor hyperactivity with impaired contractility	Urge incontinence combined with poor bladder emptying is quite common in the most frail elderly people	May include causes of both overflow and urge incontinence

- Incontinence with coughing, sneezing, laughing, or standing up (stress incontinence)
- Frequency of daytime and nighttime urination. Urinating more than 8 times during 24 hours suggests excess flow, which may be due to medications (especially diuretics), diabetes, congestive heart failure, or poor emptying. Rising to urinate 2 or more times at night (nocturia) may be due to poor bladder emptying, low functional bladder capacity, bladder spasms, or daytime fluid retention.
- Trouble starting the urine stream or dribbling at the end of urination. Slow urine stream, hesitancy, interrupted voiding, straining, and terminal dribbling suggest overflow incontinence.

Other questions you should ask include:

- "When did you first have incontinence?" Recent acute onset suggests reversible causes, which should be aggressively pursued.
- "What medicines do you take? Did you have any new medication just before your incontinence started?" Medications that commonly contribute to incontinence include diuretics, anticholinergics, cholinergic agonists, psychotropics, narcotic analgesics, alpha-adrenergic blockers, calcium channel blockers, and alcoholic or caffeinated beverages.
- "What other medical problems do you have?" *(Brain 2)*
- "Do you have any trouble walking?" *(Brain 3)*
- "How does your bladder control problem affect your daily life?"

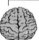

2 - Chronic conditions that commonly contribute to incontinence include diabetes mellitus, congestive heart failure, constipation, neurologic illness (stroke, Parkinson's disease, multiple sclerosis, Alzheimer's disease), venous insufficiency, and frequent urinary tract infections.

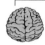

3 - The get-up-and-go test (see Chapter 33) will quickly assess whether mobility is adequate for normal toilet use.

Time	Did you urinate in the toilet? (record amount)	Was the urge to urinate present? Y = yes N = no	Did you have a leaking episode? L = large S = small	Activity at the time of leaking	Amount and type of fluid intake
6-7 am					
7-8 am					
9-10 am					

Figure 1: Voiding dairy (partial).

Incontinence may affect activities of daily living, social, emotional, and interpersonal functioning (e.g., sexual relationship), and self concept. Note the number of times incontinence pads or protective clothing have to be changed.
- For women, "How many children did you have? Vaginal deliveries?"
- "Have you had any operations on your abdomen or pelvis?"
- Have you had any treatment for this problem before now?"
- "What treatment do you know about for incontinence? Is there a kind of treatment you would prefer?"

Voiding Diary

Have patients complete a 48-hour voiding diary *(Figure 1)*. It can give valuable information about baseline frequency and severity as well as timing and circumstances of UI and continent voids. Ask the patient to record normal voids, all fluid intake, incontinent episodes, and potential precipitators, such as exercise, caffeine, or alcohol consumption. Also include voided volume if possible. For cognitively impaired patients, a caregiver will need to keep the diary.

Physical Examination

- General observation (e.g., alertness, cognition, functional status)
- Vital signs
- Screening examination of the heart and lungs *(Red Flag 1)*
- Abdomen and rectal exam (bladder by palpation, prostate size and tenderness; anal sphincter tone and sensation; masses; stool impaction)
- Pelvic exam (atrophic vaginitis, cystocele, uterine prolapse, vaginal discharge, pelvic mass, perineal irritation). Assess pelvic muscle strength in female patients by having them contract the muscles around the vagina.
- Musculoskeletal: Are mobility and manual dexterity sufficient for toilet use?

1 - Rales in the lungs, S_3 heart sound, and peripheral edema suggest congestive heart failure, which may contribute to incontinence by causing excess flow.

- Neurologic: Cognition, sensation, motor function, vibration sense, deep tendon reflexes *(Brain 4)*

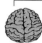

4 - Testing for perianal sensation and anal sphincter tone is important for assessing lumbosacral innervation. Anal wink is often absent in normal elderly people, however.

Additional Testing

Urinalysis should always be done. Other work-up depends on symptoms. If dysuria is present, a urine culture is indicated (urinary tract infection). If polyuria is present, serum glucose should be checked. If poor emptying, a serum B_{12} level is indicated. If mass is felt on prostate exam, have prostate-specific antigen (PSA) test performed. If a pelvic mass is suspected on exam, pelvic ultrasound or other imaging is indicated *(Red Flag 2)*.

2 - Hematuria should always be evaluated. It may be due to either benign or malignant causes. Work-up may include intravenous pyelogram, urine cytology, and cystoscopy.

Post-void residual volume *(Definition 1)* should be done if there is any question of adequacy of bladder emptying. Urodynamic testing is not routinely indicated. Refer for this testing if surgery is planned, when diagnosis is unclear, or when initial therapy fails.

1 - **Post-void residual volume:** A measure of impaired emptying. To measure post-void residual, instruct the patient to void normally into toilet. Within 5–10 minutes, measure the residual urine in the bladder by ultrasound or straight catheterization. High post-void residual urine (> 100 ml) implies impaired emptying. Overflow incontinence may occur at volumes over 400 ml.

Putting It All Together

Patients may present with acute or chronic incontinence. If incontinence is acute, the priority should be diagnosing reversible causes, such as urinary tract infections or medications. When incontinence is chronic, identify the type of incontinence and look for reversible contributors. Chronic illness, such as diabetes or congestive heart failure, will often be contributing. Functional impairments, such as unstable gait or cognitive impairment, may also play a major role *(Red Flag 3)*.

3 - Occasionally, serious conditions, such as bladder tumor or pelvic abscess, present as incontinence.

Management

General Principles

Treatment of urinary incontinence may be behavioral, pharmacologic, surgical, or a combination of these. Referral to a gynecologist or urologist is indicated in the case of urinary retention, hematuria, abnormal neurologic examination, pelvic prolapse, failure of initial treatment, or if surgery is being considered. Always maximize treatment of contributing medical problems, such as congestive heart failure or diabetes. When mobility or dexterity is impaired, refer to physical or occupational therapists for strength training, gait training, and assistive devices. Have the patient maintain adequate fluid intake but distribute intake throughout the day and avoid large intake. Instruct the patient to avoid caffeinated and alcoholic beverages. The patient should minimize evening intake of fluids if nocturnal UI is bothersome.

Behavioral Treatment

"Bladder retraining" is very successful for cognitively intact, motivated patients. It usually takes several weeks to see substantial results, so be sure to schedule frequent follow-up to monitor progress, discuss problems, and offer encouragement. Elements of bladder retraining include:

- Scheduled voiding while awake, usually every 2–3 hours

- Pelvic floor muscle (Kegel) exercises to strengthen levator muscles and increase urethral sphincter tone *(Brain 5)*

Pharmacologic Treatment

Discontinue potentially contributing medications if possible. For urge incontinence, anticholinergic medications are the most effective option. For stress incontinence, alpha-adrenergic agonists can be helpful. Estrogen, either systemic or topical, also may be useful for some patients with incontinence. For overflow incontinence due to prostate enlargement, alpha blockers (prazosin and terazosin) and anti-androgens (finasteride) often help.

Surgery

For stress incontinence, bladder suspension surgery has the highest cure rates but also causes the most complications. Injection of periurethral bulking agents such as collagen is sometimes successful for sphincter insufficiency. For men with postprostatectomy stress incontinence, artificial sphincter devices are often effective.

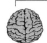

5 - Teaching Kegel exercises:
- During the bimanual part of the pelvic examination, explain to the patient that you are going to assess the strength of the muscles that help keep the bladder closed. Ask the patient to squeeze her vaginal muscles around your finger.
- Instruct the patient to slowly contract to a count of 5, hold for a count of 5, then slowly relax to a count of 5. The goal will be to hold the contraction for 10 seconds, although many women will be unable to sustain the contraction that long at first.
- Recommend ten repetitions 3 times per day initially. Over time, increase the frequency of exercises up to 10 times per day if possible.

Selected Readings

1. Busby-Whithead J, Johnson TM: Urinary incontinence. Clin Geriatr Med 14:285–296, 1998.
2. Fantl JA, Newman DK, Colling J, et al: Urinary Incontinence in Adults: Acute and Chronic Management. Clinical Practice Guideline No. 2. Rockville, MD, US Department of Health and Human Services, 1996, AHCPR publication 96-0682.
3. Ouslander JG, Schnelle JF, Uman G, et al: Predictors of successful prompted voiding among incontinent nursing home residents. JAMA 273:1366–1370, 1995.
4. Resnick NM: Geriatric incontinence. Urol Clin North Am 23:55–74, 1996.
5. Retzky SS, Rogers RM: Urinary incontinence in women. Clin Symp 47:3, 1995.
6. Wein AJ: Pharmacology of incontinence. Urol Clin North Am 22:557–77, 1995.

64. Vomiting and Diarrhea in Children

David R. Mack, MD

Synopsis

Vomiting is an unpleasant gastrointestinal motor activity with physical expulsion of stomach contents through the mouth. It can occur in an acute or chronic manner. The causes of vomiting in children are broad and thus require a thorough history and physical examination. Regurgitation in infants is not true vomiting, but results from inappropriate transient relaxation of the lower esophageal sphincter. The emesis of regurgitation occurs to a variable extent in all infants, is effortless, and will generally disappear with advancing age *(Brain 1)*. Children with bilious vomiting or vomiting associated with alteration in neurologic examination need immediate evaluation. Severe dehydration is a medical emergency that may occur with both vomiting and diarrhea and requires immediate referral to a hospital setting. Most causes of acute diarrhea are due to infections of either the intestines or other organs in close proximity. In contrast, the causes of chronic diarrhea vary considerably with the age of the patient. Chronic diarrhea should be thoroughly evaluated because it may suggest the presence of significant organic disease and necessitate referral to a pediatric gastrointestinal disease specialist.

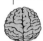

1 - The infant with uncomplicated regurgitation will have formula emanating nonforcefully from the mouth, but is otherwise a happy child who is growing well. Regurgitation in infants generally disappears around 12–18 months, but sometimes consequences of regurgitation, like all forms of gastroesophageal reflux, include poor growth, respiratory symptomatology, or inflammation of the esophagus, which may require surgical intervention. The questions in the history section will help to elucidate if the vomiting may have an organic origin that needs further evaluation or intervention.

Differential Diagnosis

Acute Vomiting

- Gastroenteritis (e.g., viral, bacterial, food poisoning)
- Nonintestinal infections (e.g., upper respiratory tract infections, urinary tract infections, blood)
- Malrotation with volvulus *(Red Flag 1)*
- Appendicitis, intussusception (see Chapter 11)
- Metabolic *(Red Flag 2)*
- Central nervous system *(Red Flag 3)*
- Other (e.g., pancreatitis, cholecystitis, hepatitis)

1 - In malrotation with midgut volvulus, bilious vomiting typically occurs 24–48 hours after birth with abdominal distention of the upper abdomen. Visible peristaltic waves may be present. Signs of vascular obstruction (i.e., melena, currant jelly stools) are followed by sepsis, perforation, and peritonitis.

Chronic Vomiting

- Gastroesophageal reflux ± esophagitis
- Respiratory (e.g., asthma, sinusitis)
- Gastritis, duodenitis or ileitis (e.g., infections, food related)
- Pyloric stenosis *(Red Flag 4)*
- Overfeeding, feeding disorders, eating disorders
- Infections of the urinary system
- Poisoning (e.g., lead)
- Other (e.g., pregnancy, pancreatitis, endocrine, anatomic obstructions)

2 - Abnormal amounts of substances whose presence in the brain triggers vomiting (e.g., lactic acid, ketones, urea, ammonia) may accumulate. They may form as a result of the abnormal cellular processes that an infant or child is born with (inborn errors of metabolism). Many present in the newborn period, but occasionally infections can provoke their onset.

Acute Diarrhea

- Infectious diarrhea (e.g., viral, bacterial, parasitic)
- Extraintestinal infections (e.g., otitis media, pneumonia, blood, urinary tract infections)
- Induced by antibiotics or other drugs
- Other enterocolitides *(Red Flag 5)*

Chronic Diarrhea

- **Toddler's diarrhea** *(Definition 1)*
- Food related:
    Milk and soy protein hypersensitivity *(Definition 2)*
    Lactose intolerance (see Chapter 11)
    Celiac disease *(Definition 3)*
- Allergy
- **Encopresis** *(Definition 4)*
- Other (hormone disorders, liver disorders, exocrine pancreatic disorders)

History

Vomiting

Questions likely will have to be addressed to the parent or caregiver.

"Tell me about the vomiting."

- Onset, duration, severity
- Bilious vomiting *(Red Flag 6)*
- Bloody (bright red versus coffee-ground color)
- Temporal pattern (e.g., early morning, postprandial, relationship to diet, specific foods)
- Previous episodes, previous surgery
- Neurologic symptoms (see Red Flag 2)
- Thirst, urinary frequency, fluid intake *(Table 1)*
- Medications, drugs, nonprescription pharmaceuticals, supplements, or preparations

"Tell me about other problems your child is having."

- Growth, appetite, energy, weight loss, fever
- Jaundice, stool color, urine color *(Brain 2)*
- Nausea, diarrhea, abdominal pain, headache
- Frequent infections *(Brain 3)*
- Skin rash, chronic rhinitis, hoarse voice
- Wheezing, recurrent pneumonia, apnea, cyanosis
- Swallowing difficulties (e.g., pain, liquids versus solids)
- Difficulties with breast-feeding (if appropriate)
- Previous trauma *(Red Flag 7)*

"Tell me about the family."

- History of peptic ulcer disease, pancreatitis, inflammatory bowel disease
- Medications in household
- Contacts with similar symptoms in caregivers *(Brain 4)*
- Travel, food handling, pets

 3 - Increased pressure inside the fixed confines of the skull will lead to vomiting. Acutely, infections are usually the cause of inflammation of either the coverings of the brain (meningitis) or brain tissue (encephalitis). Chronically, conditions that can lead to vomiting include excessive accumulation of cerebrospinal fluid (hydrocephalus), abnormal growth of cells (tumors), or abnormal collection of body waste products (e.g., after the liver fails).

 4 - Patients will have nonbilious, projectile, postprandial vomiting beginning after 3 weeks of age (range 1 week to 5 months). On physical exam, a 2 cm, mobile, olive-shaped mass will be palpable and is best palpated from the left side above and to the right of the umbilicus in midepigastrium beneath the liver edge. The typical electrolyte disturbance is hypochloremic metabolic alkalosis.

 5 - Hematochezia (passage of bright red blood in the stools) in the newborn infant requires urgent consultation for inflammation of the intestines, which is associated with necrosis of the intestines in newborns (necrotizing enterocolitis), lack of ganglion cells of the colon (Hirschsprung's enterocolitis), maternally acquired *Salmonella*, and formula hypersensitivity.

 1 - Toddler's diarrhea (chronic nonspecific diarrhea): Condition in children usually between the ages of 1 and 4 years, who pass between 4 and 10 watery stools per day, but do not have nocturnal diarrhea. Otherwise, these children appear well with a normal physical examination. Improvement in consistency and number of stools can be obtained by increasing fat and fiber in the diet and reducing simple sugar carbohydrates (e.g., fruit juices, soft drinks).

 2 - Milk and soy protein hypersensitivity (cow's milk allergy): An immunologic reaction to the ingestion of cow's milk or soy proteins. It may or may not involve IgE antibody. The gastrointestinal manifestations include recurrent vomiting, food refusal, irritability, diarrhea, rectal bleeding, and malabsorption. Systemic manifestations may include failure to thrive, atopic dermatitis, chronic rhinitis, and secretory otitis. Infants will generally outgrow this by age 3 years.

Table 1. Clinical Features of Dehydration

Severity	% Water Loss (< 1 year old)	% Water Loss (> 1 year old)	Clinical Signs
Minimal	5	3	Thirst, mild oliguria, dry mucous membranes
Moderate	10	6	Loss of skin turgor, severe thirst, sunken eyeballs and fontanelle
Severe	15	9	Low blood pressure, poor circulation, central nervouse system changes, fever

Diarrhea

"Tell me about the diarrhea."

- Onset, duration, size of stools, mucus present, color
- Consistency and number of stools
- Odor, greasy, floating *(Brain 5)*
- Previous episodes
- Hematochezia (blood in stool) or melena *(Brain 6)*
- Perianal irritation from diarrhea *(Brain 7)*
- Diet (e.g., breast milk only, milk)
- Medications (prescription and nonprescription), other drugs

"Tell me about other problems your child is having."

- **Tenesmus, urgency** *(Definition 5)*
- Fever, abdominal pain or distention, vomiting
- Growth, appetite, energy, weight loss, body image
- Irritability, fussiness, decreased energy, decreased appetite
- Urinary symptoms
- Respiratory symptoms

"Tell me about the family."

- History of inflammatory bowel disease, irritable bowel syndrome, lactose intolerance, cystic fibrosis, celiac disease, liver disease
- Other children who have problems growing
- Medications in household
- Contacts with persons having similar symptoms (e.g., caregivers, siblings)
- Travel, food handling, pets

Physical Examination

- General observation (alertness, toxic appearing, body habitus)
- Vital signs including temperature, height, and weight
- **Anterior fontanelle** sunken or raised *(Definition 6)*
- Eyes (e.g., sclera, optic disk, retina)
- Oral (e.g., hydration, lesions)
- Neck (e.g., nodes, thyroid)
- Abdominal (e.g., distention, masses, tenderness, peristaltic movements, organomegaly)
- Perianal (e.g., erythema, skin tags, fissures, fistulas) (see Chapter 23)

3 - Celiac disease: Small bowel inflammation due to a permanent sensitivity to dietary gluten. Children present after gluten-containing cereals introduced into the diet (usually around 6–24 months of age). The common symptoms are poor weight gain, diarrhea, and irritability. The common signs are muscle wasting, abdominal distention, height or weight < 25th percentile, and finger clubbing. Screening is available through blood tests, but confirmation requires a small bowel biopsy.

4 - Encopresis: Involuntary passage of stool. Whereas children with true diarrhea are able to hold stool until they reach a toilet, children with significant constipation may have their colon become so dilated that there is uncontrolled flow of stool around the fecal impaction (overflow incontinence). The loose stools in the underwear are misinterpreted as diarrhea.

6 - Dark green vomitus is a strong indication of the intestinal tract obstruction below the point where the bile is secreted into the duodenum (i.e., ampulla of Vater) and requires emergency attention.

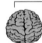

2 - Bilirubin is formed from hemoglobin during normal or abnormal destruction of erythrocytes. Most bilirubin is normally excreted through the bowels after being processed in the liver. If the processing in the liver or secretion into the bowels is affected, more bilirubin than normal is found in the blood, urine, and tissues of the body and less is found in the intestinal contents of the bowel. Therefore, patients will have a yellowish color to their skin (i.e., jaundice) or the white part of the eye (i.e., sclera), the urine will be tea-colored, and stools will be pale.

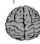

3 - Most bacterial and viral infections will resolve within 2 weeks, but parasitic infections may persist longer (e.g., *Giardia lamblia*). Sometimes after a viral infection of the small bowel (i.e., post-viral enteropathy), normal absorption will be decreased for a period of time. This can be exacerbated by high-carbohydrate diets or prolonged fasting. If children have numerous or unusual infections of the bowel, consider immune deficiencies.

- Pulmonary (e.g., breathing pattern, abnormal breath sounds, air entry)
- Skin (e.g., pigmentation, discoloration, rashes)
- Finger clubbing (see Chapter 22)
- Edema *(Brain 8)*
- Neurologic (e.g., alertness, tone, developmental level, nuchal rigidity, reflexes)
- Nipples of breast-feeding mothers (i.e., cracks and fissures)

Testing

Acute onset of vomiting or diarrhea with evidence of moderate and severe dehydration necessitates obtaining:

- Serum electrolytes (so that the proper water and electrolyte replacement fluid may be initiated)
- Stool specimen for presence of reducing sugars or microscopic blood (clues to the diagnosis when infection is suspected)
- Metabolic studies (if patient has altered mental state)
- Complete blood count (CBC) if the emesis or fecal discharge contains blood. This can help determine the significance of the blood loss and whether there is a bleeding disorder or infectious etiologies.
- C-reactive protein (CRP) (when an acute inflammatory process is suspected)
- Erythrocyte sedimentation rate (ESR). Elevated ESR plus elevated CRP suggests a more chronic condition.

Some bacterial intestinal infections (e.g., *Escherichia coli* O157:H7) are associated with the development of renal failure up to 2 weeks following the onset of bloody diarrhea. Therefore, in this circumstance, this child would also need to have:

- Serum electrolytes, blood ureanitrogen (BUN) and creatinine
- A CBC, both acutely and 2 weeks later

Newborns and young infants with acute onset of bloody diarrhea need consideration for the culturing of other body fluids in addition to stool. Abdominal radiographs may be needed:

- In the neonatal period, for some conditions (see Red Flag 5)
- For a child with bilious vomiting, but additional imaging studies (e.g., ultrasound, barium examinations) may be required to determine whether intestinal obstruction is present *(Consultation and Referral 1)*.

For vomiting and diarrhea of a chronic nature, plan to obtain:

- A CBC and ESR
- Serum electrolytes and albumin
- Urinalysis
- Stool for ova and parasite testing

For patients with chronic vomiting, an upper gastrointestinal barium examination with a small bowel series to evaluate anatomy is useful prior to referral to a pediatric gastroenterologist. Endoscopic examination has largely superseded barium examinations for mucosal diseases of the intestinal tract.

7 - Shaken baby syndrome is a form of child abuse associated with acute subdural hematoma caused by the forceful shaking of an infant, which causes rupture of bridging cortical veins. These children have symptomatology of increased intracranial pressure. Examination may show bulging fontanelle, retinal hemorrhages, and evidence of previous abuse.

4 - Children in daycare are much more likely to develop infections than children whose primary caregiver is a parent at home.

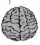
5 - Stools that have increased amounts of fat (i.e., steatorrhea) will be noted to have these qualities.

6 - Hematochezia may result from significant upper gastrointestinal bleeding as well as colitis.

7 - Infections of the small intestine (predominantly viral and parasitic) yield reducing sugar positivity (i.e., Clinitest positive) on stool testing. The carbohydrates are fermentable by the normal bacteria of the large bowel yielding stool pH < 4 and causing erythema of the skin around the anus. Colonic infections are more likely to be of bacterial origin with stools containing blood and mucus with tenesmus and urgency. Stool testing yields microscopic blood loss, but normal pH and no reducing sugars.

5 - Tenesmus: A painful spasm of the anal sphincter that is involuntary and may lead to the passage of little fecal matter.

Urgency: The desire to evacuate the bowel that may be so severe that there is inability to refrain from the passage of fecal material. Both are associated with inflammation of the colon.

6 - Anterior fontanelle: The diamond-shaped membranous interval at the junction of the coronal, sagittal, and metopic sutures of the skull where the frontal angles of the parietal bones meet the two ununited halves of the frontal skull bones. The usual size is 2 x 2 cm and closes around 18 months of age. Prior to its closure, its examination can relay important information. Best examined when the patient is held upright, asleep, or feeding, it is normally slightly depressed and pulsatile. A bulging fontanelle is a reliable indicator of increased intracranial pressure. A depressed fontanelle is a sign of dehydration.

Other testing is largely directed by history, physical examination, patient age, and screening tests *(Consultation and Referral 2)*.

Putting It All Together

Vomiting and diarrhea are very common problems in children. In the acute setting, these are usually caused by self-limited infections. Careful attention must be paid to hydration of the patient. Children with bilious or bloody vomiting or bloody diarrhea can have a much more serious problem and require consultation. Of great concern are those children who appear toxic or have altered neurologic status. These patients need emergent evaluation.

With a more chronic problem, a detailed history and physical examination are of great importance. Knowledge of benign conditions (e.g., constipation with encopresis, toddler's diarrhea, regurgitation in an infant) that occur at different ages will be helpful to direct care. Chronic gastrointestinal problems associated with any additional features, including poor growth, need to have a definitive diagnosis made prior to any therapies being introduced.

Management

Oral rehydration therapy is the preferred treatment for fluid and electrolyte losses caused by diarrhea in children who have mild-to-moderate dehydration. Children who have diarrhea and are not dehydrated should continue to be fed age-appropriate diets. Children who require rehydration should be fed age-appropriate diets as soon as they have been rehydrated. As a general rule, pharmacologic agents should not be used to treat acute diarrhea. Children with bilious vomiting should refrain from eating or drinking and should have intravenous therapy, a nasogastric tube for gastric drainage, and referral. Children who experience massive gastrointestinal bleeding need to be stabilized and then transferred immediately to a facility for management by endoscopists and surgeons skilled in pediatric care.

For those children in whom benign conditions are suspected and therapy is introduced (e.g., change in formula, change to increased fat and fiber, reduction in simple sugars), follow-up in 2 weeks is indicated to ensure that the problem has resolved itself. If it has not, referral should be considered. Because a great number of children who are referred to a pediatric gastroenterologist suffer from constipation and encopresis (which can be mistaken for diarrhea), attention to bowel habits during well-child checks should be part of routine care.

Selected Readings

1. Antonson DL, Madison JK: Eating disorders and obesity. In Wylie R, Hyams JS (eds): Pediatric Gastrointestinal Disease, 2nd ed. Philadelphia, W.B. Saunders, 1999, pp 73–87.
2. Branski D, Lerner A, Lebenthal E: Chronic diarrhea and malabsorption. Pediatr Clin North Am 43:307–331, 1996.

8 - Extracellular fluid accumulation in body tissues (i.e., edema) in the absence of heart disease may be associated with hypoalbuminemia. Hypoalbuminemia is usually due to increased body losses from either the kidney (i.e., nephrotic syndrome) or intestinal conditions (i.e., protein-losing enteropathy).

1 - Consultation should be considered for children with severe dehydration, bilious vomiting, significant intestinal bleeding, altered neurologic status, and toxic appearance on examination.

2 - Consultation should be considered for children with bloody stools lasting longer than 2 weeks and for children with vomiting or diarrhea that has lasted for 2 weeks despite treatment.

3. Li BUK, Sferra TJ: Vomiting. In Wylie R, Hyams JS (eds): Pediatric Gastrointestinal Disease, 2nd ed. Philadelphia, W.B. Saunders, 1999, pp 14–31.
4. Murray KF, Christie DL: Vomiting. Pediatr Rev 19:337–341, 1998.
5. Provisional Committee on Quality Improvement, Subcommittee on Acute Gastroenteritis: Practice parameter: The management of acute gastroenteritis in young children. Pediatrics 97:424–437, 1996.
6. Vanderhoof J: Chronic diarrhea. Pediatr Rev 19:418–422, 1998.

65. Casting, Splinting, and Taping

Christopher C. Madden, MD

Synopsis

Immobilization of acute fractures dates back to 2600 B.C., when splints were constructed from tree bark. Casting and splinting immobilization are used to immobilize acute stable fractures, reduced dislocations, and various soft tissue injuries and overuse syndromes. Although lightweight removable splints, removable cast-boots, and other orthotic devices have assumed greater importance, casting and splinting with plaster of paris and fiberglass remain useful.

Taping is another form of protection for soft tissue and joint injuries. Taping can minimize pain and swelling while offering support and protection. Taping also can play a part in the acute treatment, rehabilitation, and prevention of multiple musculoskeletal injuries. Although physicians may perform taping, it is often left to the expertise of physical therapists and athletic trainers.

Indications

Casting and Splinting

Casts and splints can be used appropriately in many similar situations, but there are some clear advantages and disadvantages of each. Casts provide better overall immobilization and protection of acute fractures, and they cannot be removed by a noncompliant patient. However, casts are associated with a higher rate of complications, including pressure sores, circulatory problems, neuropraxia, and, on rare occasions, infections. Splint advocates point out that a properly fashioned splint can offer similar immobilization, is more quickly and easily constructed, and may be safer in the setting of progressive swelling. Splints offer less overall injury protection and give the patient the option for easy removal. Follow-up is an important issue to consider, and many emergency department and urgent care physicians insist on splinting and leaving the application of a long-term cast to the physician who will be primarily caring for the injury.

The three most common casts used by primary care physicians are the short-arm, short-arm thumb spica, and short-leg casts. Common splints include the radial and ulnar gutter, posterior elbow and ankle, ankle stirrup brace (e.g., Aircast Air-Stirrup), thumb spica, and sugar tong. Specific indications are reviewed in *Tables 1* and *2*. Material needed is included in *Table 3*.

Taping

The main goal of taping is to restrict undesired motion. Taping can be functional, prophylactic, or rehabilitative (e.g., enhancing proprioception). *Table 4* outlines the most common taping techniques.

Procedure

Casting

A thorough neurovascular examination of the injured extremity should be performed before casting or splinting *(Red Flag 1)*.

Plaster of paris and fiberglass work equally well for casting. Plaster casts are cheaper, more easily molded, and have low allergenicity. However, plaster is heavier and cannot get wet. Fiberglass casts are more expensive, lighter, may have superior strength and durability, have a quicker drying time, and are relatively water-resistant.

Before casting, make sure all materials are available (see Table 3). The general technique of applying lower *(Figure 1)* or upper *(Figure 2)* extremity casts is the same. Initially, a stockinette is placed over the extremity, leaving a generous amount of excess to fold over later (see Figure 1A). Cotton padding is then applied evenly in a perpendicular fashion, overlapping 50% with each pass (see Figure 1B). The padding can be torn and restarted to avoid kinks. Extra padding should be applied to bony prominences, but avoid too much padding. The plaster or fiberglass should then be soaked for 5–10 seconds in room-temperature water. Warmer water may cause a higher temperature reaction and may burn the patient *(Red Flag 2)*. Remove excess water by gently squeezing the roll at both ends—never wring it out. Apply the plaster or fiberglass rolls by following the direction of the padding, once again overlapping approximately 50% with each turn. Many physicians apply casts in a distal to proximal manner. Rolls should be applied lightly around the limb using gentle pressure applied with the palm to mold the plaster (see Figure 1D). Pressure applied with fingers can create cast ridges, which can later cause pressure sores. Fiberglass can be evened by using small tucks as the extremity tapers (see Figure 2B and 2C). Three to six layers of plaster, or three to four of fiberglass should be applied. When nearing both ends of the cast, the stockinette should be folded over and covered with a few rounds of cast material. After placing the final layers, the cast can be smoothed with wetted hands (rubber gloves), once again being careful not to indent the cast. Ensure that the cast conforms to the contours of the extremity while holding it in an adequate position. The cast will set up quickly, but 24–48 hours should be allowed before exposing the cast to any external force.

Short-Arm Cast

This chapter is not intended to serve as the sole reference for independent casting. The following information should be reviewed with a knowledgeable health professional, and casting should be appropriately supervised.

Short-arm cast construction usually requires a 2- or 3-inch stockinette, two rolls of 2- or 3-inch cast padding, and two to three rolls of 3- or 4-inch plaster bandage. If using fiberglass, use 2- or 3-inch roles. The wrist should be immobilized in 15–20° of extension. A functional position is achieved by having the patient pretend that he or she is holding a can, making sure the elbow is flexed 90°. The cast should extend from 1–2 fingerbreadths distal to the flexion crease of the elbow to the distal palmar flexion crease of the hand (over metacarpal phalangeal joints). The cast should follow this crease obliquely and should stop just proximal to the knuckles. Full motion at the metacarpal phalangeal joints should be permitted. The thumb spica cast is a slight modification of the short-arm cast involving additional immobilization of the thumb to the interphalangeal joint.

1 - Always examine the injured extremity carefully for neural and vascular injuries. Document appropriate history and physical examination findings. Worrisome symptoms include numbness, tingling, and paresthesias in the affected extremity. Abnormal physical exam findings may include pale skin color, capillary refill > 2 seconds, decreased peripheral pulses, and abnormal sensation with pinprick and light touch.

2 - As plaster of paris is moistened, heat is generated. Use room temperature water to avoid a reaction that may burn the patient.

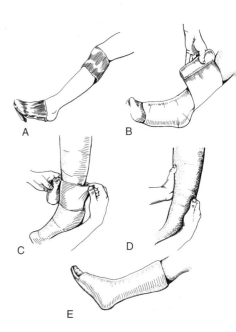

Figure 1: Casting principles of the lower extremiti
(From Simon R, Koenigsknecht S: Fracture principles. In Emergency Orthopedics: The Extremities. Stamford, CT, Appleto & Lange, 1996, with permission.)

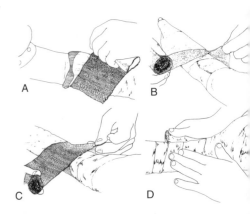

Figure 2: Casting principles of the upper extremitie
(From Simon R, Koenigsknecht S: Fracture principles. In Emergen Orthopedics: The Extremities. Stamford, CT, Appleton & Lange, 1996, with permission.)

Table 1. Cast Indications

Cast	Indications	Illustration
Short-arm	Stable fractures of distal radius, ulna, carpal, and metacarpal bones Stable wrist sprains and other soft tissue injuries	
Short-arm thumb spica	Stable thumb metacarpal, scaphoid, or trapezium fractures 1st metacarpal phalangeal dislocations or sprains (ulnar and radial collateral liagments)	
Short-leg	Stable ankle, calcaneus, tarsal, and metatarsal fractures Stable ligamentous injuries to the ankle and foot (e.g., midfoot sprain) Chronic nonresolving tendinopathy (tendinitis or tendinosis)	

From Simon R, Koenigsknecht S: Fracture principles. In Emergency Orthopedics: The Extremities. Stamford, CT, Appleton & Lange, 1996, with permission.

Short-Leg Cast

Short-leg casts require 4-inch stockinette, three or four rolls of 4-inch cast padding, and three rolls of 5-inch plaster or 4-inch fiberglass bandage. The cast can be applied with the patient in a prone position or sitting with the toes resting on a cast stand. The knee is flexed 90°, and the ankle is most often immobilized at 90°, but this can vary with the injury. The cast extends distally from just below the knee, usually including the fibular head, to the base of the toes. The metatarsal heads should be included.

Patients should be counseled about potential complications of casting **(Red Flag 3)**.

Splinting

Splinting is performed in a similar manner to casting. Splints are constructed from plaster or fiberglass rolls normally used for casting. Prepadded fiberglass splints that can be cut to the desired length are now available.

Three-inch rolls of fiberglass or 4-inch rolls of plaster work well for most upper extremity splints. Four- or 5-inch rolls of fiberglass or 5- or 6-inch rolls of plaster work for most lower extremity splints. Stockinettes or cotton padding may be applied in a similar fashion to casting for most splints. Plaster splints require up to 12 layers for adequate strength. Fiberglass splints offer good strength with 8–12 layers.

3 - Patients should be educated to watch closely for symptoms of ischemia resulting from a tight cast. Increasing pain, changing skin color, and cold or numb digits should be reported to a physician immediately. Objects should never be inserted inside a cast to relieve itching because of the potential for skin damage and infection. Care should be taken to avoid getting even fiberglass casts wet; skin maceration and infection can result from inadequate drying. Other complications include pressure sores, burns, compartment syndromes, nerve palsies, and thromboemblic events. Most physicians recheck circumferential casts within 24 hours and at regular intervals thereafter.

Table 2. Splint Indications

Splint	Indication	Illustration
Radial gutter*	Stable 2nd and 3rd phalangeal and metacarpal fractures	
Ulnar gutter*	Stable 4th and 5th phalangeal and metacarpal fractures	
Posterior elbow	Undisplaced radial head fractures Supracondylar humerus fractures Small, minimally displaced fractures of cornoid of olecranon process Immobilization after elbow dislocation Temporary support for more complicated fractures Pain control after elbow sprain	
Posterior ankle	Temporary support for distal tibia and fibula fractures Temporary support for other ankle and foot fractures Temporary support for Achilles tendon tears	
Aircast ankle stirrup†	Ankle sprains (grades 2 and 3) Small avulsion fractures of malleoli	
Thumb spica**	Stable thumb metacarpal, scaphoid, or trapezium fractures 1st metacarpophalangeal dislocations or sprains (ulnar or radial collateral ligaments)	
Sugar tong*	Some distal forearm fractures, especially distal radius (e.g., Colles')	

* Figure from Simon R, Koenigsknecht S: Fracture principles. In Emergency Orthopedics: The Extremities. Stamford, CT, Appleton & Lange, 1996, with permission.
† Figures from Fandel D, Frette T: Splinting and bracing. In Mellion M, Walsh M, Madden C, et al (eds): The Team Physician's Handbook, 3rd ed. Philadelphia, Hanley & Belfus, 2002, pp 546–565, with permission.
** Figures from Concannon MJ, Hurov J: Hand Pearls. Philadelphia, Hanley & Belfus, 2002, with permission.

Table 3. Cast Materials

• Rubber gloves	• Soft cotton (Webril)	• Assistant
• Patient drape	• Plaster of paris or synthetic material (fiberglass)	• Leg or foot stand
• Physician gown		• Felt padding
• Show covers	• Water source	• Slings
• Stockinette (2-, 3-, and 4-inch)*	• Elastic (Ace) bandages	• Scissors

*Stockinette is a tubular fabric (like a thin sock) that is fitted snugly over an extremity before cast padding is applied.

Adapted from Eathorne S, McKeag D: Cast immobilization. In Pfenninger J, Fowler G (eds): Procedures for Primary Care Physicians. St. Louis, Mosby, 1994.

Necessary splint length can be determined by measuring a single layer along the extremity. The plaster or fiberglass should then be rolled over itself until desired thickness is achieved. Padding can be applied over the stockinette on the extremity, or it can be laid directly over the wet cast material. Make sure the padding is longer and wider than the splint. The splint is then fashioned into the appropriate position depending on the injury, utilizing the same positional and smoothing techniques as with casting. While the material is setting, an elastic (Ace) bandage is wrapped around the splint and the limb. The joint should be maintained in the desired position throughout this process.

Taping

Quality taping requires much skill and should be performed by well-trained health professionals such as physical therapists and athletic trainers. Nonetheless, knowledge of taping basics often proves helpful.

Select a good quality athletic tape with adequate tensile strength to provide necessary support. Skin should be shaved, cleaned, and dried. Adhesive spray or another taping base (e.g., tincture of benzoin) can be applied for better adhesion. Underwrap (thin, nonadhesive padding) can be applied for sensitive skin. Watch closely for any allergic reactions to the materials or tape. The joint is placed in a functional position that minimally stresses injured structures. Injured ligaments should be in a shortened position. Anchor strips of tape are placed proximal and distal to the injury. Strips of tape are applied in a sequential order, each piece having a distinct purpose. Strips should bridge across the injury, duplicating the anatomy needing support. Overlap successive strips by at least 50% in a weave-like fashion to add strength. Tape should be applied smoothly and firmly, flowing with the contour of the limb. When completed, check function and comfort.

Table 4. Taping Techniques

Taping Technique	Indications	Illustration
Buddy taping	Finger sprains Minor fractures or phalanges	
Thumb figure-of-eight	Hyperflexion injuries to 1st MCP joint	
Wrist taping	Wrist sprains Dorsal impingement	
Elbow taping	Elbow hyperextension Varus and valgus injuries	
Hip or groin spica	Groin strain	
Medial or lateral knee taping	Collateral ligament sprain	
Patellofemoral (McConnel) taping	Patellofemoral pain syndromes Patellar tendinitis	

(continued on following page)

Table 4. Taping Techniques (continued)

Taping Technique	Indications	Illustration
Ankle taping	Ankle sprains: treatment and prevention	
Arch figure-of-eight	Arch sprains Plantar fasciitis	

All images except for groin spica are from Fandel D, Frette T: Taping and bracing. In Mellion M, Walsh M, Madden C, et al (eds): The Team Physician's Handbook, 3rd ed. Philadelphia, Hanley & Belfus, 2002, pp 546–565, with permission.

Selected Readings

1. Eathorne S, McKeag D: Cast immobilization. In Pfenninger J, Fowler G (eds): Procedures for Primary Care Physicians. St. Louis, Mosby, 1994.
2. Fandel D, Frette T: Taping and bracing. In Mellion M, Walsh M, Madden C, et al (eds): The Team Physician's Handbook, 3rd ed. Philadelphia, Hanley & Belfus, 2002, pp 546–565.
3. Harkess J, Ramsey W: Definitive treatment of fractures. In Bucholz RW, Heckman JD, Beaty JH, Kasser JR (eds): Rockwood, Green, and Wilkins' Fractures, 5th ed. Philadelphia, Lippincott Williams & Wilkins, 2002.
4. Simon R, Koenigsknecht S: Fracture principles. In Simon R, Koenigsknecht S (eds): Emergency Orthopedics: The Extremities, 4th ed. New York, McGraw-Hill, 2001.

66. Injections

Louise M. LaFramboise, PhD, RN

Synopsis

Parenteral administration involves injection of medications into a body tissue such as subcutaneous tissue, muscle, or veins. Parenteral administration provides for more rapid, systemic distribution of medications than oral administration and may also be beneficial when patients are vomiting, cannot swallow, or are restricted from taking oral fluids. This chapter discusses intradermal, subcutaneous, and intramuscular routes of parenteral administration.

Parenteral administration provides almost complete absorption of medications (provided there is adequate circulation and no tissue damage), so an accurate measure of the amount of drug provided is possible. A significant concern about administering medications parenterally is the potential for infection created by introducing a needle through the skin. For this reason, aseptic technique should be used for all injections.

Overview of Syringes and Needles

Many different syringe types are available. The most common are tuberculin, insulin, hypodermic, and prefilled *(Figures 1 and 2)*. Tuberculin syringes measure in hundredths of a cubic centimeter (cc) and hold 1 ml. They are commonly used for allergy injections, immunizations, and purified protein derivative (PPD) testing. They provide small, accurate dosing.

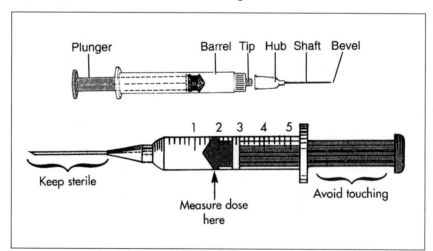

Figure 1: Parts of a syringe.
(From Elkin MK, Perry AG, Potter PA: Nursing Interventions and Clinical Skills, 2nd ed. St. Louis, Mosby, 2000, p 448, with permission)

Insulin syringes measure in units (U). Low-dose syringes hold a maximum of 50 U, whereas standard syringes measure a maximum of 100 units. The 50-unit syringe also holds 0.5 cc, and the 100-unit syringe holds 1 cc.

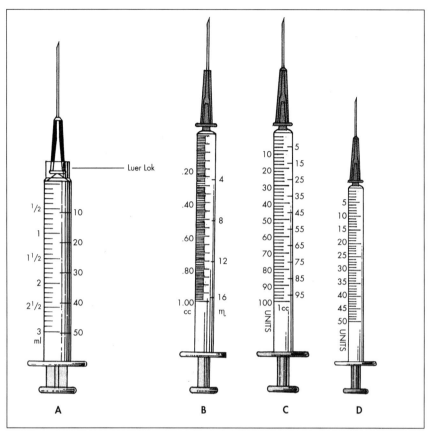

Figure 2: Types of syringes. *A*, Hypodermic syringe with 3-cc capacity. *B*, Tuberculin syringe for doses of less than 1 cc. *C*, A 100-U insulin syringe. *D*, A 50-U (low dose), insulin syringe. (From Elkin MK, Perry AG, Potter PA: Nursing Interventions and Clinical Skills, 2nd ed. St. Louis, Mosby, 2000, p 448, with permission)

Hypodermic syringes measure in both cubic centimeters (cc) and minim increments. Syringes are marked in either 0.1-cc or 0.2-cc increments. Sizes range from 3 cc to 5 cc for injection purposes but larger sizes are available for other purposes (e.g., 10 cc, 20 cc, 60 cc).

Most prefilled syringes hold 0.5–2 cc of medication and come with the appropriate needles attached. Examples of prefilled medications include opioid analgesics, anaphylactic kits (e.g., EpiPen), antibiotics, and anti-coagulants.

Needles are available in multiple gauges and lengths. The gauge or lumen of the needle can range from 30 (smallest) to 18 (largest) for injection purposes. Length of the needle will range from ⅜ inch to 2 inches. Factors that affect needle and syringe choice include the viscosity and quantity of the medication to be administered, route of administration, and body size of the recipient.

Procedure

Overview for All Injections

To prepare for an injection, assemble the equipment (syringes, needles, alcohol wipes, medication, and gloves), and verify the medication.

Before giving the injection, accurately identify the patient, determine allergies, and select the appropriate site. When selecting the site, avoid **(Red Flag 1)** areas that are burned, scarred, or atrophied or have signs of inflammation, chronic lymphedema, or impaired blood flow. Caution should be used when giving an injection to a patient who takes anticoagulants or has a bleeding disorder.

After selecting the injection site, clean the site and the area around it about 2 inches in diameter with an alcohol wipe using a circular motion and moving from the inside to the outside. Let the site air dry. Hold the skin of the injection site taut by pinching up the skin (subcutaneous) or by spreading the skin between your thumb and index finger (intradermal and intramuscular). With the needle bevel up, insert the needle at the appropriate angle and to the appropriate depth **(Table 1)**. With subcutaneous and intramuscular injections, you should go quickly through the skin in a dart-like motion and usually insert the needle up to the hub.

If you are giving an intramuscular injection, you should **aspirate (Definition 1)** to determine that you have not entered a vein. If blood enters the syringe upon aspiration, remove the needle from the patient and discard the syringe and medication. Prepare a new syringe and begin again. Blood entering the syringe indicates the needle is in a vein, which is not the appropriate route of administration for an intramuscular injection. With subcutaneous and intradermal injections, this step is not necessary. Inject the medication slowly to minimize patient discomfort.

With intradermal injections, if the needle is correctly positioned, injecting the medication will form a tense white wheal. A wheal should not be apparent with subcutaneous and intramuscular injections. After the medication has been injected, hold the skin with your gloved finger at the insertion site and remove the needle with a swift, straight, backward motion. It is not necessary to massage the site after the injection has been given.

Recapping needles is generally not recommended. However, to maintain the sterility of a needle prior to its use or to avoid injuring others prior to discarding the needle, recapping is sometimes necessary. To avoid a needle stick, the recommended procedure for recapping is to use the scoop technique. Lay the needle cap down on the counter and scoop it up with the needle **(Figure 3)**. Do not use your hand to hold the cap in place because the likelihood of a needle stick is great.

Intradermal Injection

Intradermal administration of a medication is used primarily for skin testing, such as for tuberculosis and allergies. Medications administered in this manner are usually very potent so it is important that they be administered into the dermis **(Figure 4)** rather than the subcutaneous tissues where they may be absorbed more readily into the systemic circulation.

Equipment needed includes a 1-ml syringe (or a tuberculin syringe) and a short (⅜–⅝ inch), small-gauge (25–27) needle. The needle is inserted at a 5–15° angle into the layer just under the epidermis, and the fluid is injected to produce a small bleb just under the skin. The site for PPD testing is usually the area that lies between 3 and 4 fingerwidths below the antecubital space and a handwidth above the wrist. The site for allergy testing is usually the inner forearm, upper arm, upper chest, or upper back **(Figure 5)**. It is most important that the site chosen for an intradermal injection is clear so that results can be accurately interpreted.

1 - These areas should be avoided when giving injections to prevent further tissue injury and delayed medication absorption. A patient with prolonged coagulation time has a greater potential for hematoma formation. Pressure should be held on the injection site for several minutes to minimize hematoma formation.

1 - Aspirate: To pull back on the plunger of the syringe, creating a suction, to check for a blood return. If blood is aspirated into the syringe, it indicates potential intravenous placement of the needle. If blood is aspirated into the syringe, the needle should be removed and the medication discarded. A new syringe of medication should be prepared for administration.

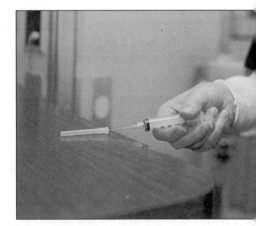

Figure 3: The scoop technique for recapping needles. (From Elkin MK, Perry AG, Potter PA: Nursing Interventions and Clinical Skills, 2nd ed. St. Louis, Mosby, 2000, p 451, with permission.)

Table I. Injection Guide

Type	Indications	Equipment	Appropriate Administration Sites	Considerations	Recommended Fluid Amount	Angle	Depth
Intradermal	Skin testing such as tuberculin screening or allergy testing	Tuberculin syringe with ⅜–⅝ inch, 25–27-gauge needle	Inner forearm, Upper arm, Upper chest, Upper back	Site should be lightly pigmented, free of lesions, and hairless	0.01–0.10 cc	5°–15°	No more than ⅛ inch below the skin
Subcutaneous (SQ)	Medication administration into the SQ tissue	2–3 cc syringe with ⅜–1 inch, 24–27-gauge needle, Insulin syringe for insulin administration	Upper outer arm, Lower abdomen, Upper outer thigh, Upper back, Flank region	Fluid administered should be isotonic, nonirritating, nonviscous, and water-soluble	0.50–1.0 cc	Average size adult: 45° Obese adult: 45°–90° Thin adult, elderly, child: < 45°	After choosing the correct angle for amount of SQ tissue, insert the needle completely
Intramuscular	Administration of irritating or viscous drugs deep into the muscle tissue	2–3-cc syringe with 1½–2 inch, 18–22-gauge needle	Deltoid, Ventrogluteal, Dorsogluteal, Vastus lateralis, Rectus femoris	For medications very irritating to SQ and dermal tissues, Z-track method should be used	Deltoid up to 1.5 cc All other sites up to 3 cc	Average size adult: 90° Thin or obese adult or child: adjust needle length, angle or both as needed	Insert the needle completely

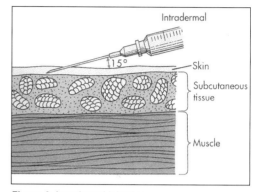

Figure 4: Intradermal injection.
(From Elkin MK, Perry AG, Potter PA: Nursing Interventions and Clinical Skills, 2nd ed. St. Louis, Mosby, 2000, p 451, with permission.)

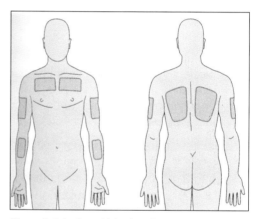

Figure 5: Intradermal injection sites.
(From Leahy JM, Kizilay PE: Foundations of Nursing Practice: A Nursing Process Approach. Philadelphia, W.B. Saunders, 1998, with permission.)

Subcutaneous Injection

Subcutaneous medication administration involves small doses (usually 0.5–1.0 cc) to avoid irritation and development of sterile abscesses. Absorption of a medication through the subcutaneous tissue is slower than absorption from a muscle because of a smaller blood supply. For medications such as anticoagulants and insulin, the slower absorption allows for more gradual effect of the medication.

Equipment needed includes a syringe that can hold up to 2 cc of medication and a short (⅜ inch to 1 inch), small-gauge (24–27) needle. The angle of insertion for a subcutaneous injection is dependent on the size and weight of the individual. For an average-sized adult, a 45° angle is used. If the client is obese, a 90° angle may be used. If the client is very thin, elderly, or a child, an angle of less than 45° may be best. To administer a subcutaneous injection, first select the site *(Figure 6)*. Sites include upper outer arm, lower abdomen, upper outer thigh, upper back, and flank region.

Intramuscular Injection

Intramuscular (IM) injections involve insertion of a needle deep into a muscle where medication will be absorbed more rapidly. The amount of medication that can be administered into one intramuscular site is 3 cc. For children, older adults, and very thin adults, 2 cc may be the maximum amount tolerated.

Because muscles lie deeper than the subcutaneous tissues, a longer needle is required. Equipment needed includes a syringe that can hold up to 3 cc of medication and a longer (1½–2 inch), larger gauge (18–22) needle. To administer an IM injection, first select the site *(Figure 7)*. Sites include the deltoid, ventrogluteal, dorsogluteal, vastus lateralis, and rectus femoris muscles.

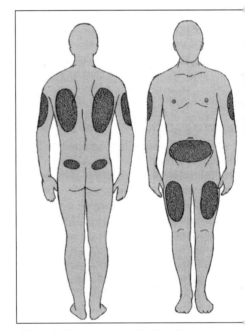

Figure 6: Subcutaneous injection sites.
(From Elkin MK, Perry AG, Potter PA: Nursing Interventions and Clinical Skill, 2nd ed. St. Louis, Mosby, with permission.)

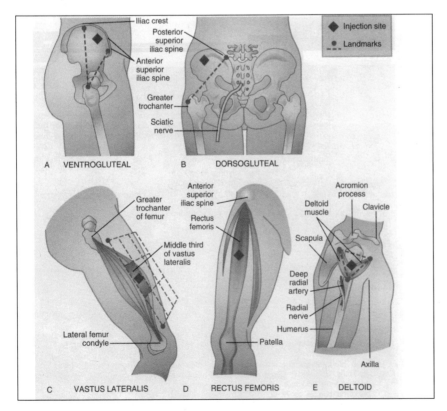

Figure 7: Intramuscular injection sites.
(From Leahy JM, Kizilay PE: Foundations of Nursing Practice: A Nursing Process Approach. Philadelphia, W.B. Saunders, 1998, with permission.)

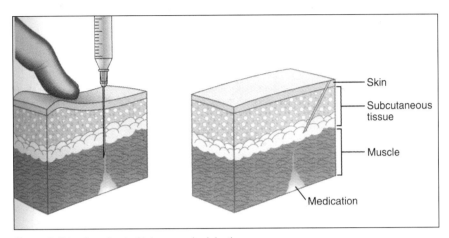

Figure 8: Z-track method of intramuscular injection.

(From Leahy JM, Kizilay PE: Foundations of Nursing Practice: A Nursing Process Approach. Philadelphia, W.B. Saunders, 1998, with permission.)

For medications that are very irritating to the subcutaneous and dermal tissues, the injection should be given deep into a well-developed muscle (commonly the dorsogluteal) using a special technique called *Z-track*. This involves pulling the skin and tissues 2.5–3.5 cm (1–1.5 inches) to the side prior to inserting the needle. After the injection is given, the needle should be held in place for about 10 seconds. The needle should then be withdrawn quickly and the skin released immediately to seal the medication in the muscle *(Figure 8)*.

Because they are given deep in the muscle, IM injections have the greatest potential for complications. Most complications can be avoided by using proper injection technique. Complications that may occur include:

- **Nerve injury:** If an injection is given too close to a nerve or if the needle strikes a nerve, the patient will complain of significant pain either at the time of injection or during medication administration. Some medications normally cause burning during administration, which is usually a different sensation than that felt with nerve injury. If the nerve has been injured, monitor for numbness and tingling distal to the injection site. Using landmarks to clearly identify muscle location is the best method for avoiding nerve injury.
- **Intravenous administration:** An IM injection is intended for deposition into the muscle, not a vein. Venous administration of a medication results in decreased bioavailability of the medication. Some drugs are inactivated and excreted after the first pass through the liver. With IM administration, the drug is leeched out more slowly, resulting in improved efficacy of the medication. Additionally, the base in which the medication is prepared may not be appropriate for direct venous administration. Aspirating before injecting is the best method for avoiding accidental venous administration of an IM medication.
- **Hematoma formation:** It is possible to pass through a vein during needle insertion. When the needle is withdrawn, a tract is formed in the vein that allows blood to leak out into the tissues. To minimize hematoma formation, monitor for blood droplet formation at the insertion site when the needle is withdrawn. Holding pressure on the site for a few minutes will minimize hematoma formation.

Selected Readings

1. Elkin MK, Perry AG, Potter PA: Nursing Interventions and Clinical Skills, 2nd ed. St. Louis, Mosby, 2000.
2. Leahy JM, Kizilay PE: Foundations of Nursing Practice: A Nursing Process Approach. Philadelphia, W.B. Saunders, 1998.

67. Joint Aspiration and Injection

Jeffrey D. Harrison, MD

Synopsis

Joint aspiration and injection can provide both diagnostic information and therapeutic treatments. Fluid from almost any joint in the body can be aspirated. Once a joint space has been entered, both medication and analgesics can be instilled to provide symptom relief. This procedure has a high degree of sensitivity and specificity for infection, crystal-induced arthropathy, and fracture.

Indications

The diagnostic indication for this procedure is to determine if a **joint effusion (Definition 1)** is from an infectious, rheumatic, traumatic, or crystal-induced etiology. This procedure also can be used diagnostically to differentiate various causes of painful conditions (e.g., costochondritis versus coronary artery disease as a cause of chest pain).

1 - Effusion: Fluid from the blood vessels or lymphatics that escapes into the tissues or a cavity.

Any joint with an unexplained monoarthritis should be considered for immediate aspiration because of the risk of infection. Delay in initiating antibiotic treatment can have profound effects on the long-term function of the joint.

Therapeutic indications include the relief of pain in a grossly swollen joint, the removal of exudative fluid from a septic joint, and the instillation of lidocaine or steroids into an acutely inflamed joint **(Brain 1)**.

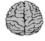

1 - Steroids act to modify the vascular inflammatory response to injury, inhibit destructive enzymes, and ameliorate the action of inflammatory cells. Injectable steroids maximize local anti-inflammatory benefits while minimizing systemic adverse reactions. The potency and duration of action of steroid preparations vary widely.

Contraindications to joint aspiration include overlying cellulitis, bacteremia, over-anticoagulation, and an uncooperative patient. Steroid injections should not be performed if a weight-bearing joint has been injected 3 times in the preceding 12 months or if the joint is unstable. In the case where an infection is suspected in a prosthetic joint the orthopedist who placed the prosthesis should be consulted.

Procedure

Joint aspiration and injection should be done wearing gloves and following sterile technique. There is not a consensus as to whether extensive sterile draping should be employed. Most authors agree that sterile gloves and use of an alcohol or povidone-iodine wipe are adequate preparation for most joint aspirations. In patients at higher risk for infection, such as patients who are immunosuppressed or have diabetes, more extensive draping and preparation are prudent.

The equipment needed for this procedure includes:

- Povidone-iodine wipes or alcohol wipes
- Sterile gloves
- 22–25 gauge, 1.5-inch needles for injection
- 18–20 gauge, 1.5-inch needles for aspiration
- One 10-cc syringe for injections
- Three 50-cc syringes for aspiration
- Single-dose vials of 1% lidocaine or bupivacaine
- Corticosteroid preparations (Celestone, Kenalog, Solu-Medrol)
- Hemostat to secure needle when aspiration followed by injection

As with any procedure, the risks and benefits should first be explained to the patient. Typical risks include bleeding, infection, and pain. When steroid injections are performed, added risks include **postinjection flare (Definition 2)**, **steroid arthropathy (Definition 3)**, tendon rupture, and local skin atrophy.

2 - Postinjection flare: Increased joint pain and swelling that usually begin 6–12 hours after a steroid injection. It is caused by steroid crystals that cause an inflammatory synovitis and is seen in 1–2% of individuals.

3 - Steroid arthropathy: Complication that occurs due to repeated steroid injections, resulting in joint instability due to osteonecrosis (bone death) of juxta-articular bone and weakened capsular ligaments.

Once consent has been obtained, the site for entry should be determined. It is beyond the scope of this chapter to discuss the entry points for every potential aspiration or injection that can be performed. The entry site should be marked with an indelible marker or other object (retracted pen) that will leave an indentation that will not be removed by the alcohol or povidone-iodine wipe. In the case of aspiration alone, some physicians will offer to anesthetize the area of entry with a small wheal of 1% lidocaine. If an injection is planned, draw up the appropriate volume of anesthetic or steroid to be infiltrated. Many times, an anesthetic will be co-administered with a steroid. Occasionally, an aspiration followed by an injection will be needed; in that case a syringe for aspiration and a syringe for injection will be used. A hemostat can be used to secure the needle in place when switching from the aspiration to injection syringe. This is achieved by clamping across the needle flush with the skin. Prior to any injection, the plunger on the syringe should be pulled back to assure the needle is not in a blood vessel. Fluid that is aspirated can be sent to the lab for appropriate analysis. The area of entry is covered with a Band-aid and the patient instructed to rest the area. Ice can be applied after a steroid injection to help avoid postinjection pain.

Interpretation

Fluid aspirated from a joint is commonly evaluated for its physical appearance, microscopic appearance, microbiology, and chemistries. Not every sample will require complete testing; the clinical diagnosis should help guide the decision. Joint fluid aspirate should be placed in a sterilized tube for possible culture and into a second heparinized tube for cell count, then sent to the lab. **Table 1** delineates the typical findings in normal synovial fluid as well as common pathologic findings.

Treatment is based on the clinical and fluid analysis findings. If there is any suspicion of a septic joint, parenteral antibiotics should be initiated immediately. Most crystal and rheumatic joint disorders will respond favorably to nonsteroidal anti-inflammatory drugs; local steroid injection is also advocated by some authors for these disorders. Fractures, as evidenced by fat droplets, mandate appropriate orthopedic management.

Table 1. Joint Fluid Findings

Condition	Physical Appearence	Microscopy	Microbiology	Glucose
Normal	Clear to slightly yellow	No crystals	WBC < 200/mm	Equal to blood
Rheumatologic	Clear to yellow, some turbidity	No crystals	WBC 2000–50,000, 70–85% PMNs	Normal to 30 mg < blood
Gout	Clear to yellow, some turbidity	Negative birefringent crytals (urate)	WBC 2000–50,000 40–90% PMNs	Normal to 30 mg < blood
Pseudogout	Clear to yellow, some turbidity	Positive birefringent crystals (calcium pyrophosphate)	WBC 2000–50,000, 35–85% PMNs	Equal to blood
Trauma	Grossly bloody	Fat droplets, RBCs	WBC > 5000	Equal to blood
Septic	Turbid	Gram stain positive in 30–90%	WBC > 50,000 (up to 3 million), > 90% PMNs	40 mg or more < blood

WBC = white blood cell count; PMNs = polymorphonuclear neutrophils; RBCs = red blood cells.

Selected Readings

1. Mercier L: Practical Orthopedics. St. Louis, Mosby, 1995.
2. Pfenninger JL: Joint and soft tissue aspiration and injection. In Pfenninger JL, Fowler GC (eds): Procedures for Primary Care Physicians. St. Louis, Mosby, 1994, pp 1036–1054.
3. Wilson S, Driscoll C: Joint aspiration. In Rakel R, Driscoll C (eds): Procedures for Your Practice. Montvale, NJ, Medical Economics, 1988.

68. Minor Surgery

John L. Smith, MD

Synopsis

Minor surgery is often performed in the outpatient setting by primary care physicians. It generally involves a relatively short visit and only local anesthesia. This chapter familiarizes you with the basics of these procedures so that you will have a better understanding of what you observe your preceptor doing. You may even be given opportunities to assist your preceptor. You should not attempt these procedures without the guidance of an experienced physician. The areas to be addressed are local anesthesia, wound care, biopsy of lesions, suturing, cryotherapy, electrosurgery, subungual hematomas, and wedge resections.

Local Anesthesia

See also Chapter 66 on Injections.

History

- "Have you had any allergic reactions to local anesthetics in the past?"
- "Are you aware of any bleeding disorders?" (e.g., excessive bleeding with minor cuts, easy bruising)

Supplies and Equipment

- Lidocaine, 1% or 2%, with or without epinephrine.
- Lidocaine with epinephrine is advised to help control bleeding **(Red Flag 1)**.
- 3-cc or 5-cc syringe with a 22-gauge needle
- 27- or 30-gauge needle
- Alcohol pad

1 - Epinephrine use is not advised on toes, fingers, and penis. It may cut off blood supply to the tissue and result in damage. Although many physicians are uncomfortable with epinephrine usage on the ears and nose, it is safe and quite helpful in controlling bleeding.

Technique

After an alcohol pad is wiped across the rubber port on the lidocaine bottle, a 3-cc or 5-cc syringe with a 22-gauge needle is used to draw up the lidocaine. The 22-gauge needle is then replaced by a 27- or 30-gauge needle. The needle is placed into the skin, either intradermally or into the subcutaneous tissue, and slowly injected **(Red Flag 2)**. The anesthetic may be placed directly under smaller lesions or circumferentially around larger ones in a "field block" **(Brain 1)**.

2 - Prior to injecting, pull back on the plunger and check for a flash of blood, a sign that the needle is in a blood vessel. If present, redirect the needle and recheck.

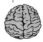

1 - Most procedures require less than 5–10 cc of lidocaine.

Wound Care

Instructions for Patients after Minor Surgical Procedures

For Simple Interrupted Sutures:

- Clean 2–3 times daily with half-strength hydrogen peroxide and water until all scabs and crusts are removed.
- Apply antibiotic ointment in a thin layer after cleaning.
- Covering is unnecessary except for draining wounds.
- The patient may shower or clean the area with soap and water but should avoid soaking in a bath or swimming.

If Steri-strips in Place:

- It is unnecessary and logistically difficult to clean and apply antibiotic ointment as noted above.
- Return to clinic if (1) signs of infection such as purulent drainage (pus) or expanding redness develop; (2) a hematoma develops; (3) the wound begins to open (which indicates "failure" of suture line occurred).

Suture Removal

- **Face:** Simple interrupted sutures, the type most commonly used on the face, should be removed in 5 days to decrease suture marks (cross-hatching). The face heals more quickly than most other areas.
- **Body:** Usually remove after 7 days to minimize scarring, but a running subcutaneous suture may be left in place for up to 10–14 days.

Subungual Hematoma *(Definition 1)*

1 - Subungual hematoma: An accumulation of blood beneath a fingernail or toenail.

History

This type of injury usually occurs following trauma to the tip of finger or toe. It usually is painful if the hematoma is large.

Physical Examination

- Nail bed will have a dark blue or black area *(Red Flag 3)*.
- The injury may cause separation of the nail from the nail bed with subsequent nail loss.

3 - A melanoma under the nail bed may resemble a subungual hematoma. Suspect melanoma if the lesion did not follow trauma or has slowly grown over time.

Technique

If larger and painful, these may be drained by one of two frequently used methods.

- Partially straighten a paper clip and heat the end with a match or lighter. Place the heated point of the paper clip over the hematoma and rotate clockwise and counterclockwise (twirling it back and forth) with mild pressure until a hole is punctured in the nail and drainage occurs.
- A battery powered pencil cautery may be used to puncture a similar hole in the nail. Lighter pressure is used because this works more quickly.

- The blood accumulation will protect the underlying nail bed from the heat to some extent. Avoid using too much pressure and poking the nail bed because this can be very painful.

Cryotherapy

Cryotherapy is an operation employing liquid nitrogen or carbon dioxide to freeze and destroy tissue. Most commonly, a cup with liquid nitrogen or a spray cannister is used. Many lesions can be treated with this technique, most commonly warts, actinic keratoses, and seborrheic keratoses or solar lentigenes *(Red Flag 4)*.

4 - It is inadvisable to freeze a nevus with suspicious characteristics because there is no way to know if melanoma exists.

Technique

- If the spray technique is used, spray the lesion until a white area of frost, or "frost ball," appears. Try to limit the freezing to 2 mm from the border of lesion so less tissue damage occurs. The length of the freeze cycle varies by type of lesion and provider *(Table 1)*.
- If liquid nitrogen is used, a large or small cotton-tipped applicator is dipped in the liquid nitrogen and held against the lesion. Pressure should be light on superficial lesions, because subcutaneous damage may occur with increased pressure.

Table 1. Cryotherapy Duration

Lesion	Cycle Length	No. of Cycles
Wart	30–45 sec	2
Seborrheic keratosis	20–30 sec	1–2
Actinic keratosis	20–30 sec	1–2
Solar lentigo	5–10 sec	1

Complications

- Hemorrhagic bullae (blood-filled blister at the area of freeze)
- Damage to adjacent tissue
- Incomplete destruction—may necessitate repeat treatment

2 - Digital block: Lidocaine placed around the base of the finger or toe to block the digital nerves. This anesthetizes the entire digit.

Wedge Resection of Toenail or Fingernail

This treatment is indicated for ingrown nails.

- Have patient recline or lie down.
- A **digital block** *(Definition 2)* is placed at the base of the digit with lidocaine *without* epinephrine.
- The digit and surrounding area are cleansed with povidone-iodine (Betadine).
- A rubber band or Penrose drain may be used as a tourniquet at the base of the digit.
- The portion of the nail to be removed is separated from the eponychia with a probe.
- A straight hemostat or elevator is gently forced under the ingrown side of the toenail to separate it from the nail bed.
- Scissors are used to cut the nail all the way to the nail fold.
- The hemostat is then clamped on the wedge of nail (all the way to the base) and rolled over in an upward direction to peel the nail off the bed and out of the fold *(Figure 1)*.

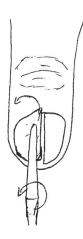
Figure 1: Removing the nail wedge.

- A probe is used to explore the proximal and lateral nail fold to insure no part of the nail remains.
- The tourniquet is removed. Antibiotic ointment is applied, and the nail bed is covered with a bulky dressing.
- A hard-soled shoe or toeless sandal may be worn for comfort.
- Patient should be directed to soak the toe twice daily in epsom salts solution for the next 4 or 5 days.

Biopsy of Lesions

The three most common techniques used for the biopsy of lesions are (1) shave biopsy; (2) elliptical biopsy; and (3) punch biopsy. Biopsies are performed to treat a lesion definitively (by removing it) or to sample a lesion to help establish a diagnosis.

For all techniques, the area to be biopsied is anesthetized (see above) and skin preparation is performed with povidone-iodine or by scrubbing with a soap solution (e.g., chlorhexidine).

Technique

Shave Biopsy *(Figure 2)*
- This technique is used most often for raised lesions.
- A scalpel or razor blade is placed almost flat against the skin and uni-directional strokes are made just beneath the base of the lesion. Forceps may be used to slightly elevate the lesion and provide countertraction if needed.
- A little pressure with a cotton-tipped applicator soaked in Drysol solution (20% aluminum chloride in alcohol) will stop the minimal bleeding and will not damage normal skin.
- Antibiotic ointment and an adhesive bandage (Band-Aid) are usually adequate as a dressing. Complications may include hyper- or hypopigmentation or hypertrophic scar.

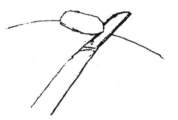

Figure 2: Shave biopsy.

Punch Biopsy
- This is most often used to sample a larger lesion, but it is occasionally used to remove a whole lesion.
- Disposable or re-useable punches may be utilized.
- Punch sizes larger than 4.0 mm may leave a closure that is not as cosmetically acceptable because of "dog-ears" (bunching up of tissue at the ends of the incision).
- The punch biopsy is performed by placing downward pressure on the punch while rolling it back and forth with the fingers. The punch needs to penetrate through the dermis and into the subcutaneous fat.
- During the procedure, the skin is spread perpendicular to the skin tension lines *(Figure 3)* with the other thumb and index finger. This creates a bit of an oval shape, which will close more easily.
- The specimen is elevated with forceps and excised through the base at the level of the adipose.
- The defect may be closed with one or two simple interrupted sutures in the skin. For larger punches, one or two deep sutures may be placed for strength.
- Sutures should be removed in 1 week.

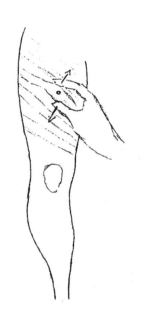

Figure 3: Traction applied perpendicular to skin tension lines.

Elliptical Biopsy
- This procedure is most often used to remove an entire lesion, including the deepest levels.
- Draw an ellipse around the lesion that has a length that is three times the width *(Figure 4)*.
- The long axis should be in the direction of the skin tension lines.
- A scalpel with a #15 blade is generally used to excise the lesion. The incision should be perpendicular to the surface of the skin and taken through the dermis to the adipose.
- The scalpel or tissue scissors may be used to remove the lesion by excising the underside at the level of the adipose.
- For most biopsies, three deep dermal (buried vertical mattress) sutures are placed with an absorbable suture to add strength to the wound over the following weeks and decrease spreading of the wound.
- A running subcutaneous suture or simple interrupted sutures are placed to approximate the more superficial layers of the skin.
- Steri-strips may be placed over the wound and ends of the suture if a running subcutaneous style was used.

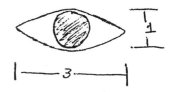

Figure 4: Relative dimensions of ellipse.

Suturing

Sutures are classified as absorbable or nonabsorbable. Absorbable suture is used in the wound and therefore cannot be removed. It takes days to weeks to absorb depending on the suture type. Nonabsorbable suture is permanent and needs to be removed *(Table 2)*.

Table 2. Suture Removal Schedule

	Tissue Reaction	Absorption	Strength Retention
Absorbable			
Chromic (coated gut)	Moderate	30 days	4 weeks
Polyglactic acid (Vicryl)	Mild	60–90 days	30% in 3 weeks
Polydioxanone (PDS)	Mild	210 days	50% in 4 weeks
Nonabsorbable			
Nylon	Very low	20% per year	
Polypropylene (Prolene)	Minimal	Never	Indefinite

Common Suture Techniques in Minor Surgery

Simple Interrupted *(Figure 5)*
- Advantages: simple; best skin edge approximation
- Disadvantages: hatchmarking on the skin after healing
- Uses: anywhere, but very good for the face because they can be removed in 5 days from this location and less hatchmarking occurs
- Most commonly used suture types: nylon and polypropylene

Running Subcutaneous Suture *(Figure 6)*
- Advantages: Because the suture is below the epidermis, it can be left for 7–14 days without the hatchmarking resulting from simple interrupted sutures; good skin approximation
- Disadvantages: if suture pulls loose when healing, the entire wound may separate

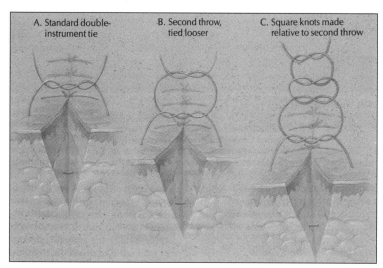

Figure 5: Simple interrupted sutures.
(From Moy R, Lee A, Zalka A: Commonly used suturing techniques in skin surgery. Am Fam Physician 44:1625–1634, 1991, with permission)

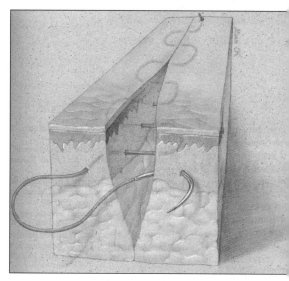

Figure 6: Running subcutaneous suture.
(From Moy R, Lee A, Zalka A: Commonly used suturing techniques in skin surgery. Am Fam Physician 44:1625–1634, 1991, with permission)

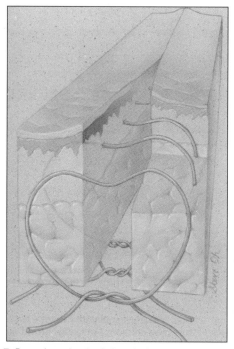

Figure 7: Deep dermal or buried vertical mattress suture.
(From Moy R, Lee A, Zalka A: Commonly used suturing techniques in skin surgery. Am Fam Physician 44:1625–1634, 1991, with permission)

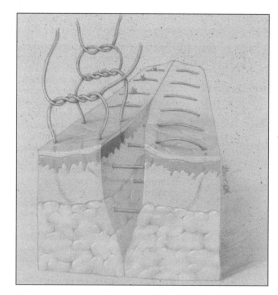

Figure 8: Vertical mattress sutures.
(From Moy R, Lee A, Zalka A: Commonly used suturing techniques in skin surgery. Am Fam Physician 44:1625–1634, 1991, with permission)

- Uses: anywhere; less often on the face because the skin edge approximation is not as good as simple interrupted sutures
- Most common suture material used: 5-0 polypropylene (pulls out nicely and causes minimal tissue reaction)

Deep Dermal (Buried Vertical Mattress) *(Figure 7)*

- Advantages: holds the wound together for a prolonged period of time; good for wounds under increased tension; should be incorporated in most repairs with the exceptions of fingers, tip of nose, and penis (thin dermal layers).

- Most common suture type: chromic on face; polydioxanone and polyglactic acid on body (stronger, lasts longer)

Vertical Mattress *(Figure 8)*
- Advantages: holds wound together well under tension and keeps skin edges everted for better approximation
- Disadvantage: increased tension on suture leads to more cross-hatching and scarring
- Most common suture types: nylon, polypropylene

Electrosurgery *(Figure 9)*

Electrosurgery is performed with numerous models of electrosurgical units. The unit called a Hyfrecator is commonly used in the primary care setting. Tissue can be removed one of two ways. In electrofulguration, the tip of the electrosurgical handpiece is held a couple millimeters from the surface of the skin or lesion, and the emitted spark produces a superficial level of tissue destruction. In electrodesiccation, the tip of the handpiece is placed in contact with the skin lesion, which causes a deeper level of tissue destruction. Electrosurgery is used to remove or treat warts, skin tags, seborrheic keratoses, telangiectasias, molluscum contagiosum, and many other skin disorders.

Procedure

Anesthetize the lesion if necessary (smaller lesions may not need anesthesia).

Wattage setting should be based on literature accompanying the electrosurgical unit, or start at a low setting and increase until desired effect is observed.

Selected Readings

1. Bass R, Abdouch I, Halm D, et al: Office Surgery: Home Study Self-Assessment Program. Edition 232. Kansas City, MO, American Academy of Family Physicians, 1998.
2. Moy R, Lee A, Zalka A: Commonly used suturing techniques in skin surgery. Am Fam Physician 44:1625–1634, 1991.
3. Pfenninger JL, Fowler GC: Procedures for Primary Care Physicians. St. Louis, Mosby, 1994.
4. Robinson JK, Arndt KA, LeBoit PE, et al: Atlas of Cutaneous Surgery. Philadelphia, W.B. Saunders, 1996.
5. Usatine RP, Moy RL: Skin Surgery: A Practical Guide. St. Louis, Mosby, 1998.

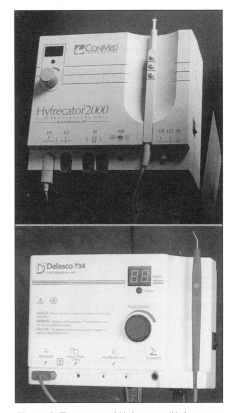

Figure 9: Two types of Hyfrecator (Hyfrecator 2000 and Delasco 734).
(From Usatine RP, Moy RL: Skin Surgery: A Practical Guide. St. Louis, Mosby, 1998, with permission.)

69. Office Laboratory Procedures

Audrey Paulman, MD

Synopsis

An in-office laboratory provides rapid turnaround of commonly ordered tests. The phrase in-office refers to tests that are actually done on the premises by the physician or medical assistant. Reference laboratory is the phrase used to designate the laboratory that performs more complex testing at a site distant from the primary care office.

In-office laboratories are regulated by the Clinical Laboratory Improvement Amendments of 1988 (CLIA), which set standards designed to improve quality in laboratory management and **proficiency testing** *(Definition 1)*. As a result of this amendment, many in-office labs chose to do only tests that are waived by CLIA to avoid the increased administrative and training costs of the more complex testing. Waived tests are those not categorized as complex by CLIA, usually simple tests with built-in **controls** *(Definition 2)* and possible over-the-counter availability (e.g., some urine pregnancy tests). Tests waived by CLIA include:

1 - Proficiency testing: A process in which individual laboratories perform testing on standard samples to document competency.

2 - Control: For a laboratory test, the performance of testing of known normal and abnormal results to confirm that the test kit is properly analyzing the sample.

- Dipstick urinalysis (test strip of urine without microscopy)
- Fecal occult blood (test for hidden blood in the stool)
- Urine pregnancy test (test to identify pregnancy)
- Erythrocyte sedimentation rate (test to screen for inflammation)
- Hemoglobin (measurement of iron in the blood)
- Spun hematocrit (measurement for anemia)
- Blood glucose (testing for sugar level in blood)

These tests require minimal training, have built-in controls, and are easy to reproduce.

Laboratory tests categorized as moderately complex include:

- Direct antigen strep (for *Streptococcus* A infection of the throat)
- Monospot (agglutination test for infectious mononucleosis)

These tests are commercially available kits with built in controls.

Another test commonly performed in the physician's office is physician-performed microscopy, which usually includes wet mounts of vaginal or cervical secretions and examination of urinary sediment.

Other testing, such as Pap smears, cultures, and more complex chemical and hematologic testing, is done by sending the patient to the reference laboratory (where specimens are collected by an independent, certified laboratory) or by in-office personnel who prepare a specimen according to the reference lab's orders for specific tests. The results are usually made available to the office by a computer printout, with critical levels called in directly to the office. Critical levels are sometimes called **red flags** or **panic levels**.

Table 1. Interpretation of Urinalysis

Test	Normal	Abnormalities May Indicate
Appearance	Clear to hazy	Cloudy urine may be infected or may have been handled improperly
Color	Yellow	Urine may be clear to dark brown or even blue in color. Orange urine may indicate dehydration or jaundice; cola-colored urine may indicate kidney disease; and blue urine probably indicates ingestion of methylene blue. **Red flag:** Bright red may represent bleeding.
Glucose	Negative Sugar in urine is reported 1+ – 4+, based on the amount of sugar in the urine: 1+ is a little; 4+ is a lot	Usually indicates elevated blood sugar. **Pitfall:** Some people have a low threshold of urine excretion and spill sugar with normal blood sugars **Panic:** Large amounts of sugar in diabetics (4+, especially when ketones are also present); ≥ 2+ in nondiabetic patients
Ketones	Negative Usually reported as small, moderate, or large	Ketones show up in diabetic ketoacidosis or when a patient is in a starvation state (NPO, vomiting, dehydration) **Panic:** Moderate to large ketones should be reported immediately.
Nitrate	Negative Abnormal nitrates are reported	Positive nitrates indicate infection **Red flag:** Positive nitrates in sick patient without suspected UTI
Blood	Negative Abnormal reports are small, moderate, and large	Blood usually shows up in kidney stones, bladder inflammation, trauma, and infection. Some contamination with menstrual blood may occur. **Red flag:** Large blood or gross hematuria should be reported immediately.
pH	4.5–8.0	The urine pH represents the acid-base balance of the patient. Medications, tubular disease, and infection affect it. pH > 7 may indicate infection, and acid urine may represent acidosis.
Odor	Faint	Infection smells bad. Diabetic ketoacidosis smells fruity.
Protein	Negative Abnormalities are reported as 1+ – 4+	Protein is not supposed to be excreted by the kidney. Although a patient may have some proteinuria with dehydration or viral infections, this should revert to negative after the patient is well. Abnormalities are caused by illness that makes the glomerulus leak, such as multiple myeloma, glomelular disease of the kidney, and diabetes. The urine protein should be further quantified with a 24-hour urine collection.
Specific gravity	1.000–1.030	The urine becomes more concentrated with dehydration and increased solute load (x-ray contrast material). Dilute urine may represent diabetes insipidus or the diuretic phase of acute tubular necrosis.
Urobilinogen	Negative 0–0.1	Elevation may indicate underlying liver disease or infectious process.

Urinalysis

The urine sample is obtained by clean catch method in the office. This requires a cleansing of the area, and the initial stream of urine is discarded to decrease the possibility of contamination from surrounding tissue. Interpretation of the urinalysis results is noted in **Table 1**.

Fecal Occult Blood

The fecal occult blood test detects gastrointestinal bleeding and aids in the screening for early colorectal cancer and polyps. Routinely, the patient obtains the sample at home and places it on a card, which is then tested in the lab. Sometimes, a physician will get a stool sample at the time of a rectal examination to help diagnose acute problems causing bleeding. Results will be:

Table 2. Hemoglobin and Hematocrit Abnormalities

Condition	Symptoms	Causes
Low hemoglobin/hematocrit	Decreased pulse pressure, poor skin turgor, dry mucouse membranes, weight loss, light-headed on arising	Bleeding, bone marrow failure, overhydration
High hemoglobin/hematocrit	Symptoms of heart failure: rales, dilated neck veins, short of breath	Addison's disease (adrenal insufficiency), severe dehydration, polycythemia (overproduction of RBCs)

RBCs = red blood cells.

- Normal: negative (i.e., no blood in the stool)
- Abnormal: positive (i.e., blood is present)

Because the test is usually done on three specimens, the report may indicate 1 out of 3 or 2 out of 3 tests are positive. If any one of the three samples is positive, the whole test is positive. False-positives may be caused by ingestion of raw red meat. Bleeding may be caused by medications such as anti-inflammatory medications, polyps, ulcers, and cancers. Vitamin C will make a test falsely negative.

Urine Pregnancy Test

Human chorionic gonadotropin (hCG) is a hormone secreted by the placenta of a fertilized egg. It becomes present about a week after conception and ceases to be secreted after delivery. It can be measured in the blood or in the urine; the CLIA-waived test is performed on urine. This test is most accurate when done on first-void urine (i.e., the first time the patient urinates in the morning). Results indicate:

- Negative: not pregnant
- Positive: pregnant

False-positives (showing a pregnancy when there is not one) may occur in some malignancies and hydatidiform mole, sometimes called a "false pregnancy," where the uterus is filled with a tumor instead of a pregnancy.

False-negative results (not showing a pregnancy when the patient is pregnant) may occur if the test was done too soon and the hCG level was not yet high enough. Repeat the test in a few days.

Urine pregnancy tests can also be used to diagnose ectopic pregnancy and threatened or actual miscarriage. In instances where the early or definitive diagnosis of pregnancy is important, a serum hCG can be performed to detect pregnancy as early as 5 days after conception.

Erythrocyte Sedimentation Rate

The erythrocyte sedimentation rate (ESR) is a screen for inflammation. The patient's blood sample is placed in a columnar tube, and the red blood cells (RBCs) are allowed to sediment, or settle, to the bottom of the tube by gravity. An elevation in this rate is a nonspecific screen for inflammation.

- Normal adult: < 20. There is some elevation in the elderly, with < 30 being acceptable in those over the age of 85.
- Normal child: < 10

Any illness that causes inflammation may elevate the ESR. Rheumatologic diseases and temporal arteritis can cause extremely high elevations. Also, infectious processes (e.g., abscess) may cause elevation, as can embolus, endocarditis, and pericarditis.

Table 3. Symptoms and Causes of Abnormal Blood Sugar

Condition	Symptoms	Causes
Low blood sugar	Confusion, irritability, nervous, restless, sweating	Addison's, alcoholism, hypothermia, insulinoma, pancreatitis, insulin, inborn erros of metabolism
High blood sugar	Fatigue, thirst, sleepiness, nausea, polyuria	Diabetes, Cushing's disease, pregnancy, hemochromatosis, medications, steroid use, epinephrine use

Spun Hematocrit

The patient's blood is obtained by fingerstick put in a tube, and spun. The hematocrit represents the percent of RBCs in a unit of blood.

- Normals:
    Adult females: 35–47%
    Adult males: 42–52%
    Children: specific by age
- Red flags: < 15%; > 60%; or any acute change

Diseases associated with abnormal hematocrits are noted in *Table 2*.

Hemoglobin

This is another method of measuring the oxygen-carrying capacity of the blood. Diseases associated with abnormal hemoglobin levels are listed in Table 2. As a rule, the hemoglobin will be one-third of the number of the hematocrit.

- Normals:
    Adult females: 12–15 g/dl
    Adult males: 14–16.5 g/dl
    Children: varies by age
- Red flags: < 5 /dl, > 20 g/dl, or any acute change

Blood Glucose

This test is usually done with a fingerstick collection.

- Normal: 70–110 mg/dl
- Elevated: > 110 mg/dl
- Diabetes: Two fasting sugars ≥ 126
- Random sugar > 200 mg/dl
- Red flags: < 40 or > 600 mg/dl

Abnormalities in glucose levels are noted in *Table 3*.

Direct Antigen *Streptococcus* Test

This is commonly referred to as a "quick strep" because the results are available before the patient leaves the office.

Table 4. Wet Mount Examination Findings

Cell/Organism	Appearance	Patient Symptoms and Signs
Yeast	Budding yeast may be mistaken for RBC's; refractile wall	Cottage cheese discharge, itching
Bacterial vaginosis	Epithelial cells with bacteria stuck on the cell wall, giving a stippled appearance called glitter cells or "clue cells" Cell walls become blurred.	Foul odor, discharge preterm labor
Trichomonas vaginitis	Motile, single-celled organisms, slightly larger than RBC's	Recurrent vaginitis (partner must be treated)
Bacteria	Rods, cocci, clumps, single	Bacteria are normally found in vaginal secretions
RBC	Doughnut-shaped	May be normal
WBC	Round, granular shape twice the size of RBC	May be normal. If increased, they represent infection.
Sperm	Smaller than a RBC or *Trichomonas*, motile, long tail	Presence indicates intercourse. Absence does not indicate no intercouse
Epithelial cells	Large, flat, irregular, with a nucleus	Normal in wet prep

RBC = red blood cell; WBC = white blood cell.

To perform the test, the patient's sore throat is swabbed, and the specimen is analyzed. For the antigen of group A *Streptococcus*, the organism responsible for strep throat, rheumatic heart disease, and post-streptococcal glomerulonephritis.

- Normal: negative
- Abnormal: positive (i.e., *Streptococcus* bacteria are present)

A patient with a positive strep screen may be in an acute or a chronic carrier state, and treatment will depend on the clinical picture.

A negative strep screen indicates either no strep or a false-negative. False-negatives may occur up to 10% of the time, so many physicians send a strep culture to the reference laboratory for confirmation of all negative strep tests.

Heterophil Agglutinin Test (Monospot)

A heterophil agglutinin test of the blood is commonly called a monospot test. This is done to detect mononucleosis, a viral infection.

- Normal: negative
- Abnormal: positive

It usually takes 3–10 days after the onset of disease for this test to be positive, and results may be positive for up to 1 year after the disease. Other viral infections or serum sickness may cause false-positives.

Physician-performed Microscopy

Wet Mounts of Vaginal Secretions

A swab is taken of the cervical or vaginal secretions during a pelvic examination. This is placed in normal saline and covered with a coverslip. The specimen may be prepared with 10% potassium

Table 5. Physician-Performed Microscopy of Urine

Findings	Normal	Abnormalities
RBCs	Less than 3/high-powered field. Urine samples with significant blood should be centrifuged and looked at under the microscope	Elevation of number of red blood cells may indicate tumor, stone, or glomerulonephritis. The RBC/WBC ratio may help determine if the process is infectious
WBCs	Less than 4/high-powered field	Large numbers of WBC usually indicate infection
Squamous cells	Less than 10 cells/high-powered field	High numbers indicate contamination in the surrounding tissue
Crystals	Small number	Abnormalities may indicate stone formation
Bacteria	Few	High numbers indicate infection
Parasites	None	Any parasites noted should be identified
Casts	Moderate clear protein	Underlying kidney disease may show with RBC or WBC casts

RBC = red blood cell; WBC = white blood cell.

hydroxide, which will remove everything but yeast from the slide. The slide is then examined under high power. Possible results are noted in *Table 4*.

Physician-performed Microscopy of Urine

This test is usually done on spun urine, with microscopic examination of the sediment only. The urine sediment is placed on a slide, covered with a coverslip, and evaluated on high power. The findings on routine urine microscopy are noted in *Table 5*.

70. Spirometry

Brian J. Finley, MD

Synopsis

Spirometry, or **pulmonary function tests** (PFTs) *(Definition 1)*, provides accurate, objective measurement of the patient's ventilatory function (i.e., how well he or she is breathing). Although spirometry is easy to perform, results can vary depending on the patient's effort *(Red Flag 1)*. The spirometry device is inexpensive and easy to use in any office. The most important factor in achieving accurate and reproducible results is having a trained person administer the test.

Indications

Spirometry is indicated for the evaluation of any patient with a breathing problem. It determines breathing fitness and disability and is used for preoperative evaluation or occupational screening. A patient does not have to present with shortness of breath to have lung problems *(Red Flag 2)*. The subjective signs of respiratory rate, **respiratory distress** *(Definition 2)*, and auscultation of the lungs may all be normal, yet the patient may still have significant lung disease. Consequently, being able to measure lung volumes and function or flow rates (the ability and speed at which the patient can move air in and out of the lungs) is essential to make the diagnosis and determine appropriate treatment.

Procedure

Spirometry is performed by having the patient take in a maximal inhalation, seal his or her lips around the mouthpiece (some also place nose plugs on the patient's nostrils), and then blow out all the air as quickly as possible. Typically, the patient is asked to repeat this sequence three times. The two best tests should not vary more than 100 ml or 5% to indicate a consistent best effort. Coughing, intra-test breathing, or less than maximal effort will invalidate the test and must be individually evaluated by the technician.

The results obtained depend on patient effort. It is critical to have a person perform the test who is trained to elicit maximal effort. This person can explain and demonstrate how to do the test and then monitor the patient's effort. The test itself takes less than a minute to perform. If asthma or reactive airway disease (RAD) is suspected, the test can be performed prior to, and 15–20 minutes after, the use of a bronchodilator to aid in the diagnosis.

1 - Pulmonary function tests (PFTs): The objective measurement of how well a person is breathing. PFTs measure how much air a person can move with each breath (called the volume) and how fast they can get that breath in and out (called the flow rate).

1 - This test is dependent on the patient's effort. A well-trained technician is necessary to encourage the patient to do his or her best and determine whether a maximal effort has been expended.

2 - Patients only develop shortness of breath when the lung problem is already in the moderate-to-severe category. Always keep in mind that those patients who present with mild symptoms of a persistent cough or tightness in the chest without any physical findings can still have lung disease. Remember the old saying, "you don't have to wheeze to have asthma and not all wheezing is asthma." Getting PFTs will help in your evaluation of these patients.

2 - Respiratory distress: Any subjective sign (coughing, shortness of breath, or wheezing) or objective symptom (e.g., nasal flaring, retractions, or tachypnea) that indicates that the patient is having problems breathing.

Interpretation

Spirometry yields either a graph or a loop diagram, depending on the type of machine used. With the new computerized machines, it is easy to get full PFTs that automatically compare a patient's measurements to normal values and calculate the results as a percentage of the predicted *(Figure 1)*.

Pulmonary function tests are interpreted as either normal, restrictive, or obstructive. Normal is defined as 80–120% of the predicted value. These predicted values are established based on a patient's position, age, height, and the altitude at which the test is being performed. Restrictive diseases, such as interstitial lung diseases (e.g., sarcoidosis, connective tissue disorders, and pulmonary vascular diseases) and bellows disorders (e.g., obesity, paralysis, pleural disease, and ascites), which are disorders outside of the lungs (extraparenchymal) that affect the lungs, inhibit the lungs' maximal expansion. This results in a proportional decrease in all volumes. However, flow rates are relatively normal. Obstructive diseases (anything that limits the ability to move air in or out of the lungs) include asthma, emphysema, and chronic bronchitis. Obstructive diseases are associated with the following findings:

- Decreased vital capacity (VC), the maximum volume that can be exhaled after maximum inhalation.
- Decreased **FEV$_1$** and **FEV$_{25-75}$** *(Definition 3)*
- Increased total lung capacity (TLC), the total volume in the lungs at the end of maximal inspiration
- Normal or slightly decreased forced vital capacity (FVC), the maximum volume of gas expired forcefully after maximal inspiration

Selected Readings

1. Crapo VD: Respiratory structure and function. In Goldman L, Bennett J (eds): Cecil Textbook of Medicine, 21st ed. Philadelphia, W.B. Saunders, 2000.
2. Goroll AH, May LA, Mulley AG: Respiratory problems. In Primary Care Medicine, 3rd ed. Philadelphia, Lippincott-Raven, 1995.
3. McCurley RS: Pulmonology. In Siberry GK, Iannone R (eds): The Harriet Lane Handbook: A Manual for Pediatric House Officers, 15th ed. St. Louis, Mosby, 2000.
4. Schuller D: Pulmonary diseases. In Carey CF, Lee HH, Woeltje KF (eds): Washington Manual of Medical Therapeutics, 29th ed. Philadelphia, Lippincott-Raven, 1998.

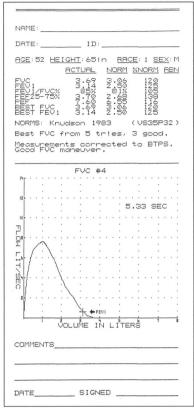

Figure 1: PFT example.

3 - FEV$_1$ (forced expired volume in 1 second): Volume of gas that can be exhaled in 1 second of a forceful expiration. This is a good indicator of how the large airways are working.

FEV$_{25-75}$: Volume of gas that can be exhaled between 25 and 75 milliseconds of a forceful expiration. This is a good indicator of how the small airways are working.

71. Tympanometry

Jeffrey L. Susman, MD

Synopsis

Tympanometry is an easily accomplished, inexpensive office procedure to assess **middle ear *(Definition 1)*** function with high sensitivity and moderate specificity. The **acoustic impedance** or **compliance *(Definition 2)*** of the tympanic membrane is measured as a function of air pressure. Although characteristic tympanograms (plots of compliance versus pressure) may suggest specific middle ear dysfunction, such results should be correlated with the physical examination and other clinical findings.

Indications

Tympanometry is indicated for the evaluation of middle ear function, ear discomfort, hearing loss, or the patency of pressure-equalization (PE) tubes. Because the physical examination alone may be equivocal, the tympanogram can be a useful adjunctive test. Tympanometry is easily performed in older children and adults, but it may be challenging to do in infants. Moreover, infants may have increased elasticity of the ear canal, falsely suggesting low compliance.

Tympanometry has a sensitivity of 90% in detecting a middle ear effusion, but a specificity of less than 80%. The negative predictive value is 77%, and the positive predictive value ranges from 49% to 99%. Thus, when the tympanogram is normal, it is probably an accurate result. Positive findings, however, depend highly on the age of the patient and skill of the examiner and should be correlated with findings on examination and **pneumatic otoscopy *(Definition 3)***.

Procedure

The tympanogram is performed by placing the appropriate-sized soft-tipped speculum of the tympanometer into the ear, taking care to obtain an adequate seal *(Figure 1)*. The ear should be examined prior to this procedure and at least partial canal patency assured. The test itself is of minimal discomfort and lasts less than 1 minute. Both ears should be tested. Small portable tympanometry units incorporated into an otoscope are available.

1 - Middle ear: The portion of the ear including the tympanic membrane (ear drum) and the tympanic cavity including the ossicles (bones that transmit sound).

2 - Acoustic impedance or compliance: During tympanometry, the ability of the ear drum to move (compliance) and opposition of flow of energy to the middle ear (impedance) are measured. A tympanogram is a display of compliance versus air pressure.

3 - Pneumatic otoscopy: Pneumatic otoscopy allows pressure to be applied through a flexible tube to assess movement of the tympanic membrane. An airtight otoscope and good seal within the canal are mandatory. Rubber-tipped specula aid in obtaining an airtight seal within the canal.

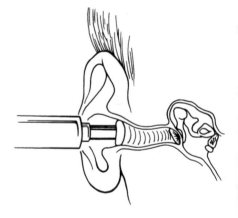
Figure 1: Performing a tympanogram. (From Forzley GJ: Tympanometry. In Pfenninger JL, Fowler GC (eds): Procedures for Primary Care Physicians. St. Louis, Mosby, 1994, with permission.)

Interpretation

Tympanometry yields a plot of compliance versus pressure and usually a measure of middle ear volume. A box usually indicates the range of normal *(Figure 2)*. A normal tympanogram (type A curve) shows a sharp peak of compliance around zero, with a normal peak occurring as low as −200 decaPascal (daPa; 1 daPa = 1.02 mm H_2O) (see Figure 2).

A "type B" curve demonstrates a flat or low-amplitude recording *(Figure 3)*. This finding is consistent with middle ear effusion, impacted cerumen, or a middle ear mass, such as a cholesteatoma. The total volume will be normal. Patients with a perforation or pressure equalization tube will also have a type B curve, but the middle ear volume will be increased. Comparing each ear will often be helpful.

Excessive negative pressure (usually greater than −200 daPa) indicates a type C curve, suggesting abnormal eustachian tube function *(Figure 4)*. With such a problem, there is not enough air entering the middle ear to repressurize it.

If the peak of the curve is above 1.5, an atrophic tympanic membrane or ossicular chain (bones in middle ear that transmit sound) disruption is suggested *(Figure 5)*.

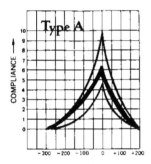

Figure 2: Type A tympanogram (normal tympanogram).
(From Northern JL: Advanced techniques for measuring middle ear function. Pediatrics 61:761–767, 1978, with permission.)

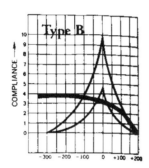

Figure 3: Type B tympanogram (middle ear effusion).
(From Northern JL: Advanced techniques for measuring middle ear function. Pediatrics 61:761–767, 1978, with permission.)

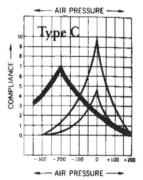

Figure 4: Type C tympanogram (abnormal eustachian tube dysfuction).
(From Northern JL: Advanced techniques for measuring middle ear function. Pediatrics 61:761–767, 1978, with permission.)

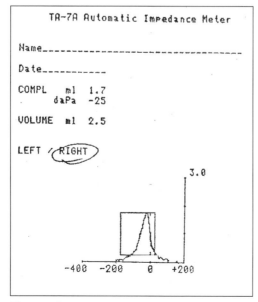

Figure 5: Tympanogram suggesting possible atrophic tympanic membrane.

Selected Readings

1. Forzley GJ: Tympanometry. In Pfenniger JL, Fowler GC (eds): Procedures for Primary Care Physicians. St. Louis, Mosby, 1994.
2. Northern JL: Advanced techniques for measuring middle ear function. Pediatrics 61:761–767, 1978.
3. Weiss J, Yates GR, Quinn LD: Acute otitis media: Making an accurate diagnosis. Am Fam Physician 53:4, 1996.
4. Wiet R, Dinces E, Rezaee A, et al: Common ENT Conditions. Home Study Self-Assessment No. 242. Kansas City, American Academy of Family Physicians, 1999.

Index

Page numbers in **boldface type** indicate complete chapters.

Climacteric, 223, 226
Clinical decision rules, 16–17
Clinical Evidence, 17–18
Clinical indicators, of disease
    definition of, 14
    predictive value of, 14, 15
    sensitivity and specificity of, 13, 14–15, 16
Clinical Laboratory Improvement Amendments of 1988, 362, 364
Clinic notes, 4–5, 6–7
Clinitest, 335
Clostridium difficile, 21
Clubbing, digital
    definition of, 149
    in pediatric patients, 65, 140
    pulmonary disease–related, 85, 136, 140
Cocaine
    as hypertension cause, 212
    as myocardial infarction cause, 126
Cochrane Library, 17–18
Codeine, as constipation cause, 122
"Coffee-ground emesis," 252
Cognex (tacrine), 222
Cognitive-behavioral therapy, 82
Cognitive impairment. *See also* Memory impairment
    dementia-related, 173
    in elderly patients, 163
    intergenerational history of, 164
    screening for, 52
Cogwheel rigidity, 219
Co-insurance, 9, 12
Colchicine, 250
Cold injuries, 308, 309, 312–313
Cold intolerance
    eating disorders–related, 232
    thyroid disease–related, 219
Cold sores, 277
Colon, infections of, 335
Colonoscopy, 66, 122, 123
Colorectal cancer
    risk factors for, 123
    screening for, 54
Colposcopy, 106, 197
Coma
    hyperosmolar, 143
    rectal temperature in, 185
Commercial insurance, 11, 12
Communication disorders, 285
    definition of, 256
    of disabled individuals, 257
Compartment syndromes, 193, 195, 341
Complementary and alternative medicine, **57–61**
COMPLETES mnemonic, for acute otitis media examination, 161
Computed tomography (CT)
    for abdominal pain evaluation, 66
    for headache evaluation, 201, 202
    for memory impairment evaluation, 221
Computerized axial tomography (CAT), for headache evaluation, 204
Condyloma, diagnostic tests for, 292
Confidentiality
    in adolescent health care, 44
    of medical information, 3–4
Congenital abnormalities, screening for, 37
Congenital heart disease, 126
Congestive heart failure (CHF), **114–120**
    coronary heart disease–related, 131
    as cough cause, 133, 137
    definition of, 127
    differentiated from chronic obstructive pulmonary disease, 109, 112
    as dyspnea cause, 147, 148
    as fatigue cause, 177
    hypertension-related, 211
    left-sided, 114–115
    as sleep disorder cause, 294
    thyroid disease–related, 219
    as urinary incontinence cause, 328, 329

Conjunctiva, examination of, 281
Conjunctivitis, 281–284
    allergic, 282
Connective tissue diseases, 245, 246
    fatigue associated with, 177
Consciousness, altered levels of, 317
Constipation, **121–125**
    as abdominal pain cause, 63, 64
    chronic, 66
    thyroid disease–related, 219
    as urinary incontinence cause, 328
Constitutional growth delay, 169
Contact precautions, for prevention of infectious disease, 21
Contraception. *See also* Oral contraception
    methods of, 93
Contraception counseling, 55, **91–93**
Contractures, Volkmann's ischemic, 193
Contusions, 192
    pulmonary, 316
COPD. *See* Chronic obstructive pulmonary disease
Core body temperature
    in children, 188
    circadian rhythm of, 188
Cornea
    abrasions of, 282
    ulcers of, 283–284
Coronary artery bypass grafting (CABG), 129
Coronary artery disease (CAD), **126–131**
    cholesterol screening in, 53
    dyslipidemia associated with, 54
    as dyspnea cause, 147, 148
    risk factors for, 53
    smoking-related, 151
Coronary heart disease (CHD), 126
    correlation with waist circumference, 213
    obesity-related, 232
Cor pulmonale, 296
Corticosteroids
    as sleep disorder cause, 294
    as soft-tissue and joint pain treatment, 250
Costochondritis, as chest pain cause, 100, 101
Cough
    in adults, **132–135**
        acute, 132
        chronic, 132, 133
    asthma-related, 84, 85, 86–87
    chronic, 136
    chronic obstructive pulmonary disease–related, 112
    complications of, 132
    croup-related, 87
    as headache cause, 201, 204
    in infants and children, **136–141**
    nocturnal, 140
        congestive heart failure–related, 117, 119
    pertussis-related, 87
    as pharyngitis cause, 299, 300
    psychogenic, 83, 140
    treatment for, 135
Cover-uncover test, 40
CPT (Current Procedural Terminology) codes, 8, 9, 12
Crackles (rales), 150, 190, 329
Cramps, muscular, thyroid disease–related, 219
Cranial nerves, areas innervated by, 158
C-reactive protein, as inflammation marker, 248
Crepitations, 194
Crohn's disease, 66
Cromoglycate, as allergic rhinitis treatment, 70
Crossed straight leg–raising test, 89
Croup, 84, 87
Crusts, cutaneous, 274
    impetigo-related, 276
Cryotherapy, 357
Crystal-induced disease. *See also* Gout; Pseudogout
    treatment for, 250
Cullen's sign, 65

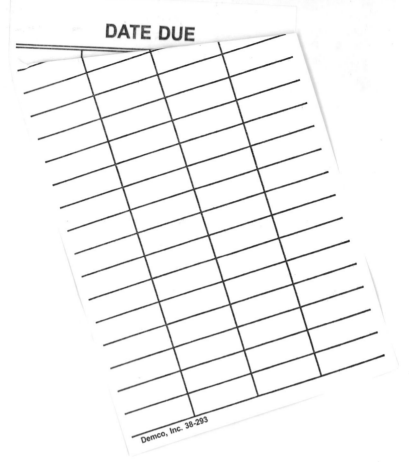

DATE DUE

Demco, Inc. 38-293